Human Genetics and Genomics

THIRD EDITION

Dedication
To Shelley, Jessica, and Katie

Human Genetics and Genomics

THIRD EDITION

Bruce R. Korf MD, PhD

Wayne H. and Sara Crews Finley Professor of Medical Genetics
Chair, Department of Genetics
University of Alabama at Birmingham, USA

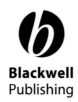

Blackwell
Publishing

1   2007

Library of Congress Cataloging-in-Publication Data
Korf, Bruce R.
   Human genetics and genomics / Bruce R. Korf. – 3rd ed.
      p.   ;   cm.
   Rev. ed. of: Human genetics / Bruce R. Korf. 2nd ed. c2000.
   Includes bibliographical references and index.
   ISBN-13: 978-0-632-04656-0 (alk. paper)
   ISBN-10: 0-632-04656-2 (alk. paper)
   1. Medical genetics – Problems, exercises, etc.   2. Human genetics – Problems, exercises, etc.
I. Korf, Bruce R. Human genetics.   II. Title.
   [DNLM: 1. Genetics, Medical–Problems and Exercises.   2. Genetic Diseases, Inborn–Problems
and Exercises.   3. Genomics–Problems and Exercises.   4. Problem-Based Learning–Problems and
Exercises. QZ 18.2 K84hu 2006]

   RB155.K666 2006
   616′.042–dc22

                                                                          2006014205

A catalogue record for this title is available from the British Library

Set in 10/12pt Berkeley by SNP Best-set Typesetter Ltd., Hong Kong
Printed and bound in Singapore by COS Printers Pte Ltd

Commissioning Editor: Martin Sugden
Editorial Assistant: Eleanor Bonnet
Development Editors: Kate Heinle and Karen Moore
Production Controller: Kate Charman
Website produced by: Meg Barton

For further information on Blackwell Publishing, visit our website:
http://www.blackwellpublishing.com

The publisher's policy is to use permanent paper from mills that operate a sustainable forestry policy,
and which has been manufactured from pulp processed using acid-free and elementary chlorine-free
practices. Furthermore, the publisher ensures that the text paper and cover board used have met
acceptable environmental accreditation standards.

Contents

Companion website: www.blackwellpublishing.com/korfgenetics

Preface

The first edition of this book was written as the Human Genome Project was just getting under way and the second edition while the project was in progress. Since then, the human genome sequence has been completed ahead of schedule. The complement of genes is smaller than many expected, but insights into both normal function and pathogenesis of disease are accumulating at the expected fast pace. The first edition was written at a time when medical genetics was identified with the study of rare disorders. Now it is increasingly being recognized that genetics contributes to all aspects of human health and disease, and that no health professional can afford to remain ignorant of the genetic approach.

Although this third edition is intended as a continuation of the spirit and approach of the first two, there have been two major changes in addition to the myriad updates necessitated by a rapidly advancing field. The first, that will be obvious to a reader familiar with the other two editions, is that this book is divided into two sections, consisting of eight didactic chapters followed by nine problem-based learning (PBL) cases. The original editions were based entirely on the PBL format. I remain committed to the PBL model and believe that it has great power to help students appreciate the importance of basic science concepts in a clinical context. Feedback about the book revealed a serious weakness in the exclusive use of PBL, however. Strict use of PBL requires that concepts be introduced as they emerge from a clinical case, but if a student is trying to master basic concepts or approaches this can lead to a disjointed narrative. Many students found it difficult to follow the flow of these basic ideas and found it especially difficult to look up information that was spread through multiple cases in the book.

The new format attempts to capture the best aspects of a classic didactic approach and the problem-based learning approach. The first eight chapters present basic concepts of gene structure and function, patterns of inheritance, chromosome structure and function, population genetics, and cancer genetics in an organized manner. The following nine chapters use the PBL format to illustrate the application of these concepts in medical practice. I hope that this will make the book a more useful study guide while retaining the power of the PBL approach to bring basic science to life.

The second major change is the addition of genomics content to the book, recognized by renaming the book "Human Genetics and Genomics." What is the difference between genetics and genomics? I think of genetics as dealing with the structure and function of individual genes, their transmission through families and in populations, and their effects on development and health in an individual. Genomics, in contrast, deals with larger sets of genes, exploring how they function in a co-ordinated manner in development and in both normal and abnormal physiology. Surely these concepts overlap, but the addition of the genomic approach to medicine, including large scale analysis of genetic variation and patterns of gene expression, is unmistakably transforming the landscape of medical practice. The new edition embraces this new approach and it seems fitting to recognize this in changing the title.

There have been many stylistic changes, such as addition of boxes to highlight clinical correlations, specific methods, ethical issues, and "hot topics." Nevertheless, the fundamental mission of the book remains unchanged: to present a set of core concepts of genetics in a way that highlights their medical application and recognizes the central role of the individual patient in medical practice.

There has never been a more exciting time to be involved in medical practice or medical research, and much of this excitement is being fired by advances in genetics and genomics. I hope that this book will help medical professionals in training appreciate the central role that genetics and genomics are playing in this new era, and perhaps will help inspire a few to join in the effort.

Acknowledgments

I am grateful to the many students and colleagues who have provided feedback about the book, especially pointing out errors or areas where improvements could be made. This new edition has benefited particularly from input from colleagues at University of Alabama School of Medicine, many of whom contributed case materials and other ideas that have been incorporated into the book. Some specific contributions deserve special mention: Dr. Phillip Wood provided material used in Chapter 1; Dr. Nathaniel Robin provided material for Chapter 3; Dr. Theresa Strong and Ms. Sandra Prucka wrote the original version of the case used in Chapter 17.

PART ONE

Basic Principles of Human Genetics

1

DNA Structure and Function

INTRODUCTION

The 20th century will likely be remembered by historians of biological science for the discovery of the structure of DNA and the mechanisms by which information coded in DNA is translated into the amino acid sequence of proteins. Although the story of modern human genetics begins about 50 years before the structure of DNA was elucidated, we will start our exploration here. We do so because everything we know about inheritance must now be viewed in the light of the underlying molecular mechanisms. We will see here how the structure of DNA sets the stage both for its replication and for its ability to direct the synthesis of proteins. We will also see that the function of the system is tightly regulated, and how variations in the structure of DNA can alter function. The story of human genetics did not begin with molecular biology, and it will not end there, as knowledge is now being integrated to explain the behavior of complex biological systems. Molecular biology, however, remains a key engine of progress in biological understanding, so it is fitting that we begin our journey here.

KEY POINTS

- DNA consists of a double helical sugar-phosphate structure with the two strands held together by hydrogen bonding between adenine and thymine or cytosine and guanine bases.
- DNA replication involves local unwinding of the double helix and copying a new strand from the base sequence of each parental strand. Replication proceeds bidirectionally from multiple start sites in the genome.
- DNA is complexed with proteins to form a highly compacted chromatin fiber in the nucleus.
- Genetic information is copied from DNA into messenger RNA in a highly regulated process that involves activation or repression of individual genes. mRNA molecules are extensively processed in the nucleus, including removal of introns and splicing together of exons, prior to export to the cytoplasm for translation into protein.
- The base sequence of mRNA is read in triplet codons to direct the assembly of amino acids into protein on ribosomes.
- Some genes are permanently repressed by methylation of some cytosine bases. These include most genes on one of two X chromosomes in cells of females and one of the two copies of genes that are said to be imprinted.

DEOXYRIBONUCLEIC ACID

Mendel described dominant and recessive inheritance before the concept of the "gene" was introduced, and long before the chemical basis of inheritance was known. Cell biologists during the late 19th and early 20th centuries had established the cell nucleus as the likely location of the genetic material, and DNA was long known to be a major chemical constituent. As the chemistry of DNA came to be understood, for a long time it was considered to be too simple a molecule – consisting of just four chemical building blocks, the bases **adenine**, **guanine**,

Methods 1.1

Mendelian inheritance in man

Dr. Victor McKusick and his colleagues at Johns Hopkins School of Medicine began to catalog genes and human genetic traits in the 1960s. The first edition of the catalog *Mendelian Inheritance in Man* was published in 1969. Multiple, subsequent print editions have appeared, and now the catalog is maintained on the world wide web by the National Center for Biotechnology Information (NCBI) as *Online Mendelian Inheritance in Man* (OMIM). The url is: http://www.ncbi.nlm.nih.gov/entrez/query.fcgi?db=OMIM

OMIM is recognized as the authoritative source of information about human genes and genetic traits. The catalog can be searched by gene, phenotype, gene locus and many other features. The catalog provides a synopsis of the gene or trait, including a summary of clinical features associated with mutations. There are links to other databases, providing access to gene and amino acid sequences, mutations, etc. Each entry has a unique, six digit number, the MIM number. Autosomal dominant traits have entries beginning with 1, recessive traits with 2, X-linked with 3, and mitochondrial with 5. Specific genes have MIM numbers that start with 6.

Throughout this book, genes or genetic traits will be annotated with their corresponding MIM number to remind the reader that more information is available on OMIM and to facilitate access to the entry.

---

thymine, and **cytosine**, along with sugar and phosphate – to account for the complexity of genetic transmission. Credit for recognition of the role of DNA in inheritance goes to the landmark experiments by Avery *et al.*, who demonstrated that a phenotype of smooth or rough colonies of the bacterium *Pneumococcus* could be transmitted from cell to cell through DNA alone. Elucidation of the structure of DNA by Watson and Crick in 1953 opened the door to understanding the mechanisms whereby this molecule functions as the agent of inheritance (Methods 1.1).

DNA Structure

DNA consists of a pair of strands of a sugar-phosphate backbone attached to a set of **pyrimidine** and **purine** bases (Figure 1.1). The sugar is **deoxyribose** – ribose missing an oxygen atom at its 2′ position. Each DNA strand consists of alternating deoxyribose molecules connected by phosphodiester bonds from the 5′ position of one deoxyribose to the 3′ position of the next.

What is the structure of DNA?

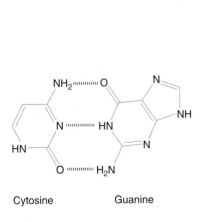

Cytosine   Guanine

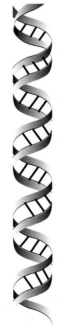

Thymine   Adenine

Figure 1.1 • Double helical structure of DNA (center). The sugar-phosphate helices are held together by hydrogen bonding between adenine and thymine bases, or guanine and cytosine bases.

Methods 1.2

Isolation of DNA

DNA, or in some cases RNA, is the starting point for most experiments aimed at study of gene structure or function. DNA can be isolated from any cell that contains a nucleus. The most commonly used tissue for human DNA isolation is peripheral blood, where white blood cells provide a readily accessible source of nucleated cells. Other commonly used tissues include cultured skin fibroblasts, epithelial cells scraped from the inner lining of the cheek and fetal cells obtained by amniocentesis or chorionic villus biopsy. Peripheral blood lymphocytes can be transformed with Epstein–Barr virus into immortalized cell lines, providing permanent access to growing cells from an individual.

Nuclear DNA is complexed with proteins, which must be removed in order for the DNA to be analyzed. For some experiments it is necessary to obtain highly purified DNA, which involves digestion or removal of the proteins. In other cases, relatively crude preparations suffice. This is the case, for example, with DNA isolated from cheek scrapings. The small amount of DNA isolated from this source is usually released from cells with minimal effort to remove proteins. This preparation is adequate for limited analysis of specific gene sequences. Crude DNA preparations can be obtained from very minute biological specimens, such as drops of dried blood, skin cells, or hair samples isolated from crime scenes for forensic analysis.

Isolation of RNA involves purification of nucleic acid from the nucleus and/or cytoplasm. This RNA can be used to study the patterns of gene expression in a particular tissue. RNA tends to be less stable than DNA, requiring special care during isolation to avoid degradation.

The strands are bound together by hydrogen bonds between adenine and thymine bases and between guanine and cytosine bases. Together these strands form a double helix. The two strands run in opposite (antiparallel) directions, so that one extends 5′ to 3′ while the other goes 3′ to 5′.

The key feature of DNA, wherein resides its ability to encode information, is in the sequence of the four bases (Methods 1.2). The number of adenine bases (A) always equals the number of thymines (T), and the number of cytosines (C) always equals the number of guanines (G). This is because A on one strand is always paired with T on the other, and C on one strand is always paired with G. The pairing is noncovalent, due to hydrogen bonding between complementary bases. G–C base pairs form three hydrogen bonds, whereas A–T pairs form two, making the G–C pairs slightly more thermodynamically stable. Because the pairs always include one purine base (A or G) and one pyrimidine base (C or T), the distance across the helix remains constant.

How are DNA molecules replicated?

DNA Replication

The complementarity of A to T and G to C provides the basis for DNA replication, a point that was recognized by Watson and Crick in their paper describing the structure of DNA. DNA replication proceeds by a localized unwinding of the double helix, with each strand serving as a template for replication of a new sister strand (Figure 1.2). Wherever a G base is found on one strand a C will be placed on the growing strand; wherever a T is found an A will be placed, etc. Bases are positioned in the newly synthesized strand by hydrogen bonding, and new phosphodiester bonds are formed in the growing strand by action of the enzyme **DNA polymerase**. This is referred to as **semiconservative replication**, because the newly synthesized DNA double helices are hybrid molecules that consist of one parental strand and one new "daughter" strand. Unwinding of the double helix is accomplished by another enzyme system, called **helicase**.

DNA replication requires growth of a strand from a pre-existing "primer" sequence. The primer sequences are provided by a process of transcription, in which a short RNA molecule is synthesized from the DNA template. We will focus on transcription in the next section when we look at the means by which genetic information is used to synthesize protein. RNA is a single-stranded nucleic acid, similar to DNA, except that the sugar molecules are ribose rather than deoxyribose, and uracil substitutes for thymine (and pairs with adenine). These short RNA primers are extended by DNA polymerase (Figure 1.3). DNA is synthesized in a 5′ (exposed phosphate on 5′ carbon of the ribose molecule) to 3′ (exposed hydroxyl on the 3′ carbon) direction.

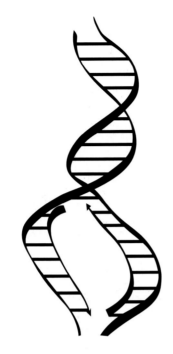

Figure 1.2 • DNA replication involves local unwinding of the double helix and copying of two daughter strands from the original parental strands.

Structure of a replication fork

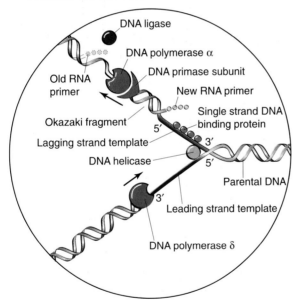

Figure 1.3 • DNA replication proceeds in a 5′ to 3′ direction. This occurs by direct addition of bases to a growing DNA strand in one direction (bottom). In the other direction, replication begins with creation of short RNA primers. DNA bases are added to the primers, and short segments, called Okazaki fragments, are ligated together. The DNA at the replication fork is unwound by a helicase enzyme. From Pritchard & Korf (2003) Medical Genetics at a Glance. Blackwell Publishing, Oxford.

For one strand, referred to as the **leading strand**, this can be accomplished continuously as the DNA unwinds. The other strand, called the **lagging strand**, is replicated in short segments, called **Okazaki fragments**, which are then enzymatically ligated together by DNA ligase. Two distinct polymerases, δ (leading strand) and α (lagging strand) replicate the DNA. The short RNA primers are ultimately removed and replaced with DNA to complete the replication process.

The human genome consists of over 3 billion base pairs of DNA packaged onto 23 pairs of chromosomes. Each chromosome consists of a single, continuous DNA molecule, encompassing tens to hundreds of millions of base pairs. If the DNA on each chromosome were to be replicated in a linear manner from one end to another the process would go on interminably – certainly too long to sustain the rates of cell division that must occur. In fact, the entire genome can be replicated in a matter of hours because replication occurs simultaneously at multiple sites along a chromosome. These origins of replication are bubble-like structures from which DNA replication proceeds bidirectionally until an adjacent bubble is reached (Figure 1.4).

Replication of human DNA

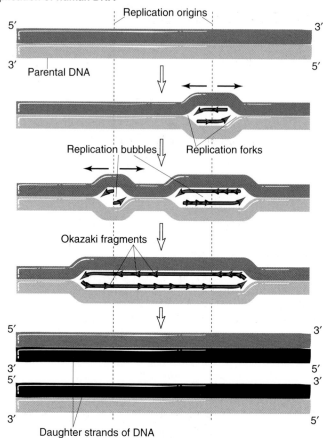

Figure 1.4 • DNA replication proceeds bidirectionally from multiple start sites. From Pritchard & Korf (2003) Medical Genetics at a Glance. Blackwell Publishing, Oxford.

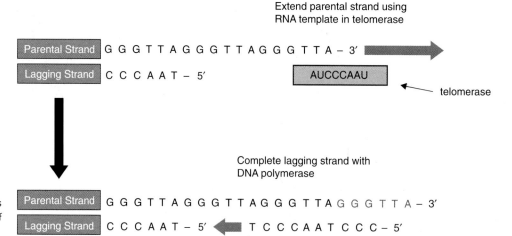

Figure 1.5 • The enzyme telomerase adds a terminal sequence to the ends of chromosomes.

One special case in DNA replication is the replication of the ends of chromosomes. Removal of the terminal RNA primer from the lagging strand at the end of a chromosome would result in shortening of the end, since there is no upstream primer for DNA polymerase to replace the short RNA primer. This problem is circumvented by action of an enzyme called **telomerase**, which uses an RNA template intrinsic to the enzyme to add a stretch of DNA onto the 3′ end of the lagging strand (Figure 1.5). The DNA sequence of the telomere is determined by the

CLINICAL SNAPSHOT 1.1

■ Dyskeratosis congenita

Eddy is a 4-year-old boy brought in by his parents because of recurrent cough. He has had two bouts of pneumonia, which were treated with antibiotics, over the past 2 months. Now he is sick again, having never stopped coughing since the last episode of pneumonia. He has also been noted by his parents to have lacked energy over the past several weeks. His examination shows a fever of 39°C and rapid respirations with frequent coughing. His breath sounds are abnormal on the right side of his chest. He also has hyperkeratotic skin with streaky hyperpigmentation. His finger and toe nails are thin and broken at the ends and his hair is sparse. A blood count shows anemia and a reduced number of white blood cells. A bone marrow aspirate is obtained, and it shows a generalized decrease in all cell lineages. A clinical diagnosis of dyskeratosis congenita is made.

Dyskeratosis congenita consists of reticulated hyperpigmentation of the skin, dystrophic hair and nails, and generalized bone marrow failure (Figure 1.6). It usually presents in childhood, often with signs of pancytopenia. There is an increased rate of spontaneous chromosome breakage seen in peripheral blood lymphocytes. Dyskeratosis congenita can be inherited as an X-linked recessive (MIM 305000), autosomal dominant (MIM 127550), or autosomal recessive (MIM 224230) trait. The X-linked form is due to mutation in a gene that encodes the protein dyskerin (MIM 300126). Dyskerin is involved in the synthesis of ribosomal RNA and also interacts with telomerase. The autosomal dominant form is due to mutation in the gene *hTERC* (MIM 602322). *hTERC* encodes the RNA component of telomerase. The gene encoding the autosomal recessive form is not yet known. The X-linked recessive form is more severe and earlier in onset than the dominant form. Both forms are associated with defective telomere functioning, leading to shortened telomeres. This likely leads to premature cell death and also explains the spontaneous chromosome breakage. The phenotype of the X-linked form may also be due, in part, to defective rRNA processing.

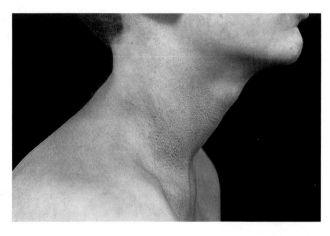

Figure 1.6 • Skin changes in an individual with dyskeratosis congenita. [Reproduced with permission from T. Burns, S. Breathnach, N. Cox, and C. Griffiths, eds, 7th edn, Rook's Textbook of Dermatology, Blackwell Publishing, Oxford.]

RNA sequence in the enzyme; for humans the sequence is GGGTTA. Each chromosome end has a tandem repeat of thousands of copies of the telomere sequence that is replicated during early development. Somatic cells may replicate without telomerase activity, resulting in a gradual shortening of the ends of the chromosomes with successive rounds of replication. This may be one of the factors that limits the number of times a cell can divide before it dies, a phenomenon known as **senescence** (Clinical Snapshot 1.1).

Chromatin

The DNA within each cell nucleus must be highly compacted to accommodate the entire genome in a very small space. The enormous stretch of DNA that composes each chromosome is actually a highly organized structure (Figure 1.7). The DNA double helix measures approx-

How is DNA packaged in the cell nucleus?

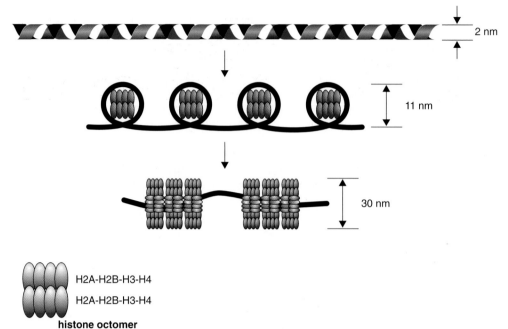

Figure 1.7 • Levels of organization of chromatin. The DNA double helix has a width of approximately 2 nm. The fundamental unit of chromatin is the nucleosome, which consists of 146 base pairs of DNA wound around a core consisting of two copies of each of the four histone proteins (H2A, H2B, H3, and H4). These are arrayed as beads on a string. The diameter of a nucleosome is 11 nm. The nucleosomes are, in turn, wound into a structure measuring 30 nm. This is further coiled and condensed to compose a metaphase chromosome.

imately 2 nm in diameter, but DNA does not exist in the nucleus in a "naked" form. It is complexed with a set of lysine- and arginine-rich proteins called histones. Two molecules of each of four major histone types – H2A, H2B, H3, and H4 – associate together with about every 146 base pairs to form a structure known as the **nucleosome**, which results in an 11-nm thick fiber. Nucleosomes are separated from one another by up to 80 base pairs, like beads on a string. This is more or less the conformation of actively transcribed chromatin but, during periods of inactivity, some regions of the genome are more highly compacted. The next level of organization is the coiling of nucleosomes into a 30-nm thick chromatin fiber held together by another histone, H1, and other nonhistone proteins. Chromatin is further compacted into the highly condensed structures comprising each chromosome, with the maximum condensation occurring during the metaphase stage of mitosis (see Chapter 6).

GENE FUNCTION

The basic tenet of molecular genetics – often referred to as "the central dogma"—is that DNA encodes RNA, which in turn encodes the amino acid sequence of proteins. It is now clear that this is a simplified view of the function of the genome. As will be seen in Chapter 4, much of the DNA sequence does not encode protein. A large proportion of the genome consists of noncoding sequences, such as repeated DNA, or encodes RNA that is not translated into protein. Nevertheless, the central dogma remains a critical principle of genome function. We will explore here the flow of information from DNA to RNA to protein.

What is the role of RNA in conveying the sequence of DNA from the nucleus to the cytoplasm?

Transcription

The process of copying the DNA sequence of a gene into **messenger RNA (mRNA)** is referred to as **transcription**. Some genes are expressed nearly ubiquitously. These are referred to as **housekeeping genes**. They include genes necessary for cell replication or metabolism. For other genes, expression is tightly controlled, with particular genes being turned on or off in particular cells at specific times in development or in response to physiological signals.

Gene expression is regulated by proteins that bind to DNA and either activate or repress

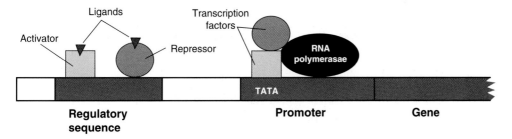

Figure 1.8 • Cis-acting elements regulating gene expression. Transcription starts at the promoter by binding of an RNA polymerase. Control of gene expression occurs via binding of transcription factors upstream of the transcription start site at the TATA box. Upstream regulatory sequences bind repressor or activator proteins, whose function is regulated by binding specific ligands.

transcription. The anatomy of elements that regulate gene transcription is shown in Figure 1.8. The **promoter region** is immediately adjacent to the transcription start site, usually within 100 base pairs. Most promoters include a base sequence of T and A bases called the TATA box. In some cases there may be multiple, alternative promoters at different sites in a gene that respond to different regulatory factors in different tissues. Regulatory sequences may occur adjacent to the promoter, or may be located thousands of base pairs away. These distantly located regulatory sequences are known as enhancers. Enhancer sequences function regardless of their orientation with respect to the gene.

DNA-binding proteins may serve as repressors or activators of transcription, and may bind to the promoter, to upstream regulatory regions, or to more distant enhancers. Activator or repressor proteins are regulated by binding of specific ligands. Ligand binding changes the confirmation of the transcription factor and may activate it or inactivate it. The ligand is typically a small molecule, such as a hormone. Many transcription factors work as a duet to form dimers. These may be homodimers of two identical proteins, or heterodimers of two different proteins. There may also be **corepressor** or **coactivator** proteins. Some transcription factors stay in the cytosol until the ligand or some other activation process occurs, at which time they move to the nucleus for activation of their target gene. In other situations, the transcription factors reside in the nucleus most of the time and may even be located at the response element sequences, but without the ligand they are inactive or even repress transcription.

Transcription begins with the attachment of the enzyme RNA polymerase to the promoter (Figure 1.9). There are three major types of RNA polymerase, designated types I, II, and III. Most gene transcription is accomplished by RNA polymerase II. Type I is involved in transcription of **rRNA** that resides in the ribosome and type III transcribes **transfer RNA (tRNA)** (see below). The polymerase reads the sequence of the DNA template strand, copying a complementary RNA molecule, which grows from the 5′ to the 3′ direction. The resulting mRNA is an exact copy of the DNA sequence, except that uracil takes the place of thymine in RNA. Soon after transcription begins, a 7-methyl guanine residue is attached to the 5′-most base, forming the "cap." Transcription proceeds through the entire coding sequence. Some genes include a sequence near the 3′ end that signals RNA cleavage at that site and enzymatic addition of 100 to 200 adenine bases, the "**poly-A tail**." Polyadenylation is characteristic of housekeeping genes, which are expressed in most cell types. Both the 5′ cap and the poly-A tail appear to function to stabilize the mRNA molecule and facilitate its export to the cytoplasm.

The DNA sequence of most genes far exceeds the length required to encode their corresponding proteins. This is accounted for by the fact that the coding sequence is broken up into segments, called **exons**, which are interrupted by segments called **introns**. Some exons may

Transcription by RNA polymerase II

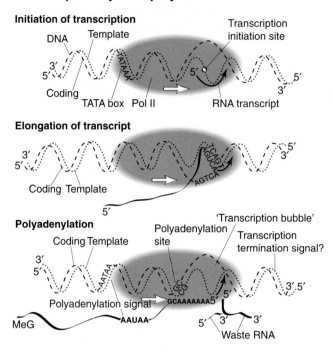

Figure 1.9 • Transcription involves copying an RNA from one stand of DNA. The reaction is catalyzed by RNA polymerase. A 7-methylguanosine cap (MeG) is added to the 5′ end of most mRNA molecules before transcription is completed. From Pritchard & Korf (2003) Medical Genetics at a Glance. Blackwell Publishing, Oxford.

Intron excision and exon splicing

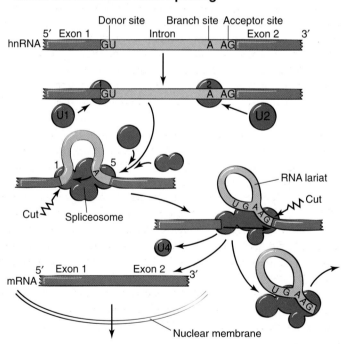

Figure 1.10 • RNA splicing begins with binding of specific ribonucleoproteins (U1 and U2) to the splice donor and acceptor. These two sites are then brought together by other components of the splicosome. The donor site is then cut and the free end of the intron binds to the branch point within the intron to form a lariat structure. Then the acceptor site is cleaved, releasing the lariat, and the exons at the two ends are ligated together. From Pritchard & Korf (2003) Medical Genetics at a Glance. Blackwell Publishing, Oxford.

be under a hundred bases long, whereas introns can be several thousand bases in length. Therefore, much of the length of a gene may be devoted to noncoding introns. The number of exons in a gene may be as few as one or two, or may number in the dozens. The processing of the RNA transcript into mature mRNA requires the removal of the introns and splicing together of the exons (Figure 1.10). This is carried out by an enzymatic process that occurs in the nucleus. The 5′ end of an intron always consists of the two bases GU, following by a con-

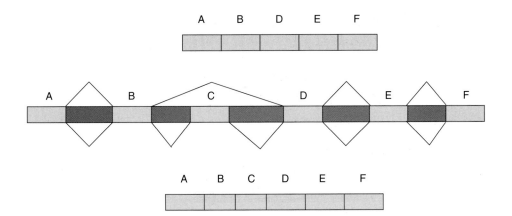

Figure 1.11 • Alternative splicing. Splicing out each intron results in inclusion of exons A–F in the mRNA. Alternatively, a splice can be made directly between exons B and D, skipping exon C. This results in production of a distinct protein, missing the amino acids encoded by exon C.

sensus sequence that is similar, but not identical, in all introns. This is the **splice donor**. The 3′ end, the **splice acceptor**, ends in AG, preceded by a consensus sequence.

The splicing process requires a complex machinery comprised of both proteins and small RNA molecules (**small nuclear RNA**, or **snRNA**), consisting of fewer than 200 bases. snRNA is also transcribed by RNA polymerase II. The splice is initiated by binding of a protein–RNA complex to the splice donor, at a point within the intron called the **branch point**, and the splice acceptor. First the DNA is cleaved at the donor site and this is attached in a 5′–2′ bond to the branch point. Then the acceptor site is cleaved, releasing a lariat structure that is subsequently degraded, and the 5′ and 3′ ends are ligated together. The splicing process also requires the function of proteins, **SR proteins**, which are involved in selecting sites for the initiation of splicing. These proteins interact with sequences known as **splice enhancers** or **silencers**. The splicing process is vulnerable to disruption by mutation, as might be predicted from its complexity.

The RNA splicing process offers a point of control of gene expression. Under the influence of control molecules present in specific cells, particular exons may be included or not included in the mRNA due to differential splicing (Figure 1.11). This results in the potential to produce multiple, different proteins from the same gene, adding greatly to the diversity of proteins encoded by the genome. Specific exons may correspond with particular functional domains of proteins, leading to the production of multiple proteins with diverse functions from the same gene. Some mRNAs are subject to RNA editing, in which a specific base may be enzymatically modified. For example, the protein apolipoprotein B exists in two forms, a 48-kDa form made in the intestine and a 100-kDa form in the liver. Both forms are the product of the same gene. In the intestine, however, the enzyme cytidine deaminase alters a C to a U at codon 2153, changing the codon from CAA (encoding glutamine) to UAA (a stop codon). This truncates the peptide, accounting for the 48-kDa form. Recently, another mechanism of post-transcritional regulation, called RNA interference, has also been identified (Hot Topics 1.1).

Translation

The mature mRNA is exported to the cytoplasm for translation into protein. During translation, the mRNA sequence is read into the amino acid sequence of a protein (Figure 1.13). The translational machinery consists of a protein–RNA complex called the **ribosome**. Ribosomes consist of a complex of proteins and specialized ribosomal RNA molecules (rRNA). The eukaryotic ribosome is comprised of two subunits, designated 60S and 40S (the "S" is a measurement of density, the Svendborg unit, reflecting how the complexes were initially characterized).

How is mRNA translated into protein?

Hot Topic 1.1   RNA INTERFERENCE

Gene regulation is not limited to control at the level of gene transcription. There is another level of control that occurs post-transcriptionally, referred to as RNA interference (RNAi). RNAi was discovered in plants, but appears to play a role in animals, including vertebrates. Its function in gene regulation is only beginning to come into focus.

The mechanisms of RNAi are illustrated in Figure 1.12. In experimental systems, and perhaps in some viral infections, RNAi begins with introduction of double-stranded RNA molecules (dsRNA), which are cleaved by the enzyme Dicer into short interfering RNA (siRNA) molecules. siRNA are 21 to 23 nucleotide, double-stranded RNAs with two unpaired bases at both ends. siRNAs separate into single strands and associate with specific proteins to form the RNA-induced silencing complex (RISC). The single-stranded siRNA binds to homologous sequences in mRNA and the RISC cleaves that RNA, thereby inactivating it.

The endogenous RNAi mechanism in animals begins with the transcription of genes that produce micro-RNAs (miRNAs), which are short RNA molecules containing segments with complementary bases that allow the molecule to form hairpin structures. The enzyme Drosha cleaves the hairpins, which are then exported to the cytoplasm, where Dicer further cleaves the hairpins into miRNA molecules that are similar to siRNAs. These associate with proteins and bind to homologous sequences, often in a region 3′ to the stop codon, referred to as the 3′ untranslated region (3′ UTR). Binding of the ribonucleoprotein complexes then inhibits translation, by as yet unknown mechanisms.

RNAi has been studied extensively in invertebrates, such as the flatworm *Caenorhabditis elegans* and the fruit fly *Drosophila*. In these organisms, interfering RNAs are involved in silencing genes during normal development. The role of RNAi in vertebrates, including humans, is just beginning to be explored, but here, too, it is likely to be involved in gene regulation. RNAi is also being exploited as an experimental tool and as an approach to therapy. dsRNA molecules can be introduced that are cleaved to produce siRNAs homologous to any gene of interest. This provides a means of selectively silencing genes in cells or tissues, allowing the function of these genes to be studied. As therapeutic tools, siRNA are being designed to silence viral genes, or to turn off genes that are activated by mutation, in genetic disorders or cancer.

Each subunit includes proteins and an rRNA molecule. The 60S subunit includes a 28S rRNA and the 40S subunit an 18S rRNA. Ribosomes can be free or associated with the **endoplasmic reticulum (ER)**, also known as the "rough ER."

The mRNA sequence is read in triplets, called **codons**, beginning at the 5′ end of the mRNA, which is always AUG, encoding methionine (although this methionine residue is often later cleaved off). Each codon corresponds with a particular complementary **anticodon**, which is part of another RNA molecule called **transfer RNA (tRNA)**. tRNA molecules bind specific amino acids defined by their anticodon sequence (Table 1.1). Protein translation therefore consists of binding of a specific tRNA to the appropriate codon, which juxtaposes the next amino acid in the growing peptide, which is enzymatically linked by an amide bond to the peptide. The process ends when a stop codon is reached (UAA, UGA, or UAG). The peptide is then released from the ribosome for transport to the appropriate site within the cell, or for secretion from the cell. A leader peptide sequence may direct the protein to its final destination in the cell; this peptide is cleaved off upon arrival. Post-translational modification, such as glycosylation, begins during the translation process and continues after translation is complete.

The process of translation consists of three phases, referred to as initiation, elongation, and termination. Initiation involves the binding of the first amino acyl tRNA, which always carries methionine, to the initiation codon, always AUG. A set of proteins, referred to as **elongation factors**, are involved in the process, which also requires ATP and GTP. The ribosome binds to the mRNA at two successive codons. One is designated the **P site** and carries the growing peptide chain. The other is the next codon, designated the **A site**. Elongation involves the binding of the next amino acyl tRNA to its anticodon at the A site. This delivers the next amino acid in the peptide chain, which is attached to the growing peptide, with peptide bond formation catalyzed by **peptidyl transferase**. The ribosome then moves on to the next codon under the action of a **translocase**, with energy provided by GTP. When a stop codon is reached, a release factor protein–GTP complex binds and the peptidyl transferase adds an OH to the end of the peptide, which is then released from the ribosome under the influence of proteins called **release factors**.

Hot Topic 1.1 RNA INTERFERENCE continued

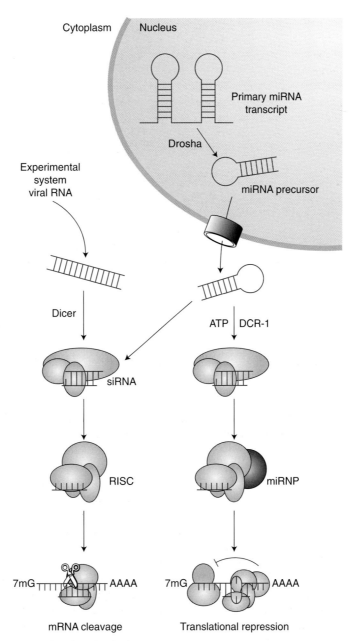

Figure 1.12 • Mechanisms of RNA interference. dsRNA may be introduced by viral infection or experimentally. siRNA is produced from dsRNA through cleavage by the enzyme Dicer. Single-stranded siRNA complexes with proteins to form the RISC, which then binds to mRNA through homologous pairing with the siRNA and cleaves the mRNA. Endogenous miRNA is transcribed and cleaved into hairpin structures in the nucleus. These are exported to the cytoplasm, where they are processed into miRNA by Dicer. The miRNA complexes with proteins and binds to mRNA, often in the 3′ UTR, and inhibits translation. (Adapted by permission from Macmillan Publishers Ltd: Meister G, Tuschl T. Mechanisms of gene silencing by double-stranded RNA. Nature 2004;431:343–349.)

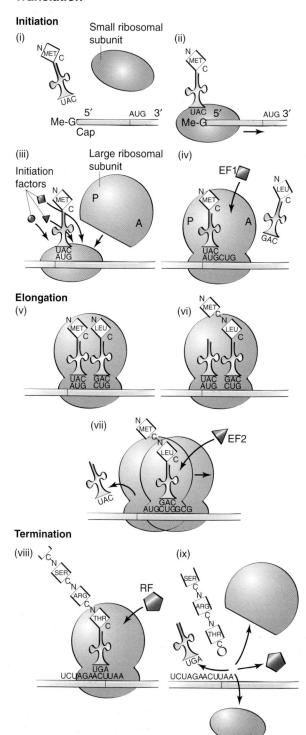

Figure 1.13 • The process of protein translation. Translation takes place at the ribosome, which binds to the mRNA. Specific amino acyl tRNA molecules bind to the mRNA by base pair complementarity between a triplet codon on the mRNA and an anticodon on the tRNA. A peptide bond is formed between the growing peptide and the next amino acyl tRNA, transferring the growing peptide and elongating it by one amino acid. This continues until a stop codon is reached. EF: elongation factor, RF: release factor. From Pritchard & Korf (2003) Medical Genetics at a Glance. Blackwell Publishing, Oxford.

How can genes be permanently inactivated?

Gene Inactivation and Imprinting

Individual genes may be reversibly activated or repressed, but there are some situations where genes or sets of genes are permanently silenced. This occurs on one of the two copies of the X chromosome in females, and on the maternal or paternal copy of a set of genes that are said to be **imprinted**. Gene silencing is accompanied by methylation of cytosine bases to

TABLE 1.1 The genetic code. A triplet codon is read from the left column, to the top row, to the full triplet in each box. Each codon corresponds with a specific amino acid, except for the three stop codons (labeled "Ter"). Most amino acids are encoded by more than one codon

	T	C	A	G
T	TTT Phe (F) TTC " TTA Leu (L) TTG "	TCT Ser (S) TCC " TCA " TCG "	TAT Tyr (Y) TAC TAA Ter TAG Ter	TGT Cys (C) TGC TGA **Ter** TGG Trp (W)
C	CTT Leu (L) CTC " CTA " CTG "	CCT Pro (P) CCC " CCA " CCG "	CAT His (H) CAC " CAA Gln (Q) CAG "	CGT Arg (R) CGC " CGA " CGG "
A	ATT I1e (I) ATC " ATA " **ATG** Met (M)	ACT Thr (T) ACC " ACA " ACG "	AAT Asn (N) AAC " AAA Lys (K) AAG "	AGT Ser (S) AGC " AGA Arg (R) AGG "
G	GTT Val (V) GTC " GTA " GTG "	GCT Ala (A) GCC " GCA " GCG "	GAT Asp (D) GAC " GAA Glu (E) GAG "	GGT Gly (G) GGC " GGA " GGG "

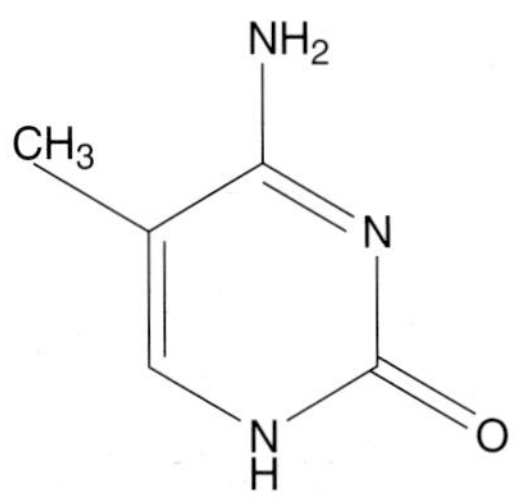

Figure 1.14 • Structure of 5-methylcytosine.

5-methylcytosine (Figure 1.14). This occurs in regions where cytosine is following by guanine (5'–CpG–3') near the promoter, sites referred to as **CpG islands**. Methylated sites bind protein complexes that remove acetyl groups from histones, leading to transcriptional repression. The silencing is continued from cell generation to generation because the enzymes responsible for methylation recognize the 5-methylcytosine on the parental strand of DNA and methylate the cytosine on the newly synthesized daughter strand (Figure 1.15).

X-chromosome inactivation provides a mechanism for equalization of gene dosage on the X chromosome in males, who have one X, and females, who have two. Most genes on one of the two X chromosomes in each cell of a female are permanently inactivated early in development (Figure 1.16). The particular X inactivated in any cell is determined at random, so that in approximately 50% of cells one X is inactivated and in the other 50% the other X is inactivated. Regions of homology between the X and Y at the two ends of the X escape inactivation. These are referred to as **pseudoautosomal regions**. The inactive X remains condensed through most of the cell cycle, and can be visualized as a densely staining body during interphase, referred to as the **Barr body**.

Initiation of inactivation is controlled from a region called the **X-inactivation center** (**Xic**). A gene within this region, known as *Xist*, is expressed on one of the two X chromosomes early in development. *Xist* encodes a 25-kb RNA that is not translated into protein, but appears to bind to sites along the X to be inactivated. Subsequently, CpG islands on this chromosome are methylated, and changes occur to histones, particularly deacetylation.

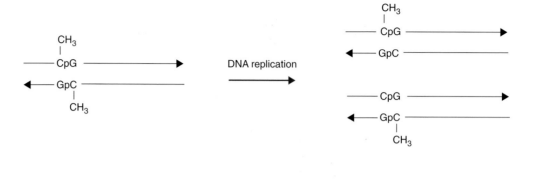

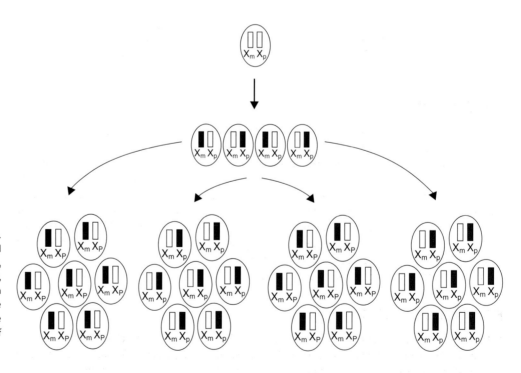

Figure 1.15 • Cytosine residues adjacent to guanines may be methylated near the 5′ ends of some genes. When the DNA is replicated, only one strand will be methylated, but then an enzyme recognizes the single methylated strand and methylates the cytosines on the opposite strand.

Figure 1.16 • X chromosome inactivation. In the zygote, both the maternally and paternally derived X chromosomes (X_m and X_p) are active. Early in development, one of the two X chromosomes in each cell is inactivated (indicated as the dark chromosome). This X chromosome remains inactive in all the descendants of that cell.

Genomic imprinting involves the silencing of either the maternal or paternal copy of a gene during early development (Figure 1.17). Like X-chromosome inactivation, imprinting is probably accomplished through methylation of specific chromosome regions. The methylation "imprint" is erased in germ cells, so the specific gene copy to be inactivated is always determined by the parent of origin, regardless of whether that particular gene copy was active or inactive in the previous generation. Genomic imprinting appears to apply only to a small subset of genes, although the full extent of imprinting is not yet known.

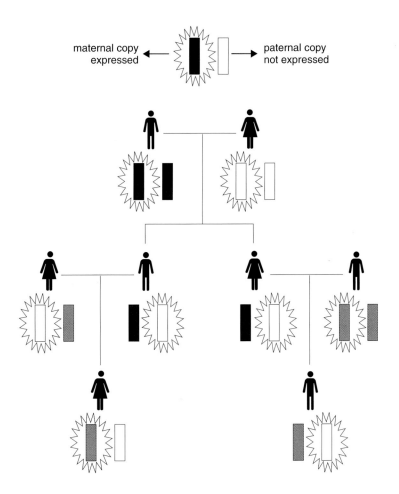

Figure 1.17 • Concept of genomic imprinting. In this example, the paternally derived copy of a gene is not expressed, whereas the maternally inherited copy is expressed. The imprint is "reset" in the germ line, so that in the next generation, the active copy of the gene depends on the parent of origin, not on whether that copy was active in the parent.

CONCLUSION

More than half a century of research in molecular biology has resulted in a detailed picture of the mechanisms of gene structure and function. Much of the remainder of this book will be devoted to exploration of the implications of dysfunction at the level of the gene or groups of genes and their interactions with the environment. We will see also that genetics research is moving to a new level of integration of basic molecular mechanisms, towards formation of a picture of how entire cells and organisms function. It is important to realize, however, that some fundamental molecular mechanisms, such as the role of small RNAs and genomic imprinting, have been discovered only within the past decade or so. Even as the effort towards larger-scale integration goes forward, there remains much to be learned about the fundamental molecular mechanisms at the level of the gene.

REVIEW QUESTIONS

1.1 The two strands of DNA separate when heated, and the temperature at which separation occurs is dependent on base content. Specifically, DNA with a higher proportion of G–C base pairs tends to "melt" at a higher temperature than molecules with a higher A–T content. Why is this?

1.2 What is the role of transcription in DNA replication?

1.3 Consider the gene sequence below. What is the base sequence of the mRNA that would be transcribed from this gene, and what is the amino acid sequence of the peptide that would be translated?

5′ – promoter – ATG GTT GAT AGT CGT TGC CGC GGG CTG TGA – 3′

3′ – promoter – TAC CAA CTA TCA GCA ACG GCG CCC GAC ACT – 5′

1.4 There are more proteins than there are genes. What are some of the mechanisms that account for this discrepancy?

1.5 A woman is heterozygous for an X-linked trait that leads to expression of two different forms of an enzyme. The two forms are separable as two distinct bands when the enzyme protein is run through an electric field by electrophoresis. If you were to test cultured skin fibroblasts and isolate enzyme, what would you expect to see? If you could isolate single fibroblasts and grow them into colonies before extracting the enzyme and subjecting it to electrophoresis what would you expect to see?

FURTHER READING

General References
Alberts B, Johnson A, Lewis J, Raff M, Roberts K, Walter P. Molecular Biology of the Cell, 4th edn., 2002, New York: Garland Science.

Lewin B. Genes VIII, 2003, Upper Saddle River, NJ: Prentice Hall.

Lodish H, Berk A, Zipursky L, Matsudaira P, Baltimore D, Darnell J. Molecular Cell Biology, 5th edn., 2004, New York: Freeman.

Chromatin Structure
Dehghani H, Dellaire G, Bazett-Jones, DP. Organization of chromatin in the interphase mammalian cell. Micron 2005;36:95–108.

X Chromosome Inactivation
Latham KE. X chromosome imprinting and inactivation in preimplantation mammalian embryos. Trends Genet 2005;21:120–127.

Imprinting
Miyoshi N, Barton SC, Kaneda M, Hajkova P, Surani MA. The continuing quest to comprehend genomic imprinting. Cytogenet Genome Res 2006;113:6–11.

Paulsen M, Ferguson-Smith AC. DNA methylation in genomic imprinting, development, and disease. J Pathol 2005;195:97–110.

Clinical Snapshot 1.1 Dyskeratosis Congenita
Bessler M, Wilson DB, Mason PJ. Dyskeratosis congenita and telomerase. Curr Opin Pediatr 2004;16:23–28.

Methods 1.1 Mendelian Inheritance in Man
Online Mendelian Inheritance in Man: http://www.ncbi.nlm.nih.gov/entrez/query.fcgi?db=OMIM

Hot Topic 1.1 RNA Interference
Hannon GJ, Rossi JJ. Unlocking the potential of the human genome with RNA interference. Nature 2004;431:371–378.

2
Genetic Variation

INTRODUCTION

The human genome contains variations in base sequence from one individual to another, on average every few hundred bases. Some sequence variants occur within areas that do not encode RNA or protein, and so have no visible effect. Others affect physical characteristics, or **phenotype**, by altering RNA or protein products. Genetic variants account for some physical differences between individuals, for example hair or eye color, body size, facial appearance, etc. Some underlie specific medical disorders. In this section, we will take a close-up look at DNA sequence variations and their effects on gene expression. Later in this book we will see how these sequence variants exert their phenotypic effects.

KEY POINTS

- DNA sequence variants are common in the population, and range from single base changes to large-scale DNA rearrangements.
- Sequence variants can be silent, or may alter the quantity or quality of the gene product.
- Mutations may occur spontaneously, or can be induced by chemical or radiation mutagens. Advanced paternal age is associated with increased rate of mutation.
- The fidelity of the DNA sequence is maintained by a DNA repair system. These enzyme systems correct errors introduced into the base sequence by mutation or during DNA replication.
- Polymorphisms are sequence variants that occur commonly in the population.
- There are four major types of base sequence polymorphisms: restriction fragment length polymorphisms, simple sequence repeats, variable number tandem repeats, and single nucleotide polymorphisms.

DNA SEQUENCE VARIANTS

There is no canonical "human DNA sequence" (Ethical Implication 2.1). Genetic variation is occurring constantly, both in germ cells and in somatic cells. Much of this variation is either repaired or is lethal to the cell. Sometimes, however, a variant will be neutral in its effect, or even convey a selective advantage. Selective advantage is the driving force of evolution at the population level, but in the individual selective advantage is the driving force of cancer.

Types of DNA Sequence Variants

DNA sequence variants can be broadly classified into single-base substitutions, rearrangements that affect small or large stretches of DNA and expansions of simple sequence repeats (Figure 2.1). The physiological effect of these changes depends on where they occur in the genome and where they occur within a specific gene.

The simplest change is a point mutation consisting of a single base substitution. This may occur as a consequence of misincorporation of a base into DNA during replication, or can be

What are the different types of DNA sequence variants?

ETHICAL IMPLICATIONS 2.1 • Eugenics

What is the "normal" DNA sequence for any particular gene? Geneticists working with experimental systems, such as the fruit fly *Drosophila*, have coined the term "wild type" to indicate the most common version of a genetic trait in the population. Most fruit flies, for example, have red eyes, so the white-eyed phenotype is consider "mutant" and red eye the "wild type" state. We will see that genetic variation is the rule, not the exception, so it is not possible to designate a "normal" or "wild type" state for most genes at the level of DNA base sequence. Some genetic variants have a profound effect on gene function and may lead to clinically evident phenotypes that may be considered "abnormal." Other variations have no detectable phenotype, or are responsible for variations such as alteration of hair or eye color that are not important medically.

It has been known for a long time that selective breeding could increase or decrease the frequency of particular genetic traits in plants and animals, knowledge that has been used to great advantage in agriculture. As the science of human hered-ity began to emerge in the late 19th century there were advocates of similar selective "breeding" in humans. Here, however, the notion of "desirable" or "undesirable" traits was in the eye of the beholder. The term "eugenics" was coined to describe the study of human traits and the application of selective breeding to increase the frequency of traits that were deemed desirable. The term has taken on sinister connotations, however, since eugenics became a tool of racist social policy. Eugenics has been invoked to deny the rights of individuals or groups to reproduce, including forced sterilization and genocide. The notion achieved its most grotesque form with the Nazi campaigns in the 1930s and 1940s to produce a "perfect" human race, largely through the mass murder of those deemed inferior.

Although modern medical genetics seeks to ameliorate or prevent the occurrence of disease due to genetic alterations, the goals are to alleviate individual suffering, not to "improve" the human race. We will see throughout this book that there are examples of genetic traits that are clearly and invariably deleterious, and others whose effects are more ambiguous, some-times being advantageous in some circumstances and disadvantageous in others. At the least, it will become clear that there is no single "correct" DNA sequence, but genetic variation occurs, throughout the human genome, from individual to individual.

a result of changes due to chemical or physical mutagens (see below). Mutation of C to T occurs fairly commonly as a result of deamination of 5-methylcytosine (Figure 2.2).

Deletions, duplications, insertions, and inversions are sequence rearrangements that may be as small as single base changes (for deletions, duplications, and insertions), or as large as millions of base pairs. The latter may be visible through the microscope when chromosomal analysis is performed. These changes occur at sites with distinctive structural features (Figure

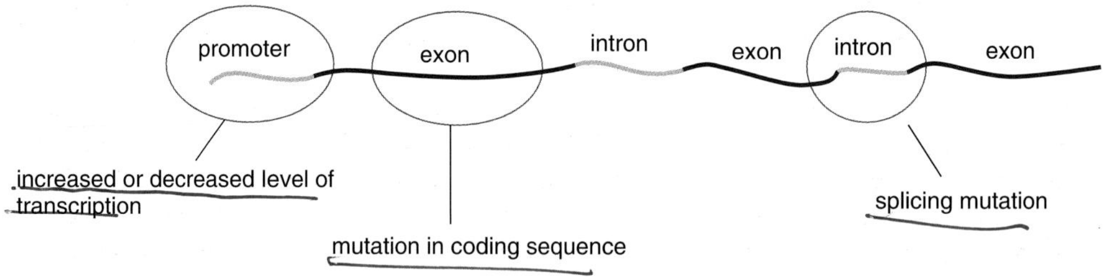

Figure 2.1 • Types of mutations. Promoter mutations lead to increased or decreased levels of transcription. Mutations within the exon cause changes of amino acid sequence or premature termination of translation. Mutations at intron–exon borders may affect the splicing process.

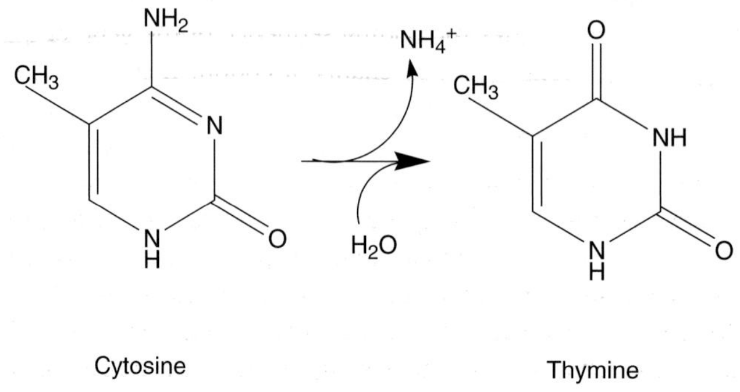

Figure 2.2 • C to T transition by deamina-tion of 5-methylcytosine to thymine.

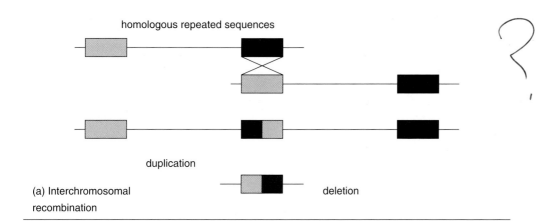

homologous repeated sequences

duplication

(a) Interchromosomal recombination

deletion

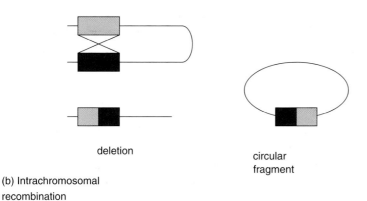

deletion

circular fragment

(b) Intrachromosomal recombination

Figure 2.3 • Mechanisms of deletion of chromosome regions flanked by repeated sequences. (a) Unequal crossing over between chromosomes during meiosis results in one copy of the chromosome with a deletion and one with a duplication. Either or both of these abnormalities may be associated with a phenotype. (b) Intrachromosomal recombination between repeated sequences produces a chromosome with a deletion and an acentric ring, which is lost from the cell.

2.3). Rearrangements involving short stretches of DNA often occur in regions of homonucleotide repeats, or at sites with repeated sequences, or sequences that can form intrastrand hairpins due to the presence of inverted repeats. These regions are prone to misreplication or to unequal crossing over events. Larger-scale deletions or duplications tend to involve sequences that are flanked by homologous repeats that may engage in unequal recombination events. Some large insertions involve repeat elements that have a potential to move about the genome. We will have more to say about these in Chapter 6.

Effects on Gene Expression

The effect of a genetic change on gene expression depends on whether the variant is located in a control region, an exon, an intron, or whether it encompasses an entire gene or group of genes.

A mutation within the promoter region or other control regions, such as an enhancer element, can alter the level of expression of the gene (Figure 2.4). Expression levels may go up or down as a consequence of the mutation, depending on whether the change affects binding of repressor or activator proteins or of the transcription initiation complex. Mutations in enhancer regions some distance from the gene can also have an effect on the level of expression. The various repressor and activator molecules are themselves gene products, so mutations in these genes can alter the expression of the target gene for those regulators.

Mutations within an exon can alter the coding sequence of the gene or may affect splicing (Figure 2.5). A single base substitution will change a codon. If the new codon encodes the same amino acid as the original, there will be no change in the protein, a **silent mutation**. If a different amino acid is encoded, the mutation is said to be **missense**. The effect on protein function depends on whether the new amino acid changes the physical and chemical properties of the protein, and whether the change occurs at a critical site along the protein. Some changes substitute amino acids with similar chemical properties, for example two nonpolar amino acids such as isoleucine and valine. These may have little or no effect on the function of the protein, representing **conservative mutations**. Other times, the substitution may alter the protein, producing a detectable, but not necessarily deleterious, change in protein function.

How do changes in base sequence affect the function of a gene product?

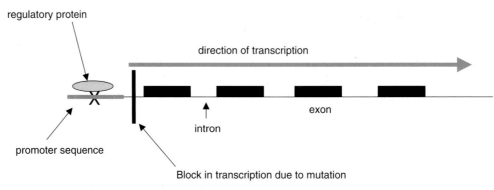

Figure 2.4 • Mutation within a promoter sequence leads to failure to initiate transcription.

TCC CAA ATC GTC CCT CGA GTT   wild type sequence
ser gln ile val pro arg val

TCC (CAG) ATC GTC CCT CGA GTT   silent mutation
ser gln ile val pro arg val

TCC CAG ATC (CTC) CCT CGA GTT   conservative mutation
ser gln ile leu pro arg val

TCC CAG ATC CTC (GCT) CGA GTT   non-conservative mutation
ser gln ile leu ala arg val

missense mutations

↳ *big difference in chemical properties of aa*

Figure 2.5 • Consequences of single base change mutations within an exon. If the amino acid is not altered, the mutation is silent. Missense mutations insert amino acids that may have an impact on protein function. A mutation that substitutes amino acids of similar chemical properties is described as conservative.

❓

What are stop mutations?

There are many sequence variants (single nucleotide polymorphisms, SNPs) between different individuals, and for that matter between homologous proteins in humans and other species, that represent such minor variants. Finally, in some cases, the amino acid change can have a profound effect on protein structure, perhaps obliterating function or leading to increased function, altered function, or aberrant response to control factors.

Some exonic mutations lead to production of a truncated peptide by introducing a premature stop codon (Figure 2.6). There are three stop codons, and mutation of an amino acid-encoding codon to a stop will have this effect. Insertion or deletion of a nonintegral multiple of three bases will cause a **frameshift**, which results in misreading of the codons until a stop is reached. Mutations within exon splice enhancer sequences can disrupt splicing, and some mutations will create a new splice donor or acceptor sequence within the exon that also can disrupt splicing. In some cases, a single base change in an exon may alter splicing in addition to disrupting the amino acid sequence, causing a stop codon, or being a silent mutation.

TCC CAA ATC GTC CCT CGA GTT   wild type sequence
ser gln ile val pro arg val

TCC CAA ATC GTC CCT (TGA) GTT   stop mutation
ser gln ile val pro stop

TCC CA(G) CAT CCT CGC TCG AGT T   frameshift insertion
ser gln his pro arg ser ser

Figure 2.6 • Mutations leading to premature termination of translation. A stop mutation changes an amino acid codon to a stop codon. A frameshift alters the amino acid sequence, and usually results in production of a stop codon.

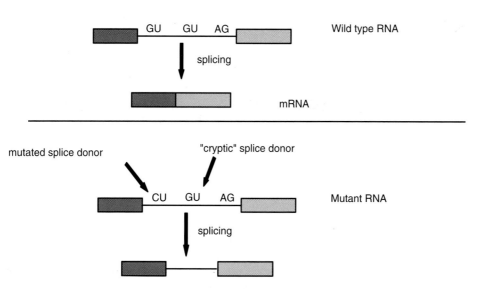

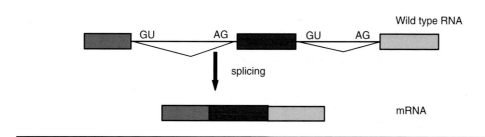

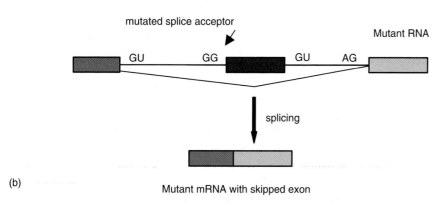

Figure 2.7 • Splicing mutations. (a) Mutation of splice donor sequence, with a cryptic splice donor (a GU followed by an "imperfect" concensus sequence that can serve as a donor if the true donor is mutated) within the intron, results in inclusion of intron sequence in the final processed mRNA. (b) Splice acceptor mutation, resulting in exon skipping.

How do mutations disrupt splicing?

Mutations within introns likewise lead to abnormal splicing (Figure 2.7). These include mutations that disrupt the splice donor, acceptor, or the branch point sequences. Sometimes these lead to inclusion of some intron sequence within the final spliced message, which will encode a meaningless amino acid sequence and often will introduce a stop codon. Other times, an exon will be skipped, so that the final spliced mRNA will be missing an exon. This can either result in a protein that is missing an essential domain (encoded by the skipped exon), or, if the two newly juxtaposed exons are not in the same reading frame, a frameshift will occur, leading to premature termination of translation. The presence of an abnormal stop codon, whether due to a single base change nonsense mutation, a frameshift, or abnormal splicing, often leads to degradation of the mutant mRNA (Hot Topics 2.1).

Longer range mutations include large deletions and chromosomal abnormalities. We will consider the latter in Chapter 6. Large deletions may encompass one or more exons of a gene, an entire gene, or a group of contiguous genes. If the deletion is entirely intragenic, the effect is similar to an exon-skipping mutation described above. Loss of the entire gene leads

Hot Topic 2.1 NONSENSE-MEDIATED DECAY

The presence of a stop codon can cause degradation of the mRNA by a process of nonsense mediated decay (NMD) (Figure 2.8). NMD occurs when a stop codon is located approximately 50 or more bases upstream of an exon splice boundary. Some components of the splicing complex remain associated with the spliced exons to form an exon junctional complex (EJC). NMD requires one round of translation. If premature termination of translation occurs prior to an EJC, the mRNA is marked for degradation. NMD does not occur when a truncating mutation occurs in the final exon, since there is no EJC beyond that point.

NMD can have significant effect on phenotypic expression. For example, a nonsense mutation in the gene *SOX10* is responsible for a disorder called Waardenburg–Shah syndrome. The condition is characterized by deafness and a white forelock, both due to abnormal neural crest cell development. Some affected individuals have, in addition, complications of peripheral neuropathy and Hirschsprung disease (lack of nerve cells in a segment of the intestine leading to intestinal obstruction). The difference is accounted for by nonsense-mediated decay. Those with uncomplicated Waardenburg–Shah syndrome have mutations at sites that lead to NMD. These individuals have no expression of the mutated copy of the SOX10 protein. Mutations responsible for the complicated form of the syndrome are at sites that do not undergo NMD. A truncated protein is produced which interferes with the function of the normal protein, causing more severe disruption of neural crest development.

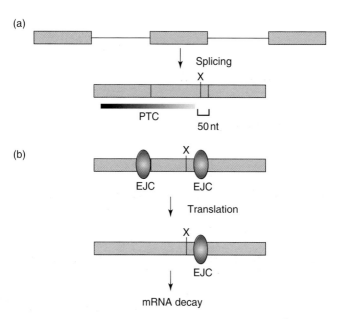

Figure 2.8 • Process of nonsense-mediated decay. (a) A stop codon (X) is located 50 or more bases upstream of splice site. (b) Part of the splicosome remains attached to the splice sites after removal of the introns, as the exon junctional complex (EJC). A single round of translation is required to displace the EJC. If this does not happen, due to presence of a stop codon, the mRNA is degraded.

to reduced levels of expression, referred to as haploinsufficiency. Deletions of contiguous genes can lead to complex phenotypes representing the combined effect of haploinsufficiency at many loci.

?

What causes gene mutation?

Causes of Mutation

As already noted, mutations often occur spontaneously due to misincorporation of a base into DNA during replication. There are proofreading and repair mechanisms that identify base mismatches, but some errors nevertheless escape detection. Some mutations occur as a result of peculiarities of DNA structure, such as the presence of repeated sequences or intrastrand homologies that allow hairpin formation. Then there are transposable genetic elements, which

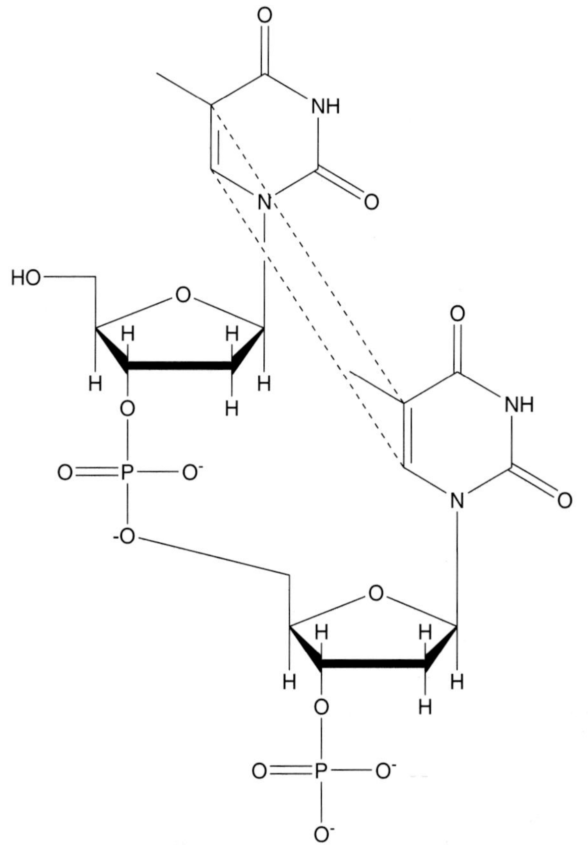

Figure 2.9 • Thymidine dimers resulting from UV exposure.

we will meet in Chapter 4, that can integrate into the chromosome and disrupt a gene. Although the genome is robust to change, it should not be a surprise that there is substantial fluidity. Not all mutations are deleterious in all situations; genome change is the engine of evolution.

It is clear, however, that there are chemical, physical, and biological circumstances that increase the likelihood of mutation. Study of these is important since mutations can lead to birth defects, genetic disorders, and cancer, and at least some of the agents that cause mutation consist of environmental exposures that might be controlled.

Mutagens alter the chemical structure of a DNA base or induce breaks in the DNA strand. Base analogs may be incorporated into DNA in the place of a normal base, for example 5-bromouracil in the place of thymine. These analogs may mispair during a subsequent round of DNA replication. Some mutations cause deamination, for example conversion of cytosine to uracil, or alkylation, leading to cross-linking of the two DNA strands. Intercalating agents fit between bases in the double helix and predispose to insertion mutations. Another class of mutations results from the production of free radicals in the nucleus, which leads to DNA strand breakage.

Ionizing radiation and ultraviolet light are two major physical mutagens. Ionizing radiation may act directly, or indirectly by increasing free radicals in the cell. A wide variety of mutations can result, including point mutations and DNA strand breaks. The major effect of UV irradiation is the dimerization of adjacent thymine bases, which can result in a deletion mutation (Figure 2.9).

Biological factors may also increase the rate of mutation. We have already encountered one example: mutations within genes that encode components of the DNA repair system. Affected individuals accumulate mutations, which leads to cell death but also to the eventual development of cancer. A more ubiquitous biological correlate of new mutation is advanced paternal age. Advanced paternal age is a risk factor for having a child with a genetic disorder due to a new mutation. Advanced maternal age does not convey similar risks; although there is an increased risk of chromosomal nondisjunction associated with advanced maternal age (see Chapter 6). The paternal age-related risk of mutation is thought to be due to the fact that male

What factors increase the rate of mutation?

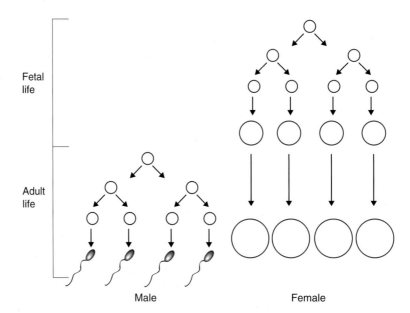

Figure 2.10 • Differences in maturation of sperm (left) and eggs (right). Sperm undergo multiple rounds of mitosis, beginning at puberty and continuing through adult life. Eggs, in contrast, complete mitotic divisions during fetal life.

germ cells continue to undergo mitotic divisions beginning in puberty and continuing throughout life (Figure 2.10). In contrast, oocytes complete all of their mitotic divisions during fetal life. Each round of DNA replication represents an opportunity for errors that result in mutation, so the older the father, the more mutations are likely to have accumulated in germ cells. The magnitude of the risk associated with advanced paternal age is small, however, and it is impossible to predict which genes might be affected, so it is difficult to provide specific counseling to a couple who may be concerned about risks.

How are errors in DNA base sequence detected and repaired?

DNA Repair

Most of the variation in base sequence never sees the light of day, as there are built-in mechanisms to repair DNA damage. Much of what is known about DNA repair was originally learned from the study of micro-organisms, such as bacteria. Similar repair pathways exist in eukaryotic cells, including human. Aberrations in DNA repair pathways underlie a set of inherited disorders (Table 2.1; Clinical Snapshot 2.1), as well as contribute to the pathogenesis of cancer.

CLINICAL SNAPSHOT 2.1

■ DNA repair disorders

Timothy is a 2-year-old referred because of unusual skin findings. He was born after a full term pregnancy and was healthy as a newborn. By the end of the first year of life, however, his parents noted that his face was becoming covered with freckles. This seemed odd for a baby, and especially odd since no one else in the family has freckles. Recently, his family spent some time at the beach and Timothy developed a severe sunburn. His parents were surprised, since they had tried to keep him out of the sun and had applied sunscreen. Now, one month later, his skin appears dry and scaly, and there are innumerable freckles on the face, arms, and trunk – all areas where he had been exposed to the sun. Timothy is in the 50th centile for height and weight, but his head is in the 20th centile. No one else in the family has had similar problems.

Timothy has signs typical for xeroderma pigmentosum (XP) (MIM 278700). The disorder usually presents in the early years of life with freckling and extreme sun sensitivity of the skin (Figure 2.11). Affected children may develop severe sunburn even with minimal ultraviolet exposure. There is a very high risk of skin cancer, with onset usually in the childhood years. There may be ocular problems due to ultraviolet light-induced damage and some children develop neurological problems, including small head size, developmental delay, deafness, ataxia, and seizures. Xeroderma pigmentosum is due to defective excision repair. Cultured cells obtained from

CLINICAL SNAPSHOT 2.1 continued

affected individuals display increased cell death on exposure to UV. At least eight distinct genes are known to be associated with XP. These genes encode proteins involved in the excision repair process. Care of persons with XP involves protection from UV exposure and careful monitoring for the development of skin cancer. The disorder is inherited as an autosomal recessive trait.

Xeroderma pigmentosum is one of a number of disorders of DNA repair or DNA replication. Some are described in Table 2.1. Most are associated with an increased risk of malignancy due to the accumulation of mutations in cells that cannot repair DNA damage. Short stature is another common feature. Management is focused on symptomatic treatment and surveillance for cancer. No primary therapy exists for any of these disorders. Each is inherited as an autosomal recessive trait.

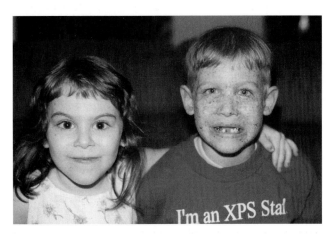

Figure 2.11 • Two children affected with xeroderma pigmentosum. Some children, such as the boy at the right, are more fair-skinned and sun-sensitive than others and develop freckling at a younger age. (Courtesy of Xeroderma Pigmentosum Society.)

TABLE 2.1 Major medical disorders resulting from mutation in the DNA repair system

Syndrome	Features	Genetic cause
Ataxia-telangiectasia MIM 208900	Ataxia, telangiectasia, immune deficiency, lymphoma	Mutations in ATM gene; cell cycle checkpoint for repair of DNA damage
Bloom syndrome MIM 210900	Short stature, photosensitive skin, risk of malignancy, increased frequency of sister chromatid exchange	Mutations in helicase gene involved in DNA replication and recombination
Werner syndrome MIM 277700	Short stature, premature aging, malignancy	Helicase gene mutations (distinct from Bloom syndrome gene)
Fanconi anemia MIM 227650	Congenital anomalies, aplastic anemia, chromosome breakage increased with alkylating agents or mitomycin C	Genetically heterogeneous
Xeroderma pigmentosum MIM 278700	Photosensitive skin, freckling, skin cancer	Defective excision repair of ultraviolet-induced DNA damage
Trichothiodystrophy MIM 234050	Abnormal skin and hair, short stature, developmental impairment	Defective excision repair of ultraviolet-induced DNA damage; possible effect on transcription
Cockayne syndrome MIM 216400	Photosensitive skin, white matter degeneration, cerebral calcification, dwarfism	Defective excision repair of ultraviolet-induced DNA damage; possible effect on transcription
Nijmegen breakage syndrome MIM 251260	Progessive microcephaly, growth retardation, immunodeficiency, and cancer predisposition	Defective response to DNA double-strand breaks

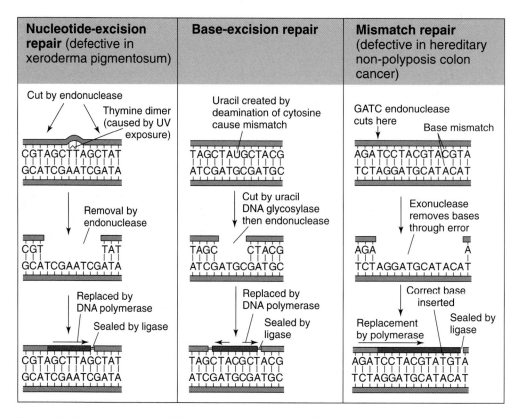

Figure 2.12 • Three major systems of DNA repair. From Pritchard & Korf (2003) Medical Genetics at a Glance, Blackwell Publishing, Oxford.

Three major systems exist for repair of three types of damage (Figure 2.12). The excision repair system removes DNA bases that have been damaged by chemicals or radiation, and then replaces the excised bases by synthesizing the short sequence using the intact strand as a template. Mismatch repair removes bases that are erroneously introduced during DNA replication that do not pair correctly. The system recognizes the short nonbase-paired segment, excises the stretch of bases from the region of the newly replicated strand, and then recopies the excised segment from the other stand. Single- and double-strand DNA breaks may occur as a result of a chemical mutagen or radiation exposure. Single-strand breaks are filled in by copying from the intact strand. Double-strand breaks are repaired by enzyme systems that juxtapose the two ends and ligate them together.

GENETIC POLYMORPHISM

Many genetic loci exhibit a high frequency of variation from individual to individual. These are referred to as polymorphisms. A polymorphism is formally defined as a locus with two or more alleles that have a population frequency of at least 1%.

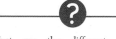

What are the different types of polymorphisms?

Types of Polymorphisms

There are four major types of DNA polymorphisms. Detection of **restriction fragment length polymorphism (RFLP)** depends on the use of enzymes called **restriction endonucleases**, which cut DNA at specific sites defined by four- to eight-base sequences. A single base change will be enough to cause failure of the enzyme to cut. An individual can therefore be homozygous for having the cutting site, homozygous for not having the site, or heterozygous, forming a two allele system (Figure 2.13). RFLPs were initially detected by Southern blotting (Methods 2.1). It is more common now to use the method of **polymerase chain reaction** (**PCR**) to detect RFLPs. In PCR, a set of short DNA sequences are used as primers to replicate a segment of DNA thousands of times (Methods 2.2).

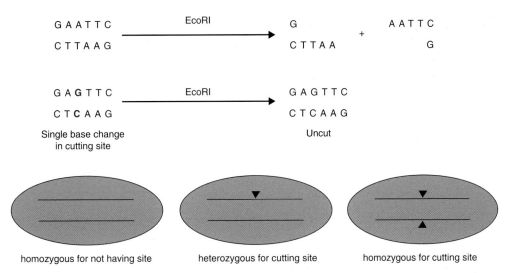

Figure 2.13 • Restriction fragment length polymorphism. The enzyme *Eco*RI recognizes the base sequence GAATTC and cuts both strands of DNA at this site (top). If a single base change occurs in the recognition site, the enzyme will not cut. An individual can have the cutting site intact on both chromosomes and be homozygous for having the site (bottom right), or can be heterozygous for the cutting site (bottom middle), or can be homozygous for not having the site. This constitutes a simple mendelian system for detecting a change of a single base of DNA.

Methods 2.1

Southern analysis

Southern analysis was one of the first approaches introduced for the analysis of DNA sequences. It is named for Edwin Southern, inventor of the technique. It is based on the principle that DNA segments with complementary base sequences will form hybrid double helices. Southern analysis is commonly used to detect a specific DNA segment against a background of a large population of different DNA sequences, such as genomic DNA (Figure 2.14).

The DNA is first cut into fragments using a restriction endonuclease. Depending on the frequency of the cutting site, a large set of fragments will be obtained, with the size of any specific fragment depending on

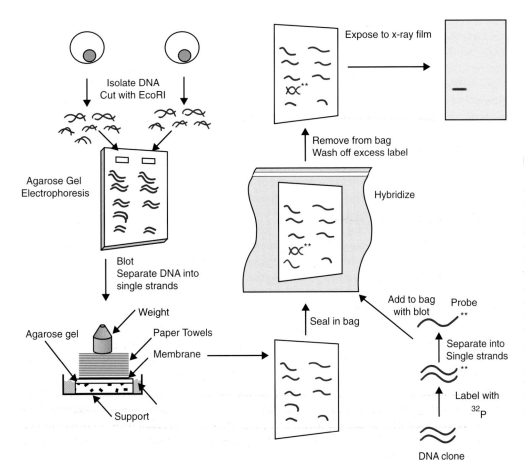

Figure 2.14 • Southern analysis. Genomic DNA is isolated (in this case from two sources of cells – one of which is missing a specific segment). The DNA is cut with a restriction endonuclease (*Eco*RI in this example) and separated by size by agarose gel electrophoresis. DNA in the gel is then blotted onto a membrane, transferring the DNA fragments, which are also separated into single strands by alkali treatment. Purified, cloned DNA corresponding with the region of interest is separated into single strands by heating and labeled with the radioactive isotope P[32]. Single-stranded "probe" DNA is then hybridized with DNA trapped in the filter. The probe binds to homologous DNA in the filter, resulting in a dark band when the radioactive probe is exposed to X-ray film. In this example, a dark band is only seen in the left lane, due to deletion from the DNA in the right lane.

Figure 2.15 • Southern blot analysis for restriction fragment length polymorphism. The *black arrows* denote constant cutting sites, and the *blue arrow* in the center a polymorphic site. The location of the cloned DNA probe is indicated. When the polymorphic site is present, the probe hybridizes with a 9-kb fragment, whereas when the polymorphic site is absent, the probe hybridizes with a 12-kb fragment. The Southern blot shown on the right is prepared by first cutting DNA with the appropriate restriction enzyme, then separating the fragments on an agarose gel, and finally by blotting these onto a membrane. The DNA in the membrane then is hybridized with radioactively labeled, cloned probe DNA. DNA in lane 1 is from an individual who is homozygous for not having the middle cutting site, and hence only a single 12-kb band is seen. The DNA in lane 2 is from an individual who is heterozygous for the polymorphic site, and therefore both a 12-kb and a 9-kb band are seen. The DNA in lane 3 is from an individual who is homozygous for having the middle site, and a single 9-kb band is seen.

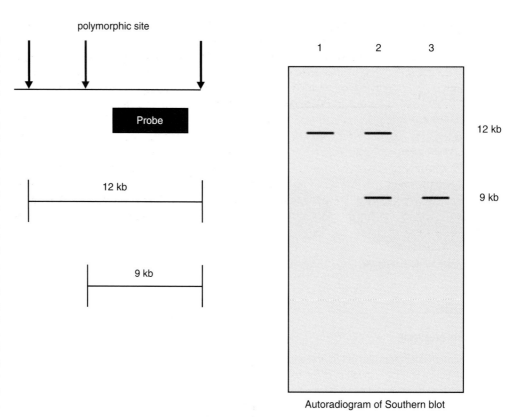

Autoradiogram of Southern blot

the distance between a pair of adjacent enzyme recognition sites. The fragments are then separated according to size by agarose gel electrophoresis. DNA is negatively charged and will migrate towards the positive terminal in an electric field. The pore sizes in the agarose slow the migration, larger molecules being more affected than smaller ones. DNA fragments are thereby separated by size, with the smaller molecules moving farther than the larger. The DNA at this point is still double stranded, but it is then separated into single strands by treatment with alkali. Single-stranded DNA in the gel is next transferred to a membrane by blotting so that the position of a fragment in the membrane is the same as its position in the gel. A labeled segment of cloned DNA is then separated into single strands and a solution containing this "probe" is exposed to the DNA in the membrane. Wherever the probe encounters homologous DNA in the membrane a stable double helix forms. The location of hybrid molecules is determined by visualization of the label. The label is often radioactivity – usually ^{32}P – and is visualized by exposing photographic film or using electronic detectors. Other labels can also be used that involve fluorescence or immunological detection systems.

Southern analysis is used to detect the presence of a specific sequence in genomic DNA. It also reveals the size of the fragment, which indicates the distance between a pair of enzyme cutting sites. If there is a restriction fragment length polymorphism the size of the fragment will be larger if the cutting site is absent and smaller if it is present (Figure 2.15).

A variation on Southern blotting, referred to as "northern blotting" detects RNA rather than DNA. In this case, RNA is isolated and separated by size by electrophoresis. The RNA is then blotted onto a membrane and hybridized with a labeled probe. Northern blotting is used to detect RNA sequences that are homologous to a cloned DNA of interest, thereby indicating the presence of the sequence among transcripts in the RNA mixture.

Methods 2.2

Polymerase chain reaction (PCR)

The polymerase chain reaction provides a means of amplifying a specific DNA sequence against a background of an entire genome (Figure 2.16). It begins with the synthesis of a pair of primers – oligonucleotides of 20 to 25 bases – that are homologous to a pair sequences that flank a region of interest. The distance between the primer binding sites is limited, usually to around 1000 bases or less. The primers are designed to bind to opposite strands of the target DNA, which is separated into single strands by heat. The primers serve as a starting point for a DNA synthesis reaction, using DNA polymerase and a supply of the four nucleotides, as the temperature of the solution is cooled. This produces a pair of hybrid molecules, which are once again separated into single strands by heating. Again the primers bind and a DNA synthesis reaction allowed to begin. The DNA polymerase is derived from a bacterium that thrives at high temperatures, allowing the same polymerase to be used in spite of multiple cycles of heating and cooling of the reaction mixture. The process is iterated multiple times, 20 or more, using an automated system, which leads to an exponential increase in the target DNA sequence. This results in over a million copies of the target sequence, sufficient to be visualized by staining the DNA following electrophoresis in an agarose gel. If the amplified sequence is cut with a restriction enzyme prior to electrophoresis, it can be used to detect the presence of a restriction fragment length polymorphism (Figure 2.17). PCR is now widely used throughout molecular genetics. We will encounter the approach throughout the remainder of this chapter and elsewhere in the book.

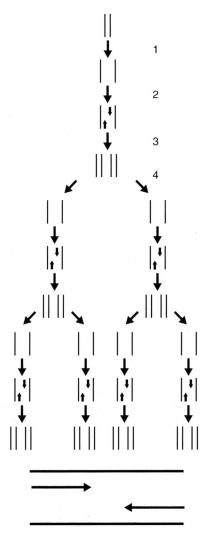

arrows indicate oligonucleotide primers bound to single-stranded DNA molecules

Figure 2.16 • Diagram of polymerase chain reaction (PCR). Strands of target DNA are separated (1) and primers allowed to bind to opposite strands (2). A DNA synthesis reaction then is allowed to proceed, copying the target DNA (3). This process is repeated cyclically (4), resulting in exponential amplification of the target sequence.

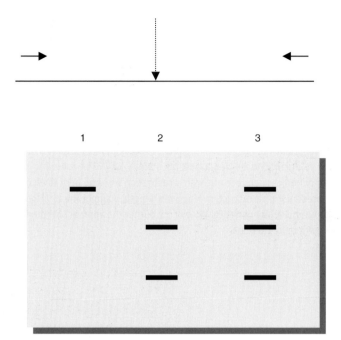

Figure 2.17 • Detection of RFLP by PCR. A segment of DNA is amplified by PCR and then cut with a restriction enzyme. The enzyme cutting site is indicated by the arrow. Fragments are then separated by size using agarose gel electrophoresis and the fragments stained in the gel. If the fragment does not cut, a single large band is seen (lane 1). If it cuts, two smaller bands are seen (lane 2). A heterozygote has all three bands (lane 3).

Simple sequence repeats comprise a second type of polymorphism. These are stretches of DNA in which a di-, tri-, or tetranucleotide sequence is repeated multiple times. The exact number of repeats can vary from individual to individual, and can be measured by PCR amplification of the segment containing the repeat and measurement of the size of the resulting fragment by electrophoresis in a polyacrylamide gel, which has sufficient resolution to detect a difference of as few as two bases (Figure 2.18). Simple sequence repeats tend to have multiple alleles, making it likely that an individual will be found to be heterozygous.

A third type of polymorphism involves short **tandem repeats**. These are repeats of tens to hundreds of bases, with the exact number of repeats being polymorphic (Figure 2.19). Short tandem repeats can be detected either with Southern blotting or PCR-based approaches.

The fourth type of polymorphism is the **single nucleotide polymorphism** (**SNP**). SNPs consist of a single base change, and may occur anywhere in a gene, including an exon, as well as between genes (Figure 2.20). SNPs occur every few hundred bases in the human genome, and several million have been identified and characterized. They are detected by a variety of approaches, most of which involve the use of PCR and sequence-specific detection systems.

Significance of Genetic Polymorphisms

What is the significance of polymorphisms in human genetics?

The term "polymorphism" does not imply whether a DNA variant will have phenotypic effect. Many polymorphisms are silent, occurring in regions that do not encode RNA or protein, but some occur within or nearby coding or regulatory sequences. These may produce medically insignificant phenotypes, or, in some cases, phenotypes that contribute to disease. We will

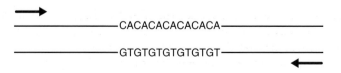

CA repeat, consisting of 7 copies of CA sequence

Figure 2.18 • Simple sequence repeat. In this case, the dinucleotide CA is repeated several times. The allele shown has 7 repeats, but other alleles might have 5, 6, 7, 8, 9, or even more copies of the CA sequence. The copy number is determined by PCR amplification of the region (*arrows* denote PCR primers in flanking DNA) and determination of the size of the product by polyacrylamide gel electrophoresis.

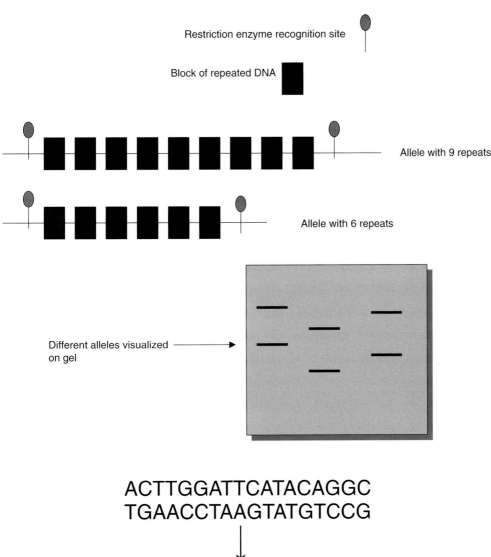

Figure 2.19 • Variable number tandem repeat polymorphism consists of multiple repeats of a block of DNA. Alleles can be detected by PCR across the region if the blocks are small, or by Southern analysis using as probe a copy of a repeat segment after the DNA is cut with an enzyme that recognizes sequences that flank the repeat region.

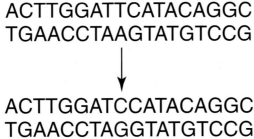

Figure 2.20 • Single nucleotide polymorphism, consisting of a single base change.

explore this further in Chapters 3 and 7. Study of genetic polymorphisms has been of critical importance in gene mapping and in searching for genes that are involved in common disorders. We will return to this in Chapter 4.

CONCLUSION

Although we speak of a "human genome sequence," in fact the genome is fluid, with constant changes occurring as cells divide. Although many of these changes are repaired, some escape repair and may persist at the level of the cell, or if they occur in the germ line, at the level of the organism. Some do not change gene function, whereas others have profound effects. The discipline of medical genetics is based on the effects of genetic variation on health and the development of diagnostic tests and interventions to deal with these changes when they impair health.

REVIEW QUESTIONS

2.1 Some silent mutations have been found to be associated with disease. Suggest a possible mechanism for this. How would you test this hypothesis?

2.2 What types of mutations are most likely to be associated with haploinsufficiency?

2.3 You are trying to find mutations in a gene and chose to look at RNA rather than DNA. The rationale is that by sequencing RNA you will see not only base substitutions, but also the effects of mutations that alter splicing. A colleague points out, however, that this strategy might miss some stop mutations. Why might this be so?

2.4 You are studying the inheritance of a gene in a family using a restriction fragment length polymorphism known to be located very near the gene. The father is known to be affected, but the child is too young to exhibit symptoms. A Southern blot is done, revealing the following pattern (Figure 2.40). You decide that the result has, in fact, revealed the underlying mutation. What kind of mutation is this?

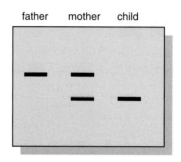

2.5 Under what circumstances might a polymorphism be associated with a pathological phenotype?

FURTHER READING

General References

Alberts B, Johnson A, Lewis J, Raff M, Roberts K, Walter P. Molecular Biology of the Cell, 4th edn., 2002, New York: Garland Science.

Lewin B. Genes VIII, 2003, Upper Saddle River, NJ: Prentice Hall.

Lodish H, Berk A, Zipursky L, Matsudaira P, Baltimore D, Darnell J. Molecular Cell Biology, 5th edn., 2004, New York: Freeman.

Guttmacher A, Collins FS. Genomic medicine – a primer. New Engl J Med 2002;347:1512–1520.

SNP Genotyping

Syvanen A-C. Accessing genetic variation: Genotyping single nucleotide polymorphisms. Nat Rev Genet 2001;2:930–942.

Regulation

Wasserman WW, Sandelin A. Applied bioinformatics for the identification of regulatory elements. Nat Rev Genet 2004;5:276–287.

DNA Repair

Sharova NP. How does a cell repair damaged DNA? Biochem 2005;70:275–291.

Clinical Snapshot 2.1 Xeroderma Pigmentosum

Norgauer J, Idzko M, Panther E, Hellstern O, Herouy Y. Xeroderma pigmentosum. Eur J Dermatol 2003;13:4–9.

Methods 2.1 Southern Blotting

DNA Learning Center animation: http://www.dnalc.org/shockwave/southan.html

Methods 2.2 PCR

DNA Learning Center Animation: http://www.dnalc.org/shockwave/pcranwhole.html

Ethics 2.1 Eugenics

Kevles, D. 1995. In the name of eugenics: Genetics and the uses of human heredity. Cambridge: Harvard University Press.

DNA Learning Center: http://www.eugenicsarchive.org/eugenics/

Hot Topics 2.1 Nonsense Mediated Decay

Inoue K, Khavavi M, Ohyama T, Hirabayashi S, Wilson J, Reggin JD, et al. Molecular mechanism for distinct neurological phenotypes conveyed by allelic truncating mutations. Nat Genet 2004;36:361–369.

3

Patterns of Inheritance

INTRODUCTION

It is likely that people have recognized that some traits – and some diseases – cluster in families long before there was any semblance of a modern concept of disease or even of medical practice. It was not until the beginning of the 20th century, however, that specific patterns of inheritance were recognized in humans. The groundwork for understanding single gene inheritance was laid by Gregor Mendel, a monk who in the 1860s experimented with pea plants at a monastery in Moravia, now the Czech Republic. Mendel's work lay unrecognized for decades, until it was discovered at the turn of the century by three botanists who performed similar experiments. Within a few years, the British physician Archibald Garrod recognized the

KEY POINTS

- An autosomal recessive trait is only expressed in individuals who are homozygous.
- An autosomal dominant trait will be expressed in homozygotes or heterozygotes. Many human autosomal dominant disorders are lethal in the homozygous state, however.
- Sex-linked traits are transmitted with the X or Y chromosome. An X-linked trait never displays male-to-male transmission.
- Pseudodominant inheritance occurs when a homozygous individual and a heterozygous individual mate. A recessive trait will thereby exhibit vertical transmission. It occurs mostly with traits that are relatively common.
- Digenic inheritance involves the occurrence of a trait in an individual who is heterozygous at two loci simultaneously.
- Penetrance is defined as the existence of a phenotype in an individual with the at-risk genotype. Nonpenetrant individuals do not express the phenotype. There may be a range of expressivity among individuals who are phenotypically affected.
- New mutations may account for sporadically-affected individuals. Some individuals are mosaic for a mutation if the mutation arose postzygotically. In some cases, the mutation is confined to the germline.
- Genomic imprinting effects may lead to a disorder only being manifest if the gene was inherited from the parent whose gene copy is expressed.
- Disorders associated with the mutational mechanism of triplet repeat expansion display the phenomenon of anticipation, where a disorder becomes more severe with each passing generation.
- Each mitochondrion contains multiple copies of a circular, double-stranded DNA molecule that encodes some of the proteins involved in oxidative phosphorylation, as well as a set of tRNAs and rRNAs.
- Mitochondrial DNA is maternally inherited, so mitochondrial traits are always passed from a female to all of her children.
- Mitochondria are passively segregated in cell division. There may be a mixture of mutant and wild type mitochondria in the same cell, which is referred to as heteroplasmy.

Methods 3.1

Taking a family history

Obtaining an accurate family history is a fundamental skill that will be increasingly crucial in the practice of medicine. It is of obvious importance if a person seeks care because of a family history of a genetic disorder. Often, however, a person will not realize the importance of a medical condition in a relative and will not volunteer the information unless it is explicitly sought. A three-generation family history, including information about siblings, parents, and grandparents, should be obtained as a standard component of medical practice. A "pedigree" should be constructed, using the symbols in Figure 3.1. Some tips for taking a complete and accurate family history are:

- If a person is seeking medical advice about a specific problem, ask specifically whether relatives have a similar problem.
- When asking about brothers and sisters, inquire whether there was ever a sibling who had died; some people will only remember to mention their living sibs.
- Inquire about neonatal deaths and miscarriages.
- Be alert to sibships in which not all sibs share the same two parents.
- Ask about consanguinity.
- Ask about the ethnic origin of different branches of the family.
- Where possible, try to obtain documentation (i.e., medical records) for important points of family history; often family members will conclude that a relative has a disorder believed to "run in the family" based on superficial information that may be inaccurate.

---

existence of families in which traits segregated in accordance with Mendel's laws, launching the discipline of medical genetics.

The study of traits determined by single genes remains the mainstay of human genetics. More than 10,000 such traits have been catalogued. From a medical point of view, many are rare, affecting fewer than one in 100,000 individuals. Some are more common, though the most common conditions tend to be determined by combinations of genes interacting with one another and with the environment. In this chapter, we will focus on patterns of genetic transmission, including Mendelian inheritance, multifactorial inheritance, and on some recently identified special cases and exceptions to the Mendelian paradigm. We will also see how modern tools of molecular genetics are beginning to reveal the mechanisms that underlie these patterns.

MENDELIAN INHERITANCE

The foundation for our modern understanding of genetic segregation is that a diploid organism contains two copies of every gene (excepting those carried on the sex chromosomes). One copy of each gene is inherited from each parent. These gene copies separate during the formation of haploid germ cells and are reunited at fertilization. The individual copies of a particular gene are called alleles. The genetic constitution of an individual with respect to a particular trait is referred to as genotype, whereas the corresponding physical manifestation of the trait is the phenotype. In human genetics, traits can be transmitted as autosomal or sex-linked, dominant or recessive. Sex is determined by the X and Y chromosomes: A male has an X and a Y chromosome and a female has two X chromosomes. Genes located on a sex chromosome are said to be sex-linked, whereas the nonsex-linked genes are referred to as autosomal. Geneticists use standard symbols to depict the inheritance of traits within a family tree, or pedigree (Methods 3.1). These symbols are illustrated in Figure 3.1.

What are the properties of autosomal recessive inheritance?

Autosomal Recessive Inheritance

The traits described by Garrod displayed the properties of recessive inheritance elucidated by Mendel. These traits are only expressed in individuals who possess two mutant gene copies

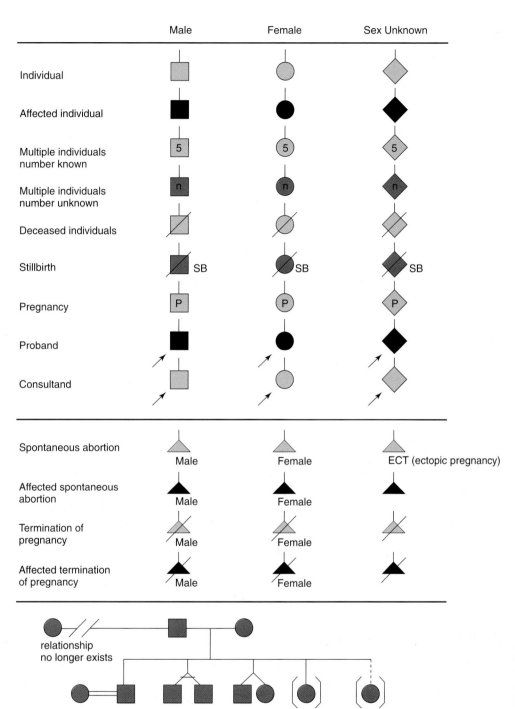

Figure 3.1 • Symbols used to draw pedigrees. (Adapted from Bennett RL, Steinhaus KA, Uhrich SB, *et al.* Recommendations for standardized human pedigree nomenclature. Pedigree Standardization Task Force of the National Society of Genetic Counselors. Am J Hum Genet 1995;56:745–752.)

(alleles) inherited from each parent (Figure 3.2). Such individuals are said to be homozygous, since both gene copies are mutated. We will see later that the specific mutation in each allele may be different, but both nevertheless are mutated. The parents are both carriers, heterozygotes, having one mutated copy and one nonmutated (wild type) copy (Figure 3.3). The parents, as a couple, face a one in four chance of each passing mutated copies to any offspring. Probably the trait has been in the family for generations, with many individuals being heterozygous carriers, but only in instances where the trait comes together in a homozygous state does the disorder surface. The likelihood of this occurring is increased if the parents are

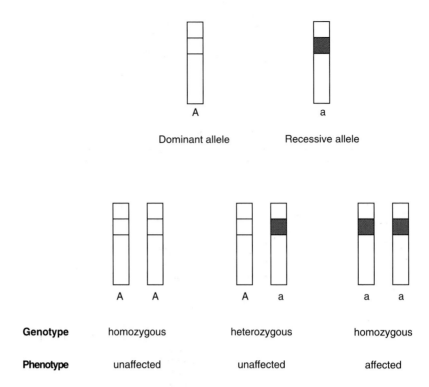

Figure 3.2 • Genotype and phenotype associated with a gene locus with dominant allele A and recessive allele a.

A	A	
	A a	
		a a

Genotype	homozygous	heterozygous	homozygous
Phenotype	unaffected	unaffected	affected

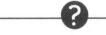

What is an inborn error of metabolism?

related to one another (consanguineous), in which case they both inherit what may be a rare recessive allele from a common ancestor (Figure 3.4). Rare recessive disorders are therefore more common in the offspring of consanguineous parents, but not all consanguineous matings result in recessive disorders and not all recessive disorders require consanguinity to be uncovered.

Garrod coined the term "inborn errors of metabolism" to describe the human genetic traits he characterized. Two of them, albinism (MIM 203100) and alkaptonuria (MIM 203500), are disorders of tyrosine metabolism (Figure 3.5). The conditions result from deficiency of specific enzymes due to mutation in the genes that encode the enzymes. Lack of enzyme activity results in buildup of a substrate, which may be toxic, and/or deficiency of a product (Figure 3.6). In albinism, there is a deficiency of the pigment melanin due to lack of activity of the enzyme tyrosinase (MIM 606933). The problem in alkaptonuria is the buildup of a toxic substance due to an enzyme deficiency. Another defect of phenylalanine metabolism, phenylketonuria (PKU) (MIM 261600) is due to deficiency of the enzyme phenylalanine

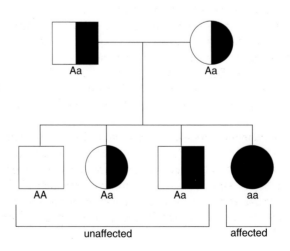

Figure 3.3 • Pedigree illustrating segregation of an autosomal recessive trait. Allele *A* is dominant, *a* is recessive.

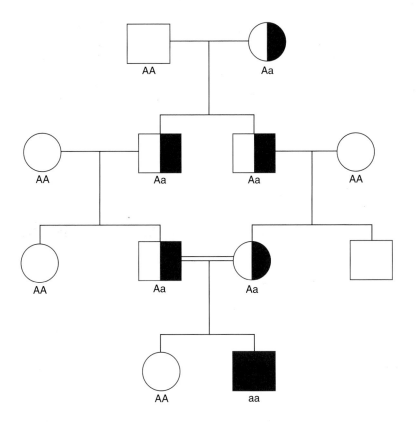

Figure 3.4 • The individual who is homozygous for *aa* has inherited the *a* allele from his great-grandmother, transmitted through both parents.

hydroxylase. Phenylalanine and its metabolites accumulate to toxic levels. There is also a deficiency of downstream products of phenylalanine, including the neurotransmitter DOPA and the pigment melanin. We will revisit PKU later in this book when we consider newborn screening.

The biochemical basis for the dominance of wild-type alleles over mutant alleles in inborn errors of metabolism can be understood by considering how enzymes function (Figure 3.7). Enzymes are proteins that catalyze chemical reactions. An enzyme is not consumed during the reaction, so only small quantities are required for a reaction to be carried out. In a person homozygous for a mutation in the gene encoding an enzyme, little or no enzyme activity is present, so he or she will manifest the abnormal phenotype. A heterozygous individual expresses 50% of the normal level of enzyme activity due to expression of the wild-type allele. This is usually sufficient to prevent phenotypic expression.

Not all recessive traits are due to enzyme deficiency. Cystic fibrosis (MIM 219700) is a recessive disorder in which there is marked thickening of secretions, especially in the lung and in ducted glands such as the pancreas. The disorder is due to mutations in a gene that encodes a chloride channel. Deficient chloride transport across the cell membrane leads to a reduction in the water content of extracellular fluid. Apparently, a 50% reduction in chloride transport in heterozygous carriers is still compatible with adequate hydration of extracellular fluid.

In general, recessive traits are associated with a reduced level of activity of a gene product in systems that have sufficient reserve function so that loss of half the activity in the heterozygous state does not perturb the system. The mutations responsible for recessive traits tend to lead either to lack of gene expression, as with promoter mutations, lack of protein production, for example due to mutations that lead to premature termination of translation, or production of a protein with reduced or absent function, such as due to amino acid substitution (Clinical Snapshot 3.1).

What is the basis for recessive inheritance?

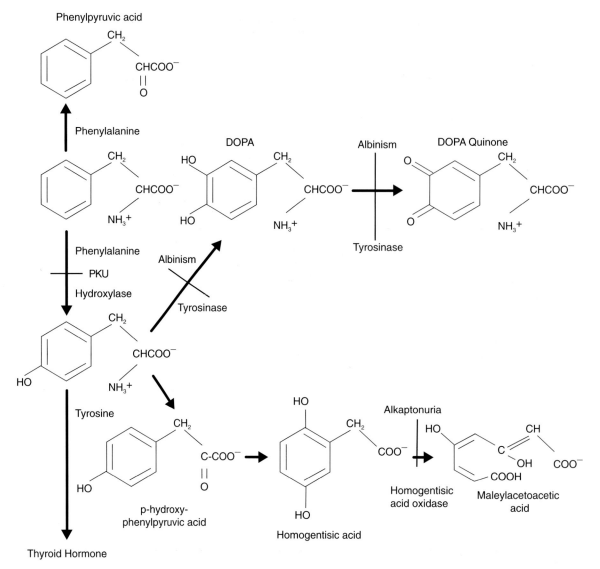

Figure 3.5 • Metabolic pathways involving tyrosine. Phenylalanine is converted to tyrosine by phenylalanine hydroxylase, the enzyme blocked in phenylketonuria. Lack of homogentisic acid oxidase leads to alkaptonuria and deficiency of tyrosinase to albinism.

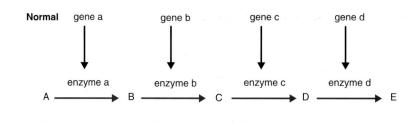

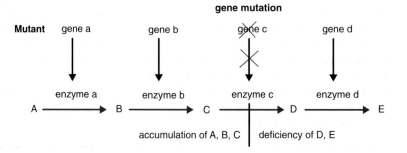

Figure 3.6 • "One gene, one enzyme" concept. Normally a specific gene directs the synthesis of each individual enzyme. Mutation of a gene leads to deficiency of the enzyme and consequent accumulation of substrate and deficiency of product.

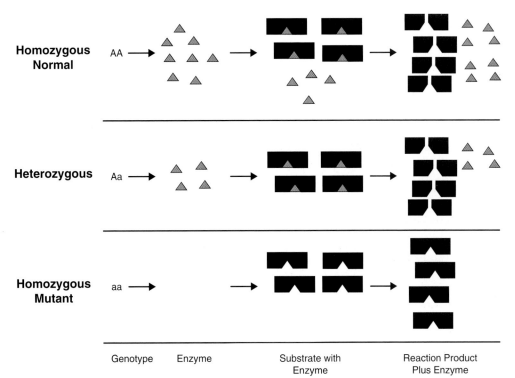

Homozygous Normal AA →

Heterozygous Aa →

Homozygous Mutant aa →

Genotype   Enzyme   Substrate with Enzyme   Reaction Product Plus Enzyme

Figure 3.7 • Model explaining recessive transmission of most enzyme deficiencies. Normally, more than sufficient enzyme is synthesized to carry out a reaction. A heterozygote still has sufficient enzyme, but a homozygote for a mutation does not make enough enzyme to complete the reaction.

CLINICAL SNAPSHOT 3.1

■ Autosomal recessive congenital deafness

Seth is 4-week-old boy who is referred to a genetics clinic for evaluation for congenital deafness. His deafness was first detected by newborn screening, and subsequently found by further testing to represent a profound sensorineural deafness. His health has been excellent and there is no known family history of deafness. A careful physical examination is performed and no congenital anomalies are noted. Genetic testing is performed looking for mutation in the GJB2 gene, and he is found to have a mutation in both alleles.

Deafness is subdivided into sensorineural and conductive causes. The former involves dysfunction in the cochlea, the auditory nerve, or in connections of the nerve to the brain. Conductive deafness is due to problems from the external ear up to the cochlea. Approximately one-third of cases of congenital sensorineural deafness are due to genetic causes and two-thirds of those are inherited in an autosomal recessive manner. In accordance with this mode of transmission, one expects to see that both parents are unaffected with the disorder, yet they face a one in four recurrence risk with each pregnancy. The most common cause of autosomal recessive congenital deafness (MIM 220290) is due to mutation in the gene *GJB2* (MIM 121011), which encodes the protein connexin26. Hexamers of connexin26 aggregate in the cell membrane to form gap junctions and are critical for the flux of potassium ions in the inner ear necessary for normal hearing (Figure 3.8). The most common mutation is a deletion of one G from a run of six in the gene which leads to a frameshift and lack of expression of the gene product. The carrier frequency of this mutation is as high as 3% in some populations. A wide variety of additional mutations may occur. Many affected individuals are compound heterozygotes, having two different mutant alleles.

CLINICAL SNAPSHOT 3.1 continued

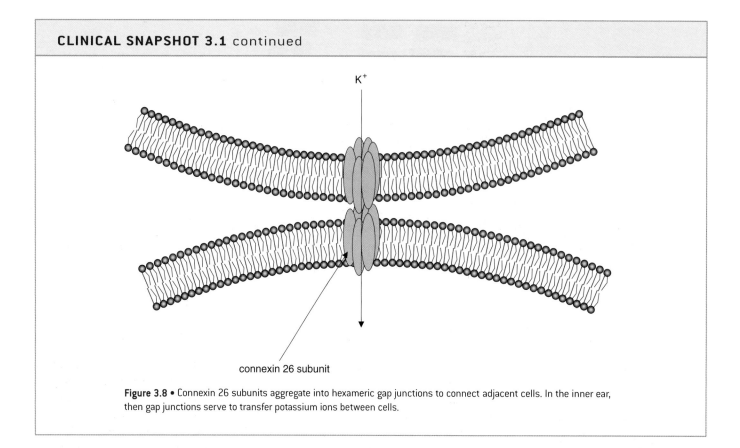

K⁺

connexin 26 subunit

Figure 3.8 • Connexin 26 subunits aggregate into hexameric gap junctions to connect adjacent cells. In the inner ear, then gap junctions serve to transfer potassium ions between cells.

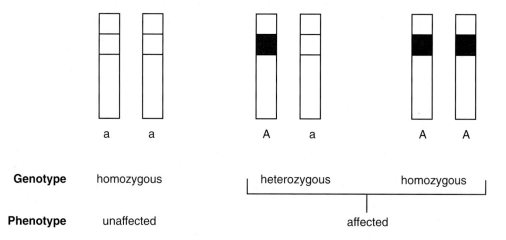

Figure 3.9 • The phenotype of a dominant allele is expressed in individuals who are either homozygous or heterozygous for the allele.

	a a	A a	A A
Genotype	homozygous	heterozygous	homozygous
Phenotype	unaffected	affected	

❓

What are the properties of autosomal dominant inheritance?

Autosomal Dominant Inheritance

Dominant traits are expressed in both the heterozygous and the homozygous states (Figure 3.9). Actually, many human dominant disorders are not "pure" dominants; the homozygote may actually be more severely affected, and even may not survive, so clinically affected individuals will be heterozygotes. For rare traits this distinction is largely academic, since usually only one of the parents carries the mutant allele (Figure 3.10). In such families, the affected individual faces a 50% risk of any offspring being affected (Ethical Implications 3.1).

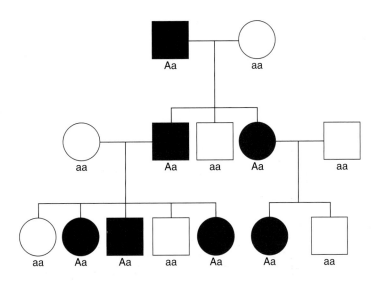

Figure 3.10 • Pedigree illustrating autosomal dominant transmission. The dominant allele *A* is passed from generation to generation.

ETHICAL IMPLICATIONS 3.1 • Family ties

One of the unique aspects of genetics as compared with other areas of medicine is that information about one family member may have an impact on other relatives. This has many implications that are important to consider when discussing family history with patients. First, relevant information may not be widely known within the family. It may be necessary to ask specific questions of relatives in order to learn of family traits that have not been openly discussed. In some cases, this may unlock family secrets that can cause discomfort or even disrupt relationships. For example, it may reveal instances where an individual stated to be the parent of a child is not the biological parent, or instances of miscarriage, termination of pregnancy, or death that have not been revealed. Second, genetic transmission of a trait may engender feelings of guilt on the part of the parent who has passed the trait on to a child. It is important to realize that taking a family history may raise such feelings, and addressing them can be helpful. Third, information learned about one member of a family may indirectly provide information about another. For example, a dominant trait known to be present in a grandparent and diagnosed by genetic testing in a child can also be assumed to be present in the parent. The parent may not wish to know of his or her diagnosis, but will probably learn of it from the child's test result. This is a risk of genetic testing that may not be obvious to the family, but should be pointed out as the possibility of testing is discussed.

Individuals with the connective tissue dysplasia Marfan syndrome (MIM 154700) have lax joints, floppy heart valves, and are prone to aortic dissection, among other problems. The disorder is due to deficient production of the protein fibrillin (MIM 134797), which is a component of connective tissue. Mutations that lead to reduction of fibrillin by 50% lead to weakening of connective tissue and signs of mild Marfan syndrome (Figure 3.11). This is referred to as haploinsufficiency. Some fibrillin mutations result in production of normal quantities of fibrillin, but the fibrillin interacts abnormally with other proteins in connective tissue. This mechanism is referred to as a dominant negative effect. The abnormal protein, in effect, "poisons" the system, leading to a more severe form of Marfan syndrome than occurs with haploinsufficiency.

Osteogenesis imperfecta (MIM 166200) is a disorder in which there is abnormal bone matrix, leading to brittle bones and frequent fractures. The condition is due to mutations in the gene that encodes components of type I collagen. Collagen is a triple helical molecule consisting of two chains of alpha$_1$(I) collagen (MIM 120150) and one of alpha$_2$(I) collagen (MIM 120160). Mutation in one allele that encodes alpha$_1$(I) can lead to disruption of 75% of collagen triple helices due to the polymeric nature of the mature molecule (Figure 3.12) – another example of a dominant negative effect.

[handwritten margin notes:]
- Too little gene product ↓ haploinsufficiency
- Abnormal product – dominant negative effect
- Gain of function

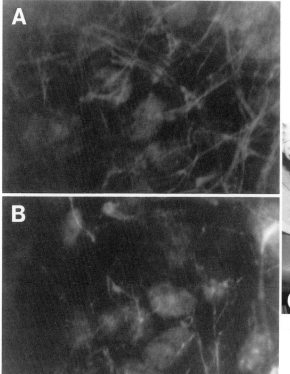

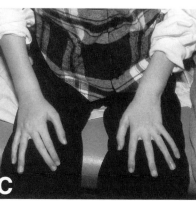

Figure 3.11 • Immunofluorescence photomicrograph of normal (A) and Marfan syndrome (B) fibroblast sample stained for fibrillin, showing deficient fibrillin in the Marfan sample. (Courtesy of Dr. Heinz Furthmayr, Department of Pathology, Stanford University.) (C) Arachnodactyly seen in a child with Marfan syndrome. (Courtesy of Dr. Ronald Lacro, Department of Cardiology, Children's Hospital, Boston.)

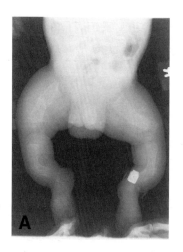

Figure 3.12 • (A) X-ray of infant with osteogenesis imperfecta, showing multiple fractures. (B) Dominant negative model. Although only one allele for alpha₁(I) procollagen is mutant (depicted by the black box over the molecule), 75% of the triple helical molecules incorporate at least one mutant protein and are degraded in the cell.

collagen triple helices

alpha₂ (1)

alpha₁ (1) wild type

alpha₁ (1) mutant

B

degraded

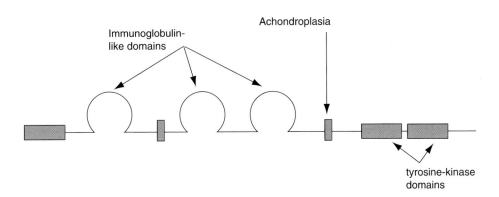

Figure 3.13 • Diagram of FGFR3 molecule, showing site of gain-of-function mutation responsible for achondroplasia.

An example of a dominant disorder due to a gain-of-function mutation is achondroplasia (MIM 100800). Achondroplasia is a form of dwarfism due to mutation in the fibroblast growth factor type 3 receptor (MIM 134934) (Figure 3.13). This is a transmembrane receptor that, when activated by binding of ligand at the cell surface, promotes the differentiation of cartilage into bone. A specific mutation in the gene for the receptor constitutively activates the system, causing premature conversion of the growth plate into bone, severely stunting growth. Gain-of-function mutations tend to be highly selective in that they require amino acid substitution at strategic sites in a protein.

The molecular basis of dominant traits tends to be diverse. One additional important mechanism of dominant inheritance is associated with a unique set of genes involved in predisposition to malignancy, referred to as tumor suppressor genes. We will defer discussion of these genes, however, until Chapter 8 where the genetics of cancer is discussed (Clinical Snapshot 3.2).

What is a gain-of-function mutation?

CLINICAL SNAPSHOT 3.2

■ Neurofibromatosis type 1 (NF1)

Amy is a 4-year-old girl brought to clinic by her parents because of multiple café-au-lait spots. These had appeared shortly after birth and have gradually increased in number. Her general health has been good, though her motor development has been slightly delayed. No one else in the family is known to have similar skin spots. On examination, she is found to have more than 20 flat, light brown skin spots – café-au-lait spots. She also has freckles in the inguinal regions and under her arms. You notice also that her right upper eyelid is swollen and her head size is greater than the 98th centile. A diagnosis of neurofibromatosis type 1 (NF1) is made.

NF1 (MIM 162200) is an autosomal dominant disorder with complete penetrance and variable expressivity. It usually presents with multiple café-au-lait spots in the early months of life. Affected individuals usually develop freckling in skin folds – under the arms and in the inguinal regions – by about 5 years of age. The disorder is named for the formation of neurofibromas, which are benign tumors that arise from the nerve sheath. These can occur on the skin, where they appear as bumps on the skin (Figure 3.14), or deeper in the body. Some larger neurofibromas, referred to as plexiform neurofibromas, involve a length of a large nerve and its branches. These can cause tissue overgrowth, as with Amy's eye, where a plexiform neurofibroma arising from nerves in the orbit has occurred. Neurofibromatosis is a gradually progressive disorder. Usually, neurofibromas do not appear until adolescence and gradually accumulate thereafter. Genetic transmission is autosomal dominant with complete penetrance. Approximately 50% of cases occur sporadically, though, due to new mutation. The expression is widely variable from one individual to another with the disorder, even among affected members of the same family. The genetic mechanism that underlies NF1 is that of a tumor suppressor, a point we will return to in Chapter 8.

CLINICAL SNAPSHOT 3.2 continued

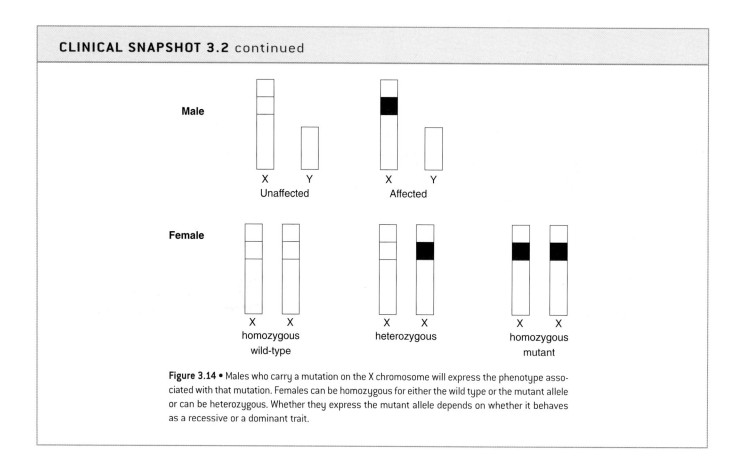

Figure 3.14 • Males who carry a mutation on the X chromosome will express the phenotype associated with that mutation. Females can be homozygous for either the wild type or the mutant allele or can be heterozygous. Whether they express the mutant allele depends on whether it behaves as a recessive or a dominant trait.

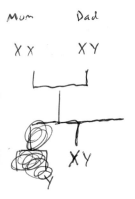

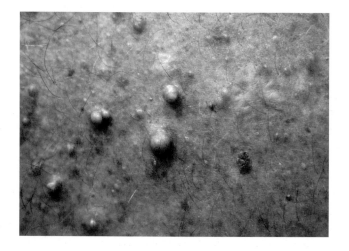

Figure 3.15 • Multiple neurofibromas on the skin of an individual with NF1.

X-linked Inheritance

What are the properties of X-linked inheritance?

The third major pattern of genetic transmission is referred to as "sex-linked," and involves genes on the X and Y chromosomes (Figure 3.15). A mutation on the X chromosome will be more likely expressed in males, who receive a single X from their mothers and a Y from their fathers. Males are said to be hemizygous for genes on the X chromosome. Females will only express the trait if they inherit it from both parents, which will occur much more rarely. A

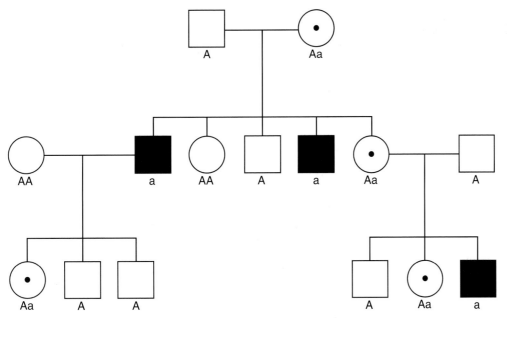

Figure 3.16 • Pedigree illustrating X-linked recessive transmission. Note the absence of male-to-male transmission.

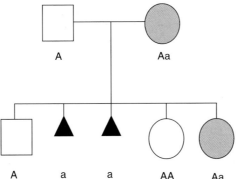

Figure 3.17 • Pedigree illustrating X-linked dominant transmission. Only females are affected. Males who inherit the mutant allele *a* die *in utero*.

female carrier for an X-linked recessive trait faces a 50% risk of transmission of the trait to any offspring. Females who inherit the trait will be carriers, whereas males who inherit the trait will be affected (Figure 3.16). Males never transmit an X-linked trait to their sons. An X-linked trait can also be transmitted as a dominant. In this case, an affected female has a 50% chance of passing the trait to any offspring, whereas males transmit the trait to all of their daughters but none of their sons. Some X-linked dominant traits are lethal in males, and therefore are only expressed in females (Figure 3.17; Clinical Snapshot 3.3).

The distinction between dominant and recessive X-linked traits is complicated by the phenomenon of X-chromosome inactivation introduced in Chapter 1. Most X-linked alleles are expressed on one of the two X chromosomes in any specific cell in a female. A female who is heterozygous for an X-linked trait will therefore express the mutant allele in approximately half her cells and the nonmutant allele in half. There may be some phenotypic expression of the trait based on the mutant allele being expressed in 50% of cells. Sometimes there is nonrandom X inactivation, that is one X chromosome is active in more than 50% of cells. This can occur by chance, or may occur if there is a structural abnormality on one X chromosome that causes a cell that expresses this X to die due to severe genetic imbalance. If nonrandom X inactivation leads to a preponderance of cells expressing an X-linked mutant gene, then the individual will express the phenotype. Another way that a female can express the phenotype of an X-linked recessive is if she has only one X chromosome. This is the case for phenotypic females with Turner syndrome, who have only 45 chromosomes and only a single sex chromosome. We will revisit Turner syndrome later in this book.

CLINICAL SNAPSHOT 3.3

▦ X-linked disorders

Emma is a 3-year-old brought to a genetics clinic because of developmental regression. She was born after an uneventful pregnancy with a normal delivery, and seemed to be well as an infant. She began to achieve her early motor milestones, getting to walk and saying a few words. Over the past year, though, she seems to have slipped in terms of development. She is much less interactive and is no longer speaking. She also has been noted to make unusual wringing movements of her hands. There is no family history of similar problems, but mother had one miscarriage before the pregnancy with Emma. Physical examination is unremarkable except that head size is in the 10th centile, whereas her pediatric records show that it was in the 50th centile a year ago. The hand wringing is readily evident. A clinical diagnosis of Rett syndrome is made.

Rett syndrome (MIM 312750) is an X-linked disorder characterized by normal early development, followed by developmental regression. Compulsive hand wringing is typical and there is a gradual decrease in head growth rate. Rett syndrome almost exclusively affects females, and has a frequency of 1 : 10,000 to 1 : 15,000 female births. It is due to mutation in a gene on the X chromosome that is lethal in affected males. The lethality leads either to death *in utero*, resulting in miscarriage, or very severe neonatal neurological problems. The gene responsible for Rett syndrome, *MECP2* (MIM 30005), binds to methylated cytosine bases and is involved in methylation-induced gene silencing. Loss of MeCp2 function leads to widespread gene dysregulation, which underlies the neurological phenotype.

Are genetic traits inherited on the Y chromosome?

Y-linked Inheritance

Pedigrees exhibiting Y-linked inheritance will show only male to male transmission, with only males being affected. Only a few such conditions exist. Mutations of Y-linked genes manifest primarily as male infertility and are therefore usually not passed on to future generations. This is changing, however, with the advent of assisted reproduction techniques that allow those with Y-linked genetic infertility to pass their genetic differences to future generations.

Of special note is the pseudoautosomal region, the small region of homology shared by the tips of the short and long arms of the X and Y chromosomes (Xp and Yp) (Figure 3.18). Very few genes reside in this region and these genes escape X chromosome inactivation. One of these is *SHOX* (MIM 312865). Heterozygous *SHOX* mutations cause Leri–Weil dyschondrosteosis (MIM 127300), a rare skeletal dysplasia that involves bilateral bowing of the forearms with dislocations of the ulna at the wrist and generalized short stature. Homozygous mutations cause the much more severe Langer mesomelic dwarfism (24970), characterized by shortening of the forearms and lower legs. Note that both of these disorders have MIM numbers

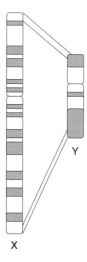

Figure 3.18 • Regions of homology on the short and long arms of the X and Y chromosome are referred to as pseudoautosomal regions. The X and Y pair in this region at their short arms. Genes in the pseudoautosomal region of the X are not subject to X chromosome inactivation.

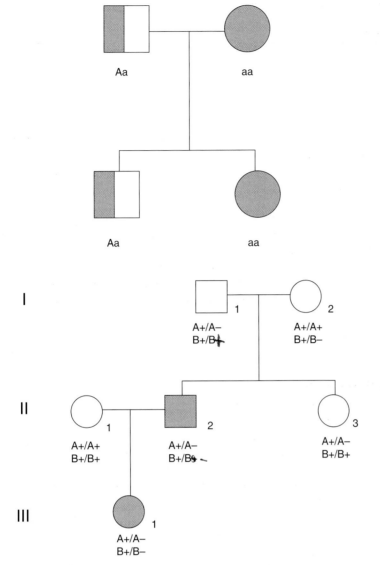

Figure 3.19 • Pseudodominant inheritance. A heterozygous male and homozygous female transmit a recessive disorder to their daughter, giving the appearance of dominant transmission. This is most likely to occur when the mutant allele is common in the population.

Heterozygous in 2 genes

Figure 3.20 • Digenic inheritance. Individual I-1 is heterozygous for a mutation in gene A (A−) and I-2 is heterozygous for a mutation in gene B (B−). One of their children, II-2, inherits A− from father and B− from mother, and, being doubly heterozygous, is affected. Sibling II-3 is only heterozygous for A− and is not affected. A child of II-2, III-1, inherits both A− and B− from her father and is also affected.

characteristic of dominant or recessive, not sex-linked traits. This is because the genes are present on both the X and Y chromosomes, and hence behave like autosomal traits.

Pseudodominant Inheritance

Pseudodominant inheritance refers to the observation of apparent parent-to-child transmission of a known autosomal recessive trait (Figure 3.19). Pseudodominant inheritance occurs when a condition is common and is compatible with reproduction. Vertical transmission occurs when one parent is homozygous and the other is heterozygous. An example is hemochromatosis (MIM 235200), a disorder in which there is excessive absorption of iron. Iron deposits in tissues such as the heart, liver, and pancreas, where it is toxic. Hemochromatosis is an autosomal recessive trait with a carrier frequency as high as one in ten in individuals of Celtic ancestry. In this population it would not be rare for a homozygous individual to have a heterozygous partner.

Digenic Inheritance

Digenic inheritance is a relatively recently recognized form of genetic transmission. It was first noted in families with the eye disorder retinitis pigmentosa (RP) (MIM 268000), in children of parents who each carried a mutation in different RP-associated genes, *ROM1* (MIM 180721) and *peripherin* (MIM 170170) (Figure 3.20). Both parents had normal vision, as one

What is meant by pseudodominance?

What is digenic inheritance?

would expect, since *ROM1* and *peripherin* typically cause RP only when an individual is homozygous for mutated alleles. Offspring who were double heterozygotes, however, developed RP.

With digenic inheritance, normal parents, one of whom carries a gene "A" mutation and the other a gene "B" mutation, will have a one in four risk of having a child who inherits both gene "A" and gene "B" mutations and will express the mutant phenotype. For the affected generation inheritance may appear like autosomal recessive (affected sibs, unaffected parents, one in four recurrence risk). An affected child will have a one in four chance of passing on both alleles (gene "A" and "B" mutations), but transmission will appear as vertical (dominant).

Known examples of digenic inheritance include RP, holoprosencephaly (MIM 236100), hereditary hearing impairment (MIM 220290), Antley–Bixler syndrome (MIM 207410) (abnormal formation of the skull and facial features, developmental delay), and autosomal dominant familial exudative vitreoretinopathy (MIM 137780). A variation on this theme has been discovered in some individuals with Bardet–Biedl syndrome (MIM 209900). This disorder is characterized by obesity, retinitis pigmentosum, and renal anomalies, among other features, and is inherited as an autosomal recessive trait. There are several distinct genes that can cause Bardet–Biedl syndrome. In some cases, the disorder requires homozygosity for mutation at one locus together with heterozygosity at another. This has been referred to as "triallelic inheritance." In effect, the heterozygous locus is serving as a modifier of the expression of the homozygous one. More conditions displaying digenic inheritance will likely be identified in the coming years. Furthermore, it is important to recognize that digenic inheritance is really the simplest form of complex genetic inheritance. As research continues, we will see many genetic diseases with two, three, four, or even more different genes interacting to produce a specific phenotype or disease.

Penetrance and Expressivity

Not all individuals who have the genotype that is associated with a specific phenotype will express the phenotype. In such individuals, the phenotype is said to be nonpenetrant. Nonpenetrance has been demonstrated to occur with many genetic traits and can be most easily inferred when a grandparent and child have a disorder that does not appear to be expressed in the parent (Figure 3.21). In deciding whether a person is nonpenetrant for a genetic trait, it is important to define the phenotype carefully. Some individuals will be very mildly affected, so the phenotype might escape detection unless a careful examination is performed.

Sometimes a rate of penetrance will be specified for a disorder. This rate applies to a population, not to an individual. For example, if 60% of individuals who carry a mutant gene express the phenotype, the rate of penetrance is 60%. A particular individual, however, either expresses the phenotype or does not. The individual is either penetrant or nonpenetrant; it does not make sense to speak in terms of *partial penetrance*, although the person may have mild expression of the trait.

What is the difference between penetrance and expressivity?

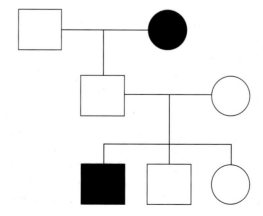

Figure 3.21 • Example of nonpenetrance, in which an autosomal dominant trait is expressed in a grandparent and child but not in the parent. The unaffected parent must carry the mutant gene and is said to be *nonpenetrant*.

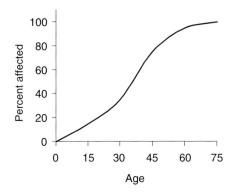

Figure 3.22 • Age-dependent penetrance. The likelihood of being affected increases with age.

Some disorders display age-dependent penetrance. These are typically adult-onset disorders, where the likelihood of a phenotype in a person with the mutation increases with age. An example is Huntington disease, a dominantly inherited neurodegenerative disorder in which there is a progressive dementia and movement disorder. Virtually all mutation carriers will express the disorder if they live long enough, but children are very rarely affected (Figure 3.22). It is important to realize that clinical evaluation of young children at risk for disorders that display age-dependent penetrance does not provide a reliable indication of whether they have inherited the disorder.

Penetrance sometimes is confused with another genetic term, expressivity. Expressivity refers to the degree of phenotypic expression of a genetic trait. Many genetic traits exhibit a wide range of expressivity, which means that the characteristics of affected individuals differ from person to person. This is illustrated by the autosomal dominant disorder neurofibromatosis type 1 (NF1)(MIM 162200). Affected individuals develop tumors along peripheral nerves, as well as patches of brown pigmentation on the skin (café-au-lait spots). Other features include bone deformities, learning disabilities, and brain tumors, but manifestations vary widely from person to person, even within the same family. Some have innumerable skin tumors and life-threatening malignant growths, whereas others have only a few skin spots. NF1 exhibits a wide range of expressivity, yet the penetrance is high: virtually all persons who carry the NF1 gene mutation express at least some signs of the disorder.

Genetic Heterogeneity

We have already encountered situations in which a single phenotype is caused by mutation in multiple distinct genes (e.g., retinitis pigmentosum, deafness). This is an example of locus heterogeneity. It reflects the fact that genes whose products participate in specific biological pathways or functions can result in similar phenotypes when mutated. Often, it is not possible to determine which gene is responsible for a phenotype solely by analyzing the phenotype. This is the case, for example, with deafness. There are dozens of genes that can cause deafness, and the phenotype for most of these is the same – lack of hearing. In some cases there may be distinct, but overlapping phenotypes. For example, Pendred syndrome (MIM 274600) causes deafness and goiter, whereas Waardenburg syndrome (MIM 193500) causes deafness and characteristic facial features.

There is a second form of genetic heterogeneity, referred to as allelic heterogeneity. A specific phenotype may result from mutation in a specific gene, but the exact mutation may differ from one affected individual to another. Sometimes the phenotypes due to specific mutations can be distinguished from one another, sometimes not. Indeed, in some cases, different mutations in the same gene can give totally different conditions. For example, specific mutations in the RET (MIM 164761) gene give rise to Hirschsprung disease (MIM 142263), a disorder in which there is aberrant migration of ganglion cells in the intestine that leads to intestinal obstruction. Other mutations in this same gene cause a form of multiple endocrine neoplasia (MEN II, phenochromocytoma, medullary thyroid carcinoma) (MIM 171400). Allelic heterogeneity is very common in genetic disorders. In autosomal recessive disorders, the two mutant alleles may differ from one another, referred to as compound heterozygosity. To some extent, allelic heterogeneity contributes to variable expression of a specific phenotype. Another major

What is meant by allelic and gene locus heterogeneity?

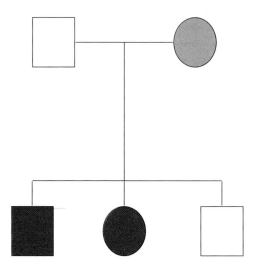

Figure 3.23 • The mother of the two affected children is a mosaic for the mutation. She does not show signs of the disorder, or signs may be exceptionally mild or limited to a restricted region of the body. If she is a germline mosaic, only egg cells would carry the mutation.

contributor is the occurrence of genetic modifiers, that is alleles at other loci that contribute to expression of the phenotype.

Mutation and Mosaicism

How do sporadic cases arise by mutation, and what is mosaicism?

Some mutations have existed in the population a long time, and segregate through families for multiple generations. There are instances, however, where an individual represents the first occurrence of a new mutation in the family. This is especially apparent in completely penetrant dominant traits, where a child may be affected but neither parent displays the phenotype. It is presumed that the mutation has occurred in the sperm or egg cell that formed the child. We have considered the phenomenon of new mutation in Chapter 2. It was noted there that there is a slightly increased risk of new mutation as a function of advanced paternal, but not maternal, age.

There are two special instances of new mutation that deserve mention (Figure 3.23). One is germline mosaicism, in which the mutation occurs during germ cell development and may involve multiple sperm or egg cells. This is of importance because an individual with germline mosaicism is at risk of having more than one affected child in spite of not being affected with the trait him or herself. The other phenomenon is somatic mosaicism. Here, the mutation occurs during early embryonic development, so the individual has multiple cells with or without the mutation. Such individuals may express mild manifestations of the phenotype, or may express the phenotype in a restricted region of the body. If the mutation is present in the germline, there is a risk of having affected children.

Genomic Imprinting

What are the genetic implications of genomic imprinting?

We have encountered the phenomenon of genomic imprinting in Chapter 1, wherein some genes are expressed only from the maternal or paternal copy. If a mutant gene is imprinted, the phenotype will be expressed only in offspring who inherit the gene from the parent whose copy is expressed. That parent, however, may not be affected if he or she inherited the mutation from the parent whose copy is not expressed. For example, familial paragangliomas (MIM 168000) are inherited as an autosomal dominant trait with an imprinting effect. The tumors arise from autonomic ganglia located at various sites in the body. The trait tends to be expressed only when inherited from the father. The responsible gene, SDHD (succinate dehydrogenase complex subunit D, MIM 602690) is inactivated in the female germline and therefore only expressed from the paternal copy. Looking at a pedigree (Figure 3.24), the trait appears to skip generations if it is transmitted from a female.

Triplet Repeat Disorders and Anticipation

It has long been recognized that there is a set of genetic disorders in which signs and symptoms tend to be more severe and have earlier age of onset from generation to generation. This

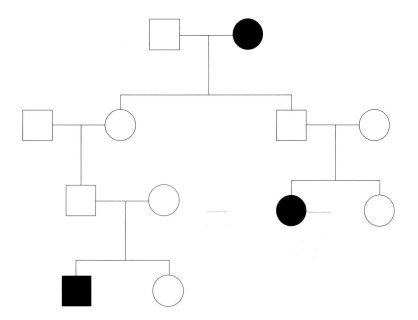

Figure 3.24 • Pedigree of family with hereditary paragangliomas, in which the mutant gene is only expressed if inherited from the father. Examples of apparent nonpenetrance are due to inheritance of the mutation from a female.

phenomenon is referred to as anticipation. An example is the muscle disorder myotonic dystrophy (MIM 160900). Affected individuals have muscle weakness and difficulty with muscle relaxation after a sustained period of contraction. The condition is transmitted as an autosomal dominant and tends to become more severe as the gene mutation is passed from generation to generation.

The basis for anticipation was unknown for a long time, and some doubted that the phenomenon was real, attributing it to bias of ascertainment – the disorder in a family would go unnoticed until it was brought to attention by a severely affected, young family member. The true explanation came to light with the discovery of a group of disorders associated with triplet repeat expansions in a variety of genes.

Many genes include regions of simple sequence repeats – dinucleotides, trinucleotides, etc. The exact number of repeats in a specific gene may differ from one individual to another, usually with no impact on gene function. There is a subset of these genes, however, with trinucleotide repeats in which expansion of the number of repeats beyond a threshold leads to abnormal gene function (Figure 3.25). In myotonic dystrophy the repeat expansion occurs near the 3′ end of the gene. The region with the triplet repeat encodes a segment of mRNA that binds a nuclear protein. Expansion of the CTG (represented as CUG in the RNA) repeat in this region causes binding of excessive protein, leading to dysfunction of this gene product, which encodes a muscle cell membrane ion channel, as well as of other gene products encoded by RNA molecules that would normally bind this nuclear protein.

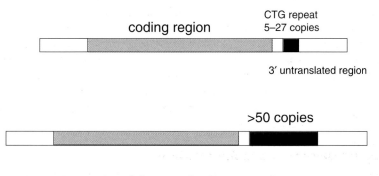

Myotonic Dystrophy

Figure 3.25 • There is a CTG repeat expansion in the 3′ untranslated region of the gene that encodes the protein involved in myotonic dystrophy. The repeat may be 5 to 27 copies in the general population, but having an expansion in excess of 50 copies is associated with myotonic dystrophy.

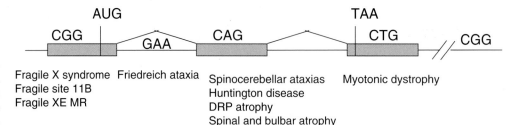

Figure 3.26 • Generic gene with three exons and two introns showing the location of triplet repeats in genes associated with neurological disorders. Each of these disorders is due to a repeat expansion in a different gene.

All known triplet repeat expansion disorders affect the nervous system (Figure 3.26). Fragile X syndrome (MIM 309550) is a form of X-linked mental retardation in which there is deficient production of a protein due to a CGG expansion near the promoter region that causes hypermethylation and consequent silencing of the gene (Hot Topic 3.1). There is a set of disorders, including Huntington disease (MIM 143100) and various forms of spinocerebellar ataxia (multiple MIM), that are due to CAG expansion in an exon within different genes that leads to a polyglutamine repeat expansion in the encoded proteins. Friedreich ataxia (MIM 229300) is due to a GAA repeat expansion within an intron, which causes abnormal mRNA processing. It is the only one of the triplet repeat expansion disorders that is inherited as an autosomal recessive trait.

How does triplet repeat expansion lead to anticipation? Understanding this requires knowledge of two points. First, the larger the repeat the more severe the disorder and the earlier the age of onset. Second, the larger the repeat, the more unstable it is, and hence the greater the chance that it will expand further as it is passed from generation to generation. This is illustrated for myotonic dystrophy in Figure 3.28.

Hot Topic 3.1　FRAGILE X-ASSOCIATED TREMOR ATAXIA SYNDROME

Fragile X syndrome is a form of X-linked mental retardation. It is called fragile X because of a tendency for the tip of the long arm of the X chromosome to be broken off from the chromosome when chromosomes are analyzed cytologically. It is due to a triplet repeat expansion in the gene *FMR1*. The expansion involves a CGG repeat near the promoter region of the gene. Normally, there are approximately 15 to 45 copies of the CGG repeat, with no phenotypic consequence. Individuals with fragile X syndrome have more than 200 repeats. This expansion is associated with methylation of the promoter region and inactivation of the gene. The FMR1 protein is an RNA-binding protein, though it is unknown how deficiency of this protein leads to abnormal brain function.

Fragile X syndrome is most often expressed in males, but some females express the phenotype if a high proportion of activated X chromosomes contain the expanded allele. Expansion to full mutation occurs from pre-existing premutation alleles. These alleles contain 55 to 200 repeats. The expanded size tends to be unstable during meiosis, leading to expansion to full mutation. Expansion occurs only in female meiosis, so premutation males do not transmit full mutation alleles to their daughters.

Premutation female carriers do not have features of fragile X syndrome, but those with expansions greater than 100 repeats can have abnormal phenotypes. These include psychiatric disturbances and premature ovarian failure. The mechanisms that underlie these changes are not known. Premutation males do not have these phenotypes, but recently a premutation phenotype, known as fragile X-associated tremor and ataxia syndrome (FXTAS), has been described that affects adult premutation males and some females. The syndrome includes intention tremor, ataxia, peripheral neuropathy, and dementia. Affected individuals usually are grandfathers of males affected with fragile X syndrome. Because of this, the condition was not recognized as being due to the *FMR1* gene for a long time.

The mechanisms of FXTAS appear to be different from those of fragile X syndrome. Males with fragile X syndrome do not develop FXTAS, so *FMR1* gene product deficiency is probably not the mechanism. Unlike fragile X males with full mutations, the males with FXTAS express their *FMR1* gene at aberrantly *high* levels, not low levels. It has been proposed that the excessive number of CGG repeats in *FMR1* premutation transcripts binds to RNA binding proteins, depleting the pool of these proteins and preventing their interaction with other transcripts (Figure 3.27). The protein–RNA complexes are then degraded in the proteosome, leading to intranuclear inclusion bodies that are seen in the brain cells of males with FXTAS.

Hot Topic 3.1 continued

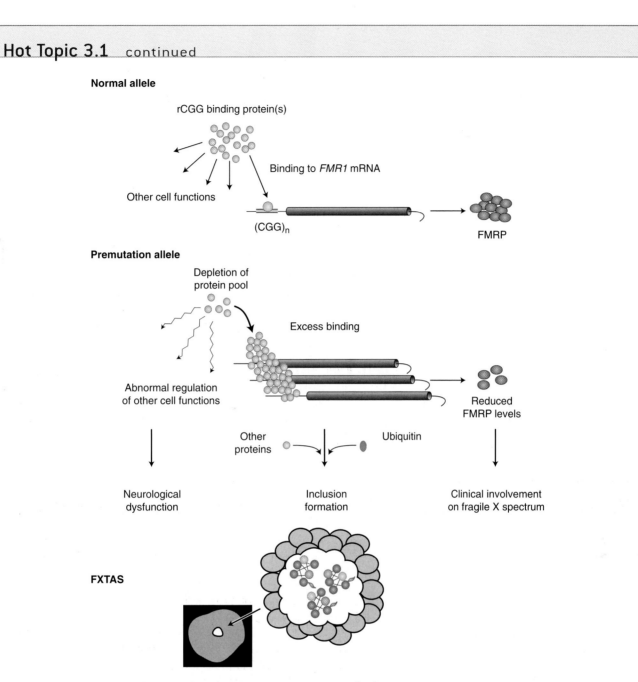

Normal allele

rCGG binding protein(s)

Binding to *FMR1* mRNA

Other cell functions

(CGG)ₙ

FMRP

Premutation allele

Depletion of
protein pool

Excess binding

Abnormal regulation
of other cell functions

Reduced
FMRP levels

Other
proteins

Ubiquitin

Neurological
dysfunction

Inclusion
formation

Clinical involvement
on fragile X spectrum

FXTAS

Figure 3.27 • Postulated mechanism of FXTAS. The normal allele (top) binds an RNA-binding protein at the CGG repeat site, and normal FMRP is produced. The binding protein also interacts with other mRNA species. In individuals with a premutation allele, increased numbers of transcripts with long CCG tracts bind excessive amounts of protein, depleting the pools required for other cellular functions. The protein-FMR1 complex is complexed with ubiquitin and is degraded in the proteosome. (Redrawn from Hagerman PJ and Hagerman RJ. The fragile X premutation: A maturing perspective. Amer J Hum Genet 2004;74:805–816.)

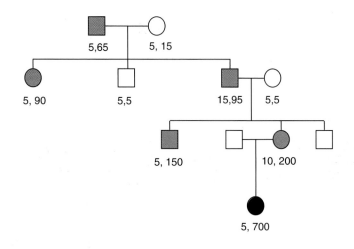

Figure 3.28 • Anticipation in myotonic dystrophy. Number of CTG repeats is indicated below each symbol. Each individual has one normal allele of 5 repeats. In the first generation, the affected individual has a 65 repeat allele that gives rise to mild myotonic dystrophy. This increases to 95 repeats in his affected son, then to 200 repeats in his affected daughter, and finally to 700 repeats in severely affected child in the last generation.

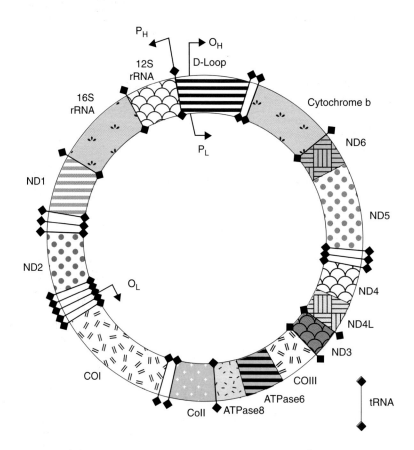

Figure 3.29 • Map of the mitocondrial genome. ND6, ND5, ND4, ND4L, ND3, ND2, and ND1 are components of complex I. COIII, COII, and COI are components of complex IV. Adenosine triphosphatase (ATPase) 6 and ATPase 8 are components of complex V. Cytochrome b is part of complex III. O_H and O_L are the origins of replication of the heavy and light strands, respectively; P_H and P_L are promoters for these strands.

What are the unique properties of mitochondrial inheritance?

MITOCHONDRIAL INHERITANCE

It used to be assumed that the entire DNA complement of a cell was contained within the nucleus, but it has become clear that this is not the case. DNA is also found within another cellular organelle, the mitochondrion. Mitochondria are responsible for the generation of adenosine triphosphate (ATP) via aerobic metabolism, and each mitochondrion contains multiple copies of a double-stranded, circular DNA molecule of 16,569 base pairs (Figure 3.29). This DNA encodes 13 peptides that are subunits of proteins required for oxidative phosphorylation. In addition, there is a complete set of 22 transfer RNAs and two ribosomal RNAs. These RNAs are involved in translation of mitochondrially encoded proteins within the mitochondrion.

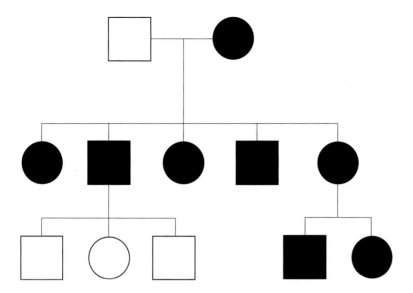

Figure 3.30 • Maternal genetic transmission. An affected woman transmits the trait to all of her children. Affected men do not pass the trait to any of their offspring.

The process of oxidative phosphorylation requires more than 60 proteins. Most are encoded in the nucleus and are transported into the mitochondrion from the cytoplasm. Only a minority of the mitochondrial proteins is encoded in the mitochondrial genome and synthesized within the mitochondrion. The structure of the mitochondrial genome bears more resemblance to prokaryotic than to eukaryotic genomes. The genes lack introns and are transcribed as polycistronic messages from two promoters. The spaces between genes consist of tRNAs, whose excision from the polycistronic message releases the individual gene transcripts. There are also two sites for initiation of DNA synthesis, one on each strand of the double helix.

A number of clinical disorders have been identified that are due to mutations within mitochondrial genes (Clinical Snapshot 3.4; Table 3.1). As might be expected, these traits are associated with failure of mitochondrial energy production. Mitochondrial DNA exhibits two critical differences from the nuclear genome that account for unusual patterns of inheritance of mitochondrial genetic traits. These are maternal transmission and heteroplasmy. A pedigree displaying maternal transmission is shown in Figure 3.30. The trait is transmitted from a mother to all of her children, but is not transmitted by males. This is due to the fact that essentially all of the mitochondria are maternally inherited. At the time of fertilization only the sperm nucleus enters the egg. Mitochondria in the sperm are shed prior to fertilization. There may be minor exceptions to this rule but, for the most part, mitochondria traits are maternally inherited.

Although all of the children of a woman with a mitochondrial mutation might be expected to inherit the mutation, there is usually a wide range of variation in expression. This is due to the phenomenon of heteroplasmy. Unlike the nuclear genome, which is represented by one complete copy per cell, there are hundreds of mitochondrial DNA molecules in each cell. These mitochondria separate passively when a cell divides, in contrast to the orderly separation of chromosomes in the nuclear genome during cell division. If some of the mitochondria contain a mutation and others do not, the result can be unequal distribution of mutant and nonmutant mitochondria to daughter cells (Figure 3.31). During egg cell production this can result in different oocytes receiving widely differing numbers of mutant or nonmutant mitochondrial DNA molecules, which translates into offspring who inherit the mutation to different degrees. In somatic cells it results in some tissues having a preponderance of mutant or nonmutant mitochondrial DNA molecules, and consequent tissue-specific effects of the mitochondrial mutation.

CONCLUSION

We have come a long way since the days of Mendel and Garrod, now having an understanding of single gene inheritance at the molecular level. With this increased understanding,

CLINICAL SNAPSHOT 3.4

■ MELAS

Evan is a 12-year-old with severe developmental delay and seizures. His seizures began around 2 years of age and have been diffi-cult to control with medication. Although his early developmental milestones were normal he has gradually lost developmental skills and has had a number of sudden episodes of neurological deficits that have been diagnosed as strokes. He has mild, diffuse muscle weakness, as well as partial loss of use of his right arm and leg since one of the strokes. A recent blood test during a stroke-like episode revealed a high lactic acid level. No one else in the family is similarly affected, though his sister has had several seizures, and his mother has a history of severe migraine headaches. A diagnosis of MELAS is made.

MELAS (MIM 540000) is an acronym for mitochondrial encephalomyopathy, lactic acidosis, and stroke-like episodes. The disorder may present at any time in life with progressive neurological deterioration and seizures. There are events in which there is sudden onset of neurological deficit that have the time course of strokes. The mechanism is not the typical vascular occlusion of strokes, though the exact pathophysiology is not known. Lactic acid tends to accumulate in the blood, especially during stroke-like episodes. Lactic acid is a byproduct of the failure of aerobic metabolism in the mitochondria. Various mitochondrial mutations can be respon-sible for MELAS. The most common is a mutation in the mitochondrial gene for leucine tRNA (MIM 590050). MELAS follows maternal transmission as expected for a mitochondrial trait, but there can be a wide range of variable expression within a family. This is accounted for by heteroplasmy for the mitochondrial mutation. Some individuals inherit only a small proportion of mutant mito-chondria and are mildly affected or entirely escape clinical signs. Others inherit a larger proportion and are more severely affected. Furthermore, the specific signs and symptoms may depend on the proportion of mutant and nonmutant mitochondria in specific tissues, such as brain or muscle.

TABLE 3.1 Major syndromes associated with mitochondrial mutations

Syndrome	Clinical features
Mitochondrial Point Mutations	
MERRF (MIM 545000)	Myoclonic epilepsy, myopathy, dementia
MELAS (MIM 540000)	Lactic acidosis, stroke-like episodes, myopathy, seizures, dementia
Leber hereditary optic neuropathy (MIM 535000)	Blindness, cardiac conduction defects
NARP (MIM 551500)	Neuropathy, ataxia, retinitis pigmentosa
Diabetes/deafness (MIM 520000)	Diabetes mellitus, deafness
Aminoglycoside-associated deafness (MIM 58000)	Sensorineural deafness following aminoglycoside exposure
Leigh syndrome (MIM 256000)	Movement disorder, respiratory dyskinesia, regression
Deletions/Duplications	
Kearns–Sayre (MIM 530000)	External ophthalmoplegia, pigmentary retinopathy, heart block, ataxia, increased cerebrospinal fluid protein
Nuclear Mutations	
MNGIE (MIM 603041)	Myopathy, neuropathy, GI disorder
Fatal infantile neuropathy (MIM 251880)	Mitochondrial DNA depletion

Reference: Shanske, AL, Shanske, S, DiMauro, S. The other human genome. Arch Pediatr Adoles Med 2001;155:1210–1216.

however, we also have a new appreciation for the complexity of genetic systems. There are no true single-gene disorders – no gene acts in isolation to determine a phenotype without inter-acting with other genes and with the environment. We will consider multifactorial traits later in this book, and traditionally these have been considered separately from monogenic traits. This distinction is beginning to blur, however. All traits are complex traits; some involve action of one or a few genes of major effect, some a larger number of genes. Understanding how these networks function remains one of the challenges in research in genetics and is likely to be translated into further advances in diagnosis and treatment.

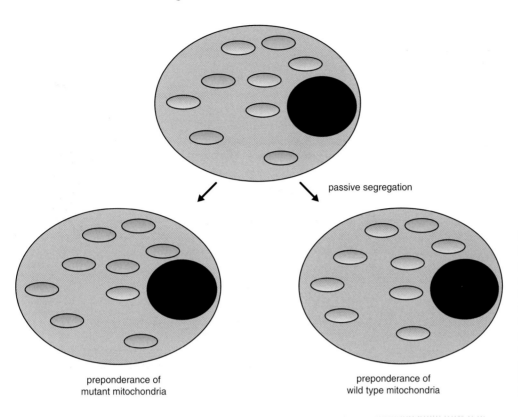

passive segregation

preponderance of
mutant mitochondria

preponderance of
wild type mitochondria

Figure 3.31 • Concept of heteroplasmy. Both wild-type (blue) and mutant (gray) mitochondria are included in the hundreds of mitochondria in a cell. These mitochondria segregate passively when the cell divides. The proportions of mutant and wild type mitochondria can change dramatically due to chance segregation. This can lead to variation in the proportion of affected mitochondria in different tissues or different individuals in a family.

REVIEW QUESTIONS

3.1 You take a family history, and obtain the pedigree below (Figure 3.1Q). How would you counsel them given this information?

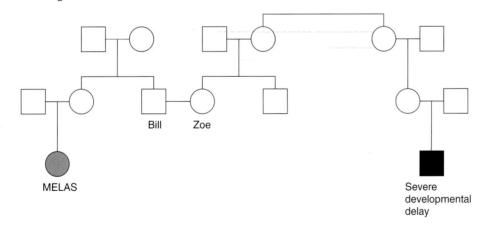

Bill Zoe

MELAS

Severe
developmental
delay

3.2 What is the most likely mode of inheritance represented in the pedigree below (Figure 3.2Q)?

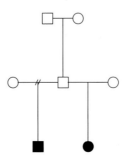

3.3 Individuals II-3 and II-4 wish to know the risk of having a child with an autosomal dominant disorder that affects I-2, II-1, and II-3 (see Figure 3.30). The penetrance of the disorder is 75%.

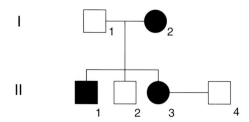

3.4 How could the following pedigrees be explained by genetic imprinting?

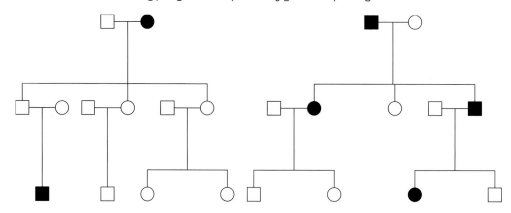

3.5 What is the genetic basis for the phenomenon of anticipation?

FURTHER READING

General References
Guttmacher A, Collins FS. Genomic medicine – a primer. New Engl J Med 2002;347:1512–1520.

Bennett RL, Steinhaus KA, Uhrich SB, O'Sullivan CK, Resta RG, Lochner-Doyle D, Markel DS, Vincent V, Hamanishi J. Recommendations for standardized human pedigree nomenclature. Pedigree Standardization Task Force of the National Society of Genetic Counselors. Am J Hum Genet 1995;56:745–752.

Badano JL, Katsanis N. Beyond Mendel: An evolving view of human genetic disease transmission. Nat Rev Genet 2002;3:779–789.

Mosaicism
Youssoufian H, Pyeritz, RE. Mechanisms and consequences of somatic mosaicism in humans. Nat Rev Genet 2002;3:748–758.

Zlotogora J. Germ line mosaicism. Hum Genet 1998;102:381–386.

Digenic Inheritance
Kajiwara K, Berson EL, Dryja TP. Digenic retinitis pigmentosa due to mutations at the unlinked peripherin/RDS and ROM1 loci. Science 1994;164:1604–1608.

Triplet Repeat Disorders
Everett CM, Wood NW. Trinucleotide repeats and neurodegenerative disease. Brain 2004;127:2385–2405.

Mitochondrial Genetics
Taylor RW, Turnbull DM. Mitochondrial DNA mutations in human disease. Nat Rev Genet 2005;6:389–402.

Clinical Snapshot 3.1 Congenital Deafness
Nance WE. The genetics of deafness. Ment Retard Develop Disabilites 2003;9:109–119.

Clinical Snapshot 3.2 NF1
Ward BA, Gutmann DH. Neurofibromatosis 1: From lab bench to clinic. Pediatr Neurol 2005;32:221–228.

Clinical Snapshot 3.3 Rett Syndrome
Weaving LS, Ellaway CJ, Gecz J, Chritodoulou J. Rett syndrome: clinical review and genetic update. J Med Genet 2005;42:1–7.

Clinical Snapshot 3.4 MELAS

Thambisetty M, Newman NJ, Glass JD, Frankel MR. A practical approach to the diagnosis and management of MELAS: case report and review. Neurologist 2002;8:302–312.

Methods 3.1 Taking a Family History

Guttmacher AE, Collins FS, Carmona RH. The family history – more important than ever. New Engl J Med 2004;351:2333–2336.

Bennett RL. The family medical history. Prim Care 2004;31:479–495.

AMA Family History Tools: http://www.ama-assn.org/ama/pub/category/2380.html

Ethical Implications 3.1 Family Ties

Taub S, Morin K, Spillman MA, Sade RM, Riddick FA. Council on Ethical and Judicial Affairs of the American Medical Association. Managing familial risk in genetic testing. Genet Test 2004;8:356–359.

Hot Topic 3.1 FXTAS

Hagerman PJ, Hagerman RJ. The fragile X permutation: A maturing perspective. Am J Hum Genet 2004;74:805–816.

4

The Human Genome

INTRODUCTION

The magnitude of the achievement represented by the sequencing of the human genome is all the more impressive when one considers that 100 years ago the genome was not known to exist. The focus during much of the 20th century was first on recognition of phenotypes, then identification of protein products responsible for those phenotypes, and finally finding the genes responsible for production of those proteins. The genome has been conceptualized by many metaphors, such as a parts list for the organism, a computer program, or even the "book of life." None of these quite capture the emerging appreciation of the complexity of the genome. We now know that only a small proportion is devoted to encoding the amino acid sequence of proteins. We also know that the genome is a dynamic system, constantly monitoring and repairing itself, and undergoing changes at multiple time scales – minutes to hours in the time-span of a cell cycle, years in the lifespan of an individual, and millennia at the level of the population and the species. We are a long way from fully appreciating the structure and function of the genome, but the availability of the complete human genome sequence has brought us to a point where the tools are at hand to explore the complexity of human biology with the promises of new appreciation for the physiology of health and disease and new approaches to diagnosis and treatment.

KEY POINTS

- Genes can be isolated by cloning in organisms such as bacteria and yeast. This provides purified DNA corresponding to a gene of interest that can be studied in detail.
- Genetic linkage analysis provides a means for mapping the genome using the frequency of recombination between loci as a measure of genetic distance.
- Linkage analysis in humans is accomplished by the calculation of LOD scores.
- A variety of DNA sequence polymorphisms can be used as markers for linkage analysis. These include restriction fragment length polymorphisms, single sequence polymorphisms, short tandem repeats, and single nucleotide polymorphisms.
- Positional cloning allows genes to be identified by first mapping the genes and then cloning the DNA within the mapped region until the gene of interest has been found.
- The Human Genome Project is an international effort that has succeeded in sequencing the human genome.
- The human genome includes around 25,000 genes, but genes comprise only about 5% of the genome. There are many RNA transcripts that are not translated into protein.
- The genome includes multiple forms of repeated sequence that are scattered through the genome.
- The ability to study the human genome has spawned new disciplines, including genomics, proteomics, and systems biology.

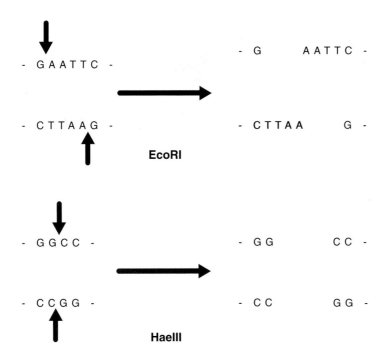

Figure 4.1 • The restriction enzyme *Eco*RI recognizes the palindromic hexamer GAATTC and cleaves asymmetrically to result in nonbase-paired ends. The enzyme *Hae*III cuts at the center of the four-base palindrome GGCC to leave blunt ends.

GENE CLONING

The possibility of determining the sequence of the human genome began with the ability to isolate specific genes. This technology, referred to as **gene cloning**, began to be developed in the 1970s. The basic goal is to isolate a specific segment of DNA so that it can be studied in great detail, including determination of its DNA sequence. DNA cloning is based on the construction of recombinant DNA molecules, inserting a fragment of interest, such as human DNA, into a vector that is capable of replication within a bacterial or yeast cell. Creation of recombinant molecules relies on the use of restriction endonucleases, already encountered in Chapter 2. Some of these enzymes leave unpaired overhangs (Figure 4.1), so mixing human DNA cut with an enzyme with vector DNA cut with the same enzyme allows hybrid molecules to form which can be "stitched" together with DNA ligase (Figure 4.2). A vector must be capable of being introduced into a host cell, such as a bacterium, and must be able to replicate itself within the host. The first vectors for such recombinant DNA experiments were plasmids, which consist of an origin of replication, one or more antibiotic resistance genes, and several unique cutting sites for various restriction enzymes that serve as points of insertion of foreign DNA.

How are individual genes isolated for study?

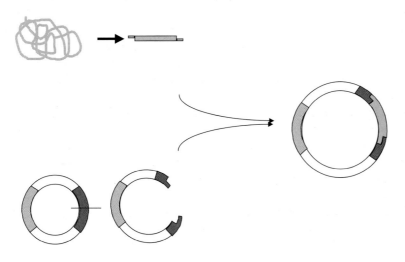

Figure 4.2 • Genomic DNA is cut into fragments with nonbased-paired ends. A plasmid cloning vector (below) is cut with the same enzyme, also producing nonbased-paired ends. Mixing the two together permits hybrid molecules to be formed, which result in a double-stranded, closed circular molecule when the ends are joined with a DNA ligase. The two genes on the plasmid are antibiotic resistance genes, one of which is interrupted by the inserted DNA.

Genomic DNA

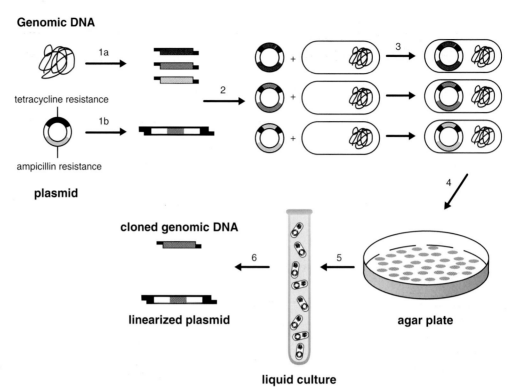

Figure 4.3 • Steps in plasmid cloning. Both genomic DNA and the plasmid are cut with the same restriction enzyme, resulting in nonbase-paired ends (steps 1a and 1b). In this example, the plasmid is cut within the tetracycline resistance gene. Individual DNA fragments attach to plasmid DNA through their complementary nonbase-paired ends and are covalently annealed with an enzyme known as a ligase (step 2). Recombinant plasmids then are taken up by bacterial cells, in which they multiply (step 3). The bacteria are grown in single-cell-derived colonies on an agar plate (step 4). Bacteria with recombinant plasmids will grow on ampicillin but not tetracycline because the inserted DNA disrupts the tetracycline resistance gene. Bacteria are picked from a single colony and grown in liquid culture (step 5). Plasmids isolated from this colony (step 6) can be treated with restriction enzyme to release their DNA insert.

TABLE 4.1 Major cloning vectors and quantity of inserted DNA that can be accommodated

Vector	Capacity
Plasmid	10 kb
Phage	23 kb
Cosmid	50 kb
P1 phage	100 kb
BAC	100–300 kb
YAC	>100 kb

What are the various types of cloning vector?

The antibiotic resistance genes allow selection of bacteria that have successfully taken up the vector. A prototypical cloning experiment is illustrated in Figure 4.3.

The plasmid vector accommodates only a small quantity of DNA (about 10,000 base pairs, or 10 kb). Other vectors have been devised that allow larger segments to be cloned (Table 4.1). Very large fragments can be cloned in **yeast artificial chromosomes** (**YACs**). A YAC consists of an origin of replication, a centromere to insure disjunction of the chromosome at cell division, a site where foreign DNA can be inserted, and telomeres to cap the ends of the chromosome (Figure 4.4). There are also selectable markers that allow isolation of yeast cells that have taken up the inserted human DNA.

Initial cloning efforts focused on genes that encoded proteins of known function. For example, the gene that encodes the enzyme tyrosinase (MIM 606933), involved in the synthesis of the skin pigment melanin, was cloned in a bacteriophage vector (Figure 4.5). First, the entire coding sequence for the gene was cloned. This was accomplished using a **cDNA library**

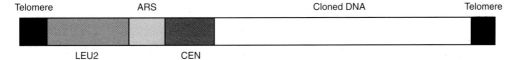

Figure 4.4 • Yeast artificial chromosome, a linear structure capable of independent replication within a yeast cell. The two ends contain telomere sequences, which are necessary to maintain the structural integrity and replication of the chromosome. The Leu2 gene (*LEU2*) is a selectable marker to identify yeast that have incorporated the recombinant chromosome. *ARS* stands for "autonomously replicating sequence" and contains an origin of replication. *CEN* is a centromere, which ensures stable division of newly replicated chromosomes to the two daughter cells. Much of the remaining material can be reserved for cloned DNA, permitting hundreds of thousands of base pairs to be cloned.

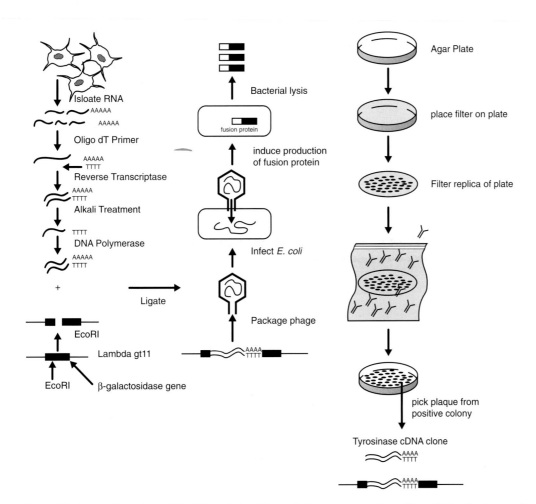

Figure 4.5 • Cloning of tyrosinase cDNA. RNA was isolated from cells that express tyrosinase. Most mRNA molecules contain a "tail" of 100 to 200 adenines at their 3′ ends ("polyA tail"). A synthetic oligo dT sequence (a string of thymidines) was bound to these polyA tails and served as a starting point (primer) for synthesis of a DNA copy of the RNA (cDNA) using the enzyme reverse transcriptase. The RNA then was digested away with alkali treatment and a second DNA copy made with the enzyme DNA polymerase, rendering the cDNA double-stranded. The phage vector lambda gt11 was digested with *Eco*RI, and cDNA molecules were ligated with the phage arms. These then were packaged into phage particles and infected into *E. coli* cells. Lambda gt11 contains a sequence for synthesis of the protein beta-galactosidase, which is located at the site into which foreign DNA is cloned. Stimulation of transcription of beta-galactosidase results in synthesis of a fusion protein consisting of part of beta-galactosidase and part of the protein encoded by the cloned sequence. After stimulation of transcription, bacteria were plated on agar and plaques of lysed bacteria were absorbed onto filters. The filters were incubated in a bag with tyrosinase antibody. The antibody became bound to tyrosinase on the filter, and the binding was detected with an immunologic staining reaction. This identified the clones containing tyrosinase cDNA, which then were isolated and used as a source of tyrosinase cDNA. (Data from Kwon BS, Haq AK, Pomerantz SH, Halaban R. Isolation and sequence of a cDNA clone from human tyrosinase that maps at the mouse c-albino locus. Proc Natl Acad Sci USA 1987;84:7473–7477.)

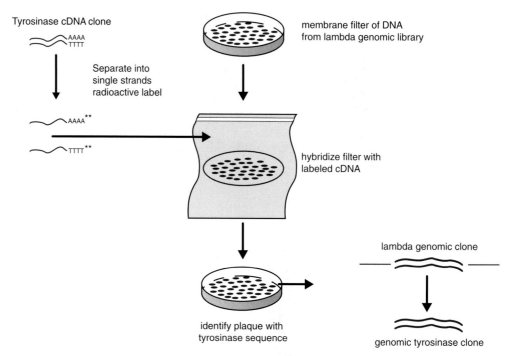

Figure 4.6 • Cloning tyrosinase genomic DNA. A membrane filter was prepared from a lambda phage library containing random fragments of genomic DNA. DNA in the filter was hybridized with labeled tyrosinase cDNA, identifying the clones containing homologous DNA. These were then isolated and used to prepare the genomic clone. (Data from Giebel LB, Strunk KM, Spritz RA. Organization and nucleotide sequences of the human tyrosinase gene and a truncated tyrosinase-related segment. Genomics 1991;9:435–445.)

obtained from cells known to synthesize large quantities of melanin. Messenger RNA was isolated from these cells and a DNA copy was made from the mRNA using the enzyme **reverse transcriptase**, which copies RNA into DNA. The resulting DNA sequences are referred to as **cDNA**. The cDNA segments were then randomly cloned into bacteriophage, which then were used to infect bacteria. The vectors were designed so that the inserted cDNA would be transcribed and translated into protein within the bacteria. Those that, by chance, had incorporated the tyrosinase cDNA could be identified using a tagged antibody to tyrosinase. The tyrosinase gene itself could then be cloned by using the cDNA to detect bacteriophage that had incorporated genomic DNA sequences rather than cDNA (Figure 4.6). The tyrosinase cDNA was radioactively labeled, separated into single strands, and used to identify homologous genomic DNA sequences in the bacteriophage-infected bacterial colonies.

A variety of similar approaches have been used with great success in cloning dozens of genes, but these approaches were limited to genes of known function. Most of the genes of medical interest are known through their associated phenotypes, and the gene products are unknown. Other approaches are necessary to identify genes involved in these disorders. Beginning in the 1980s, an approach was introduced that is referred to as **positional cloning**. This proved to be enormously successful. The approach is based on identification of a gene by cloning DNA at the site in the genome where the gene has been mapped. To understand the approach, though, we first have to look at how gene mapping was done.

GENE MAPPING

Approaches to gene mapping began to be developed during the early decades of the 20th century, initially working with plants and other experimental organisms such as the fruit fly *Drosophila* and the mouse. The basic principle is that genes are linearly arrayed on the chromosome and that the order of genes is the same from one individual to another in a species. During meiosis, however, homologous chromosomes pair and may exchange segments. Although this does not alter the order of loci on the chromosome, it does result in changes in the specific alleles that are present on a particular copy of a chromosome (Figure 4.7).

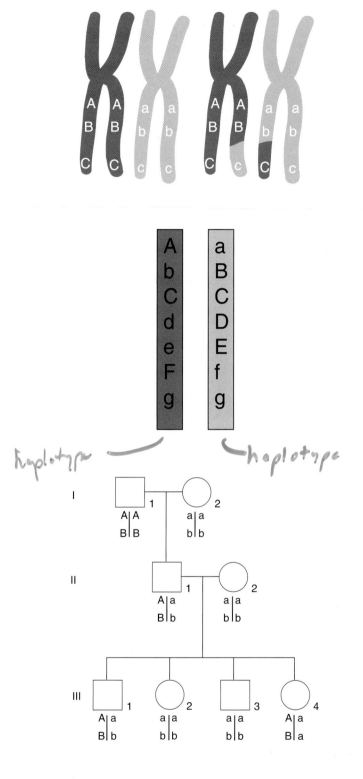

Figure 4.7 • Crossing over during meiotic pairing of homologous chromosomes. Although the relative locations of genes A, B, and C are not changed, the particular sets of alleles on the two chromosomes change. Initially, alleles *A*, *B*, and *C* were on one member of the pair, and *a*, *b*, and *c* on the other. After the crossover, *A* and *B* are together with *c*, and *a* and *b* are together with *C* on one of the two chromatids of the recombined chromosomes.

Figure 4.8 • Two haplotypes for loci A–G. Each consists of a specific set of alleles located adjacent to another on a particular copy of a specific chromosome.

Figure 4.9 • Complete linkage between a pair of loci, with no recombination between them. Individual II-1 is heterozygous at the two loci; his partner is doubly homozygous. Each offspring in generation III gets *a* and *b* from mother and either *AB* or *ab* from father. None gets the recombinant *Ab* or *aB* from father.

Linkage Analysis

The frequency of recombination between a pair of genes is a function of distance; the farther apart they are, the more often a crossover event will occur between them. If two genes are very close together, recombination between them will be rare. A particular set of alleles that are together on the same chromosome copy comprise a **haplotype** (Figure 4.8). For extremely closely linked genes, alleles that are part of a haplotype tend to remain so from generation to generation (Figure 4.9). Only rarely will new combinations be created by crossing over.

How is linkage analysis done in humans?

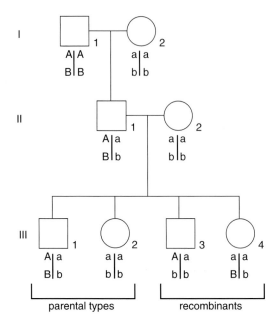

Figure 4.10 • Random segregation of alleles at two unlinked loci. Individual II-1 is doubly heterozygous and produces four types of sperm: *AB*, *Ab*, *aB*, and *ab*. Each of these four combinations is represented in one of the offspring, resulting in equal numbers of parental (nonrecombinant) and recombinant offspring.

The opposite situation is illustrated by genes that are located on different chromosomes. In this case, alleles segregate randomly to gametes. For an unlinked pair of loci, there is a 50% chance that the parental combination of alleles will be found in an offspring and a 50% chance that a nonparental combination will occur. Fifty percent **recombinant** and **nonrecombinant** genotypes is the outcome of random segregation (Figure 4.10).

Suppose that two genes are separated by a distance such that recombination occurs between them 10% of the time. On average, then, 10% of germ cells will be recombinant and 90% nonrecombinant. This expectation would be realized if a very large number of offspring were sampled. The ideal mating experiment matches a doubly heterozygous individual with a homozygous partner and samples an extremely large number of offspring. Such experiments are commonly done with fruit flies or mice but are not useful for mapping the human genome.

To circumvent this difficulty, a statistical approach has been developed to extract linkage information from smaller families. What is calculated is the relative likelihood (the odds) that a particular set of family information would be obtained if a pair of genes is linked rather than if they segregate randomly. For a family with four children, the chance of any combination of recombinant and nonrecombinant genotypes given nonlinkage (i.e., the result of random segregation) is $(1/2)(1/2)(1/2)(1/2) = 1/16$. (Note that birth order is ignored, since this factor will be the numerator and denominator of the odds ratio.) The chance of seeing any combination of recombinant and nonrecombinant genotypes if the genes are linked depends on how closely they are located. For example, if the rate of recombination between a set of genes is 10%, then the probability of a recombinant individual is 0.1 and of a nonrecombinant individual is 0.9. In a family of four (Figure 4.11), the probability of seeing one recombinant and three nonrecombinant offspring if the rate of recombination is 10% is $(0.1)(0.9)(0.9)(0.9) = 0.0729$.

In this family of four with one recombinant and four nonrecombinant combinations of alleles, which is more likely: linkage with a recombination frequency of 10% or nonlinkage? We can compare the relative likelihood of these two possibilities by creating an odds ratio. In this case, $0.0729/0.0625 = 1.167$; linkage is slightly favored over nonlinkage. The same can be done for other values of the frequency of recombination between the two genes. The frequency of recombination usually is expressed as a variable θ, the recombination fraction. At $\theta = 0$, the probability of linkage will be 0 if any recombinants occur at all, because at this value of θ, no recombination is possible. At a value of $\theta = 0.5$, the odds ratio will be 1, because 50% recombination is equivalent to nonlinkage. Between $\theta = 0$ and $\theta = 0.5$, the probability of linkage depends on family size and the number of recombinant and nonrecombinant individuals. A

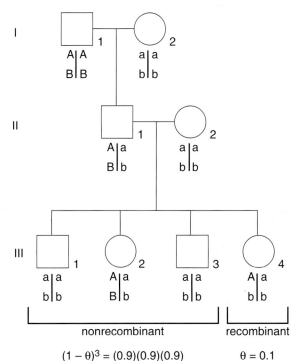

$$\text{odds ratio} = \frac{(1-\theta)^n \, \theta^r}{(1/2)^{n+r}}$$

n = number nonrecombinant offspring
r = number recombinant offspring
n+r = total number of offspring

Figure 4.11 • Calculation of odds ratio. In this sibship of four, three children are nonrecombinant and one is recombinant. The numerator of the odds ratio is the probability of seeing this number of recombinant and nonrecombinant offspring at recombination value of θ, and the denominator is the probability given random segregation (equivalent to $\theta = 0.5$). This odds ratio indicates the relative likelihood of this family's data given recombination at a set value of θ compared with random segregation. The odds ratio is computed for multiple values of θ.

family with some recombinant individuals, but fewer than expected by random segregation, will be better explained by an intermediate value of θ: If θ is too low, few or no recombinants are expected, and if θ is too high, more are expected.

Although this approach can help extract data from small families, there is a limit to what can be learned. In a family of four, chance segregation of alleles can lead to no recombinant offspring even if genes are unlinked. There is no substitute for the statistical power of large numbers. How can this be achieved?

One way is to pool data from many families – in effect, to consider many different sibships as if they were all one big sibship. In figuring the probability of linkage or nonlinkage for a family, each child is viewed as an independent statistical event, and the total probability of the recombinants and nonrecombinants in the sibship is the product of the individual probabilities for each offspring. If data from multiple sibships are obtained, the probability for each offspring can be multiplied together. This becomes unwieldy if many individuals are studied, but recall that adding logarithms is the equivalent of multiplying the numbers to which they correspond. Therefore, the odds ratio can be calculated for each sibship, the fraction converted to a logarithm, and then the log of the odds ratio added from family to family to obtain a final log of the odds ratio for the entire data set. Log of the odds is abbreviated with the acronym **lod**. Lod "scores" are calculated family by family for multiple values of θ and then are summed for each value of θ. How high does a lod score need to be to indicate probable linkage or nonlinkage of a pair of genes? Evidence for linkage generally is accepted when a lod score is 3 or greater, indicating at least a 1000:1 odds ratio favoring linkage. Lod scores of 2 or less are accepted as evidence against linkage, indicating at least a 100:1 ratio favoring nonlinkage. The value of θ at which the peak lod score is obtained is taken as the maximum likelihood value of θ (Figure 4.12).

There is one important caution that must be applied to the study of linkage by pooling data from many families. This is the possibility of genetic heterogeneity. If different genes at different locations are responsible for a trait in different families, no one marker will be linked to them all. Data favoring linkage in one family will be canceled out by data favoring nonlinkage in another, with the net result that random segregation will be favored. It is always safer to analyze linkage data from individual large families to avoid the pitfall of genetic heterogeneity.

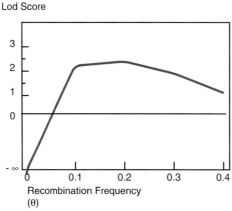

Lod Score

Recombination Frequency
(θ)

Figure 4.12 • Analysis of linkage data from five families. The number of siblings in each family, as well as the number of recombinants and nonrecombinants in each family, is shown in the table. Lod scores were computed for the indicated values of θ and summed across all the families, and then a graph of lod score versus θ was made. The lod score peaked at just less than 3 at a value of θ of 0.1. This would be the maximum likelihood estimate for θ based on these data.

					θ			
Family	Sibs	Recombinants	Nonrecombinants	0	0.1	0.2	0.3	0.4
1	3	1	2	- ∞	-0.188	0.010	0.070	0.061
2	4	0	4	1.200	1.020	0.816	0.584	0.317
3	5	1	4	- ∞	0.322	0.418	0.362	0.219
4	4	0	4	1.200	1.020	0.816	0.584	0.317
5	4	1	3	- ∞	0.066	0.214	0.216	0.141
Total				- ∞	2.240	2.274	1.816	1.055

What are the major types of genetic polymorphisms?

Genetic Polymorphism

The search for linkage requires that individuals be doubly heterozygous for the two loci that are being mapped. If one locus is associated with a phenotype such as a genetic disorder, the heterozygous individual is either affected with a dominant trait or a carrier for a recessive one. It is unlikely, however, that there will be another gene locus nearby which can also be assessed phenotypically. The advent of DNA markers, however, has provided the ability to map almost any genetic trait anywhere in the genome. The fundamental property of a useful genetic marker is that there must be at least two alleles and these alleles must be common enough so that heterozygosity is common. As we have seen in Chapter 2, the techniques of molecular genetics have revealed many different types of polymorphisms, and these have provided an extraordinarily rich map of the genome. Various web-based resources are available for selection of polymorphisms appropriate for a particular study (see http://www.ncbi.nlm.nih.gov/genome/guide/human/). If the location of a given trait is not known, the first step is to choose widely spaced markers to look for evidence of linkage. About 300 markers will cover the human genome so that there should be a marker within 10% recombination (referred to as 10 centiMorgans or 10 cM) of the trait of interest. Once this low-resolution mapping has been done, additional markers in the region of interest can be tested to achieve a high-resolution map of the region surrounding the trait.

Positional Cloning

How can genes responsible for specific phenotypes be cloned based on knowledge of their location in the genome?

As DNA polymorphisms began to become available in the early 1980s, efforts were initiated to map genes responsible for various human genetic disorders. One of the first major successes was localization of the gene for Huntington disease to the short arm of the fourth chromosome (Clinical Snapshot 4.1). Gradually, the location of many other disorders came into focus. Gene mapping began to provide tools for molecular diagnosis, since the same linkage approach that resulted in mapping a gene could also be used to track the gene mutation in a specific family. We will explore this approach later in the book. Another benefit, however, was the ability to clone the DNA for the disease gene by positional cloning.

CLINICAL SNAPSHOT 4.1

■ Huntington disease

Mark is a 45-year-old with a family history of Huntington disease. He has begun to notice abnormal movements and is concerned that he might be affected. His mother died of the disease at age 55. Recently, Mark has noted occasional sudden jerking movements of his arms or legs and he is having difficulty with his handwriting. His family has also noted that he is increasingly irritable and forgetful. His physical examination is notable only for difficulty with rapid alternating movements of his fingers. An MRI is done, which shows mild atrophy of the caudate nucleus.

Huntington disease (HD) (MIM 143100) is an autosomal dominant disorder that displays age-dependent penetrance. It rarely affects children, but the probability of manifesting signs and symptoms increases with age among those who inherit the mutation. The hallmark sign is chorea – abnormal movements that can take the form of writhing or jerking the extremities. There is also a dementia and depression. The disorder is relentlessly progressive and ultimately lethal, with death most commonly due to aspiration pneumonia as a result of abnormal control of swallowing. Suicide is also common. Abnormal movements may be treated with medications, but there is no treatment that slows the progression.

Huntington disease was one of the first disorders to be mapped using restriction fragment length polymorphisms, in 1983. The gene locus is on chromosome 4. It took ten more years to identify the gene by positional cloning. It encodes a protein, referred to as huntingtin, which is expressed in neurons. The gene includes a CAG trinucleotide repeat, with approximately 22 repeats in the general population and more than 36 in those with Huntington disease (Figure 4.13). The CAG region encodes a polyglutamine tract in the protein. The exact mechanism whereby the abnormal protein causes neurological deterioration is not known. The expanded polyglutamine region may cause abnormal folding of the protein and sequestration of other proteins in the cell. The HD mutation represents a gain of function, in that only a single mutant allele is required to achieve full expression of the disorder.

Because HD may not be clinically evident until after the reproductive years, individuals may transmit the gene before they realize that they are affected. The mapping and identification of the gene has made it possible to offer predictive testing and prenatal diagnosis. We will explore the ways in which this is done later in this book. Genetic testing must be provided with great care and sensitivity, though, since presymptomatic diagnosis of an unpreventable neurological disorder can impose a major psychological burden on the affected individual and members of the family.

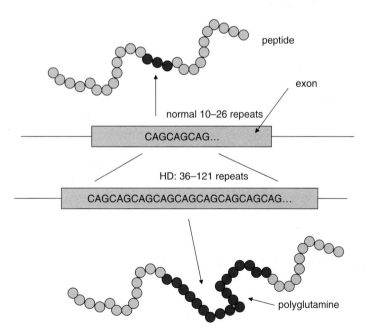

Figure 4.13 • Huntington disease results from expansion of an AG triplet repeat from a normal number of 10 to 26 repeats to greater than 36 repeats. This results in expansion of a polyglutamine sequence in the corresponding protein.

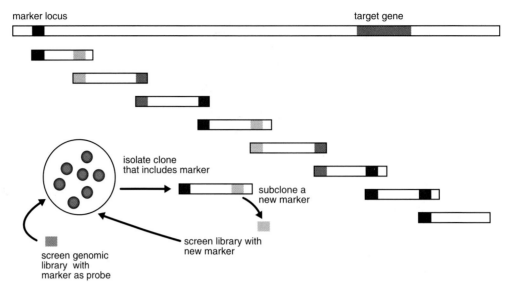

Figure 4.14 • Schematic of gene walking, in which a linked marker is used to identify a clone that includes the marker, along with additional DNA. This process is iterated until a large region of overlapping clones has been obtained. Eventually, the gene of interest will have been cloned (although it remains to be identified). A unidirectional walk is illustrated here.

The basic principle of positional cloning is to first determine the location of a gene by gene mapping and then to isolate DNA in the region and identify a segment that corresponds to the gene of interest. If one begins from a polymorphic locus that is found to be linked to the disease, one can use that locus to identify segments of DNA cloned in a vector that accommodates large inserts, such as a cosmid (which is a plasmid that is inserted into bacterial cells, like a phage) (Figure 4.14) or a YAC. Eventually the sequence of interest will be cloned. This is determined by the fact that the gene is expressed in tissues affected by the disorder and that mutations are found in affected individuals. Ultimate proof that the correct gene has been found may involve reproducing the disorder in model systems, such as a mouse model, by introduction of the mutant gene (Methods 4.1).

Methods 4.1

Animal models of human disease

Animal models offer major advantages for study of disease and test of new treatments. There are many natural animal models of human genetic disorders, but the repertoire is limited. Technologies now permit creation of a wide variety of models in many different types of organisms.

Among the most powerful are mouse models. Specific genes can be inserted into the mouse by the injection of DNA from a gene of interest into the nucleus of a fertilized oocyte (Figure 4.15). The inserted gene will integrate at random into the DNA and produce transgenic mice that express the inserted gene. It is also possible to target specific mouse genes with mutations (Figure 4.16). Embryonic stem (ES) cells are isolated from blastocysts and can be maintained in culture. A mutant version of the gene of interest is transfected into the ES cells. The gene is part of a vector that includes a selectable marker. In a small proportion of cells the inserted gene will undergo homologous recombination with the normal mouse gene and replace the normal gene with the mutant form. The selectable marker permits these cells to be isolated and they are then injected into mouse blastocysts to produce chimeric animals. The chimeric mice are mated to produce "gene knockout" animals. In some cases, the knockout proves to be lethal. To avoid this problem, conditional knockout mice can be created (Figure 4.17). In this case, the inserted gene is normal but is flanked by a pair of DNA sequences (loxP sites) that undergo homologous recombination if another gene called *cre* recombinase is activated. The *cre* recombinase is transfected into the ES cells next to a promoter that is only active in specific cell types. Activation of *cre* in these cells leads to homologous recombination between the loxP sites and excision of the inserted gene in those cells. Other cells that do not express *cre* remain unaffected. This approach permits the function of a disrupted gene to be studied in specific tissues or at specific times in development.

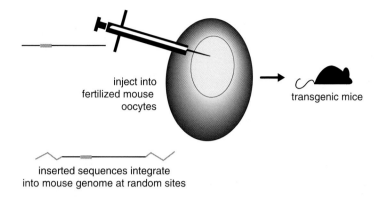

inject into
fertilized mouse
oocytes

transgenic mice

inserted sequences integrate
into mouse genome at random sites

Figure 4.15 • Production of a transgenic mouse. A gene is mutated by insertion of a synthetic oligonucleotide containing a point mutation. This gene is then injected into mouse oocytes, where inserted sequences integrate randomly into the mouse genome. A mouse grown from such an egg after fertilization will contain multiple copies of the inserted mutated gene.

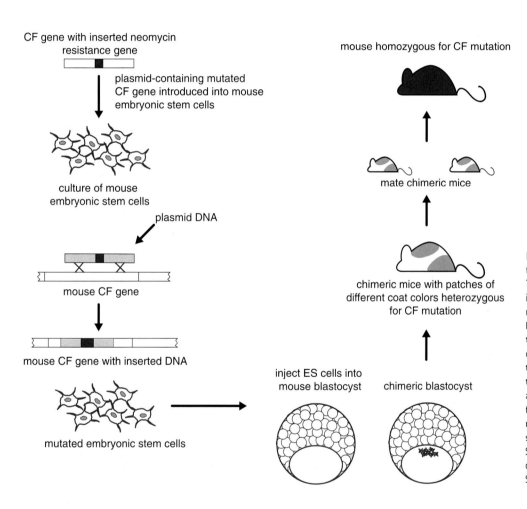

CF gene with inserted neomycin
resistance gene

plasmid-containing mutated
CF gene introduced into mouse
embryonic stem cells

culture of mouse
embryonic stem cells

plasmid DNA

mouse CF gene

mouse CF gene with inserted DNA

mutated embryonic stem cells

inject ES cells into
mouse blastocyst

chimeric blastocyst

mouse homozygous for CF mutation

mate chimeric mice

chimeric mice with patches of
different coat colors heterozygous
for CF mutation

Figure 4.16 • Creation of mouse model for cystic fibrosis by targeted knockout. The mutated CFTR gene is introduced into mouse embryonic stem cells. The mutant gene recombines with the homologous normal gene, disrupting the mouse gene. The embryonic stem cells are injected into blastocysts, which then grow into chimeric mice. Mating of the chimeric mice produces homozygous animals with the mutant CFTR gene. Data from Dorin JR, et al., Cystic fibrosis in the mouse by targeted insertional mutagenesis. Nature 1992;359:211–215; and from Snouwaert JN, et al. An animal model for cystic fibrosis made by gene targeting. Science 1992;257:1083–1088.

There are many other model organisms that are amenable to genetic manipulation. The flatworm *Caenorhabditis elegans* offers the advantage that development has been precisely cataloged from fertilization through the fully developed organism, with each cell identified. Many of the developmental pathways in higher eukaryotes are functional in *C. elegans*, permitting detailed study. The fruit fly *Drosophila* has long been a favorite organism of geneticists because of its ease of manipulation for genetic studies. Gene knockouts in *Drosophila* permit analysis of mutations in genes that are homologous to those that cause disease in humans. Another commonly used organism is the zebrafish, a small tropical fish that is nearly transparent. Mutagenized zebrafish have been used to study the effects of disruption of genes that replicate developmental and physiological defects in humans.

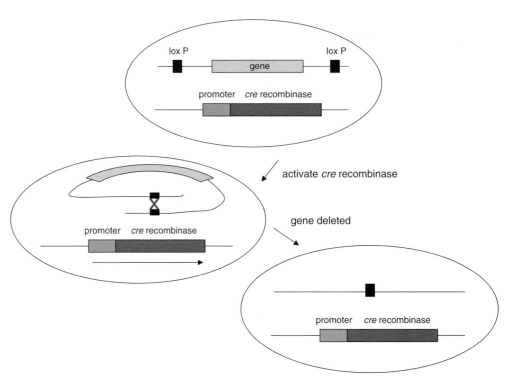

Figure 4.17 • Conditioned gene knock-out. A normal gene is replaced by a copy that is flanked by loxP sites, which are repeated sequences. A separate gene, *cre* recombinase, is inserted elsewhere adjacent to a specific promoter. When the *cre* recombinase is activated, recombination between the loxP sites results in removal of the gene. The promoter might be inducible by administration of a hormone or chemical, in which case timing of the knock-out is under control. Alternatively, it might be a tissue-specific promoter, in which case knock-out will only occur in specific tissues.

Beginning in the mid-1980s, a major series of successes led to the accumulation of genes identified by positional cloning. These include chronic granulomatous disease (MIM 306400), Duchenne muscular dystrophy (MIM 310200), cystic fibrosis (Clinical Snapshot 4.2), and neurofibromatosis type 1. This success continues to the present day, but the rate of success has been vastly increased thanks to the tools now provided by the completion of the Human Genome Project.

CLINICAL SNAPSHOT 4.2

▓ Cystic fibrosis

Emily is a 2-year-old who is being evaluated because of frequent infections and failure to thrive. She was born after a full term pregnancy with no neonatal problems. During the past 2 years, though, she has had frequent respiratory infections, including two bouts of pneumonia that required brief hospitalization. She has also had a difficult time gaining weight and her parents describe her stools as being copious and watery. Her examination reveals weight below the 3rd centile and a lack of subcutaneous fat. Her breath sounds are coarse with scattered rales and wheezes. A sweat test is ordered, which reveals an abnormally high sweat sodium and chloride levels, diagnostic of cystic fibrosis.

Cystic fibrosis (CF) (MIM 219700) is an autosomal recessive disorder characterized by markedly thickened secretions. The major site of pathology is the lung, where thickened mucous leads to blockage of small airways, creating chronic obstruction (Figure 4.18). Superimposed on this is chronic bacterial infection, including with organisms such as *Pseudomonas,* which are difficult to treat with antibiotics. This leads to progressive decline in pulmonary function. The other major feature in many patients is malabsorption, due to obstruction of pancreatic enzyme secretion. This, in turn, causes poor weight gain.

Cystic fibrosis is diagnosed by analysis of sweat for sodium and chloride levels, which are abnormally high in affected individuals. There is no definitive treatment that will reverse the physiological problems of cystic fibrosis, but there are approaches to management that can markedly improve survival and quality of life. The pulmonary symptoms are treated with antibiotics and chest

CLINICAL SNAPSHOT continued

physical therapy (pounding on the chest) to loosen secretions. Inhaled medications are available that can further break up the thick mucous. Malabsorption can be effectively treated by ingestion of pancreatic enzymes. With a carefully designed and supervised program, survival of individuals with CF now is into the 3rd and 4th decades.

The gene responsible for CF was identified by positional cloning. It is located on chromosome 7 and encodes a protein known as the cystic fibrosis transmembrane conductance regulator (CFTR) (MIM 602421). The protein functions as a chloride channel, pumping chloride ions out of the cell. Normally, water diffuses passively with the chloride to hydrate secretions, so lack of CFTR function explains the thickened secretions. There are many distinct CFTR mutations, but the most common in individuals of northern European ancestry is a deletion of three bases that removes a single phenylalanine. This mutation is designated ΔF508. Testing of *CFTR* mutations is now used as a carrier screen, a point that will be discussed in greater detail later in this book.

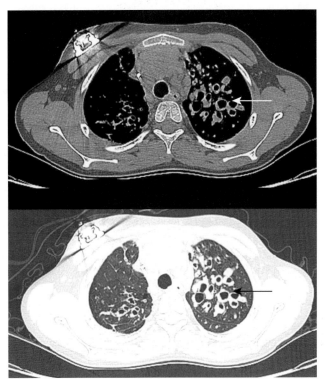

Figure 4.18 • Sagittal CT sections through the thorax of a CF patient (mediastinal windows above, lung windows below). Note prominent bronchiectasis with pooling of airway secretions (most notable in the left upper lobe, arrow), with relative sparing of the alveolar compartment. Complimentary forced expiratory volume (FEV1) for this patient was 45% of predicted. (Courtesy of Dr. J. P. Clancy, Children's Hospital, Birmingham, AL.)

THE HUMAN GENOME

The Human Genome Project was a large-scale international collaboration that began in the 1990s. The project benefited from major advances in sequencing technology that occurred over the ensuing decade. The culmination of the project, the completion of the human genome sequence, has placed major resources in the hands of the genetics community, and simultaneously raised major questions for the public such as the issues discussed in Ethical Implications 4.1.

ETHICAL IMPLICATIONS 4.1 • Genetic determinism

The publicity surrounding the Human Genome Project, and especially the announcement of the completion of the major part of the sequencing effort, has significantly raised public awareness about genetics. Along with this awareness, though, has come a heightening of expectations about medical breakthroughs that will ensue from knowledge about the human genome. This includes the promise of new diagnostic tests and treatments. It also includes the concept that genetic testing may one day be available to predict the risk of developing a wide range of common medical disorders.

Whatever role genetic testing eventually plays in determining the risk of disease, it is clear that health and disease occur as a consequence of a complex interaction of genetic and nongenetic factors. The notion that genetic factors alone are sufficient to cause an individual to develop a disease – or any trait, for that matter – is referred to as genetic determinism.

There are conditions, many of which have already been mentioned in this book, where mutations in single genes do contribute overwhelmingly to risk of disease. Everybody who is homozygous for the ΔF508 *CFTR* mutation, for example, will exhibit the signs of cystic fibrosis, although there may be differences in severity from person to person. Such differences may in part be due to action of modifying genes and in part to different environmental exposures, but it would be fair to say that having this mutation determines the CF phenotype.

This is far less the case for multifactorial disorders, however, or even for monogenic disorders with incomplete penetrance. Having a triplet repeat expansion at the Huntington disease locus does not guarantee that signs or symptoms will develop. Many people with such mutations die of other causes before manifestations of Huntington disease become apparent. Common disorders such as diabetes and hypertension have a definite genetic component, but the relative contribution of genes to predicting disease is even smaller.

Genetic determinism is a misconception that can be damaging to public perception and trust of the role of genetics in medicine. It may set up unrealistic expectations for the power of the genetic approach to prevent, diagnose, and treat disease. It also may discourage efforts to reduce exposure to environmental factors that contribute to disease and even create a sense of futility that will frustrate individual or community efforts to address risk factors. It can provide a misguided basis to discriminate against individuals for insurance coverage or employment, on the assumption that a genetic test equates with eventual development of a medical problem.

The fact that public attention has been drawn to genetics by the success of the Human Genome Project is a positive development, but it will be important to place the promise of genetics in medicine into a realistic context as public education goes forward.

What strategies were used to sequence the human genome?

Sequencing the Human Genome

The basic approach for sequencing the human genome began with cloning of fragments of human DNA in large insert vectors such as YACs or **bacterial artificial chromosomes** (**BACs**). As these were sequenced, they could be assembled as overlapping "tiles" or contigs, which covered the entire genome (Figure 4.19). The location of these sites could be referenced to a set of genetic markers that had been mapped along the human genome every million base pairs or so. Specific clones were marked with **sequence tagged sites** (**STS**), which are unique, short DNA sequences that unequivocally identify the clone. The sites of expressed genes were marked by **expressed sequence tags** (**EST**), which are unique sequences identified on cDNAs that mark expressed genes. With most of the genome covered by contigs of cloned sequence, it remained to use automated, high-speed sequencers to generate sequence data and assemble a sequence for each chromosome (Methods 4.2).

As the process of sequencing contigs proceeded, another approach was introduced by a private company. This was based on "shotgun sequencing," in which fragments were generated and sequenced at random (Figure 4.22). A computer was used to recognize overlaps in the fragments and to assemble them into contigs. This approach also made use of information about contig sequences available through the public effort.

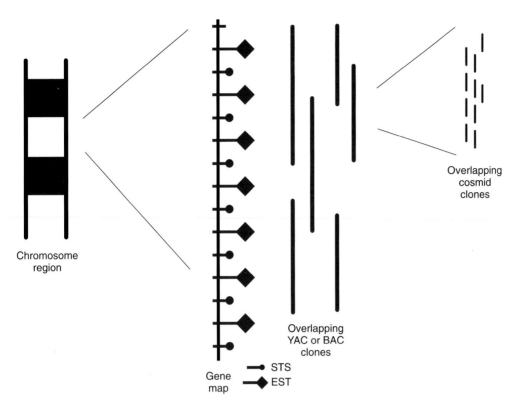

Figure 4.19 • Array of sequence tagged sites (STS) and expressed sequence tags (EST) on the gene map with physical map of yeast artificial chromosome (YAC) or bacterial artificial chromosome (BAC) and cosmid subclones.

Methods 4.2

DNA sequencing

Determination of DNA sequence has been a critical component of the study of the structure and function of individual genes, and obviously was of key importance in the Human Genome Project. The principle of the most commonly used approach is illustrated in Figure 4.20. Four separate DNA synthesis

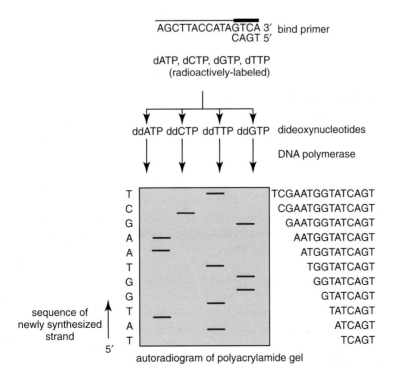

Figure 4.20 • Dideoxy DNA sequencing. Four separate reactions are performed, using the target sequence as a template. Each reaction contains a proportion of one nucleotide represented as a dideoxynucleotide. The dideoxynucleotide or the normal nucleotide can be incorporated into the growing strand, but incorporation of the dideoxynucleotide results in termination of DNA synthesis. Thus, each reaction results in a population of differently sized fragments that can be separated on a polyacrylamide gel and visualized by autoradiography. The sequence homologous to the template is read from bottom to top, 5′ to 3′, by noting the lane in which a band appears.

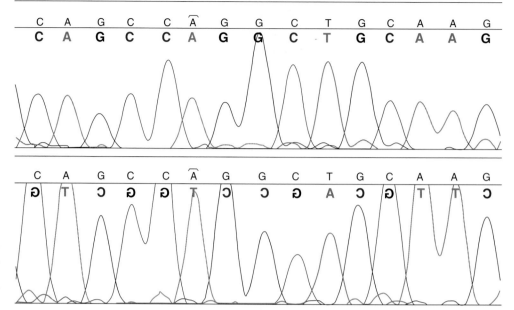

Figure 4.21 • Sequencing chromatogram. Each base is shown by a different line. The gene was sequenced bidirectionally, hence the two chromatograms shown with complementary sequences one atop the other.

reactions are set up with a primer sequence, DNA polymerase, and the four nucleotides. In each reaction, a proportion of one nucleotide is replaced by a dideoxynucleotide. When this base is incorporated into the growing DNA strand, synthesis will stop due to the lack of a free 3′ hydroxyl group. Since the reaction contains a mixture of deoxy and dideoxy nucleotides it is a matter of chance whether the dideoxy base will be incorporated at any particular site, and hence each reaction will consist of a mixture of fragments of different length. Initially, the fragments were labeled at one end with radioactivity and each reaction mixture was electrophoresed on a polyacrylamide gel side-by-side. This produced a ladder of fragments from which the DNA sequence could be read. Currently, the process is automated, and the four reactions are mixed, with the different dideoxybases labeled with a different color fluorochrome. Electrophoresis is done in tiny capillary tubes and the color is read out base-by-base (Figure 4.21).

The "first draft" of the human genome sequence was announced jointly by the public and private teams in June, 2000. Over the ensuing several years, the sequence has been refined, filling in gaps and resolving areas of uncertainty. In truth, not every base of the genome has been sequenced, and the genome may never be completely sequenced. Some areas consist of large stretches of repeated sequences that are difficult to work with and unlikely to yield much information. The entire sequence can be viewed on the internet using one of a number of genome browsers. A popular one can be found at http://genome.ucsc.edu/cgi-bin/hgGateway.

What has been learned about the human genome from the Human Genome Project?

Genome Organization

Before the Human Genome Project, a commonly heard estimate for the total number of genes was 100,000. This turns out to be a rough calculation based on there being approximately 3 billion base pairs of DNA and an average gene consists of about 30,000 base pairs. It is remarkable that this rough calculation was as close to correct as it was. The actual number of genes turns out to be 20 to 25,000, however. Although this is not a markedly more than the number of genes in "lower" organisms, such as the mouse or fruit fly, gene complexity is greater in humans. That is, individual genes consist of a larger number of domains and individual genes may encode multiple versions of a protein due to alternative splicing (See Chapter 1).

Protein-encoding sequences comprise only about 5% of the genome. A second class of genes encodes RNA that does not get translated into protein. This includes transfer and ribosomal RNAs, RNA molecules that are involved in the mRNA splicing process, and RNAs involved in gene regulation.

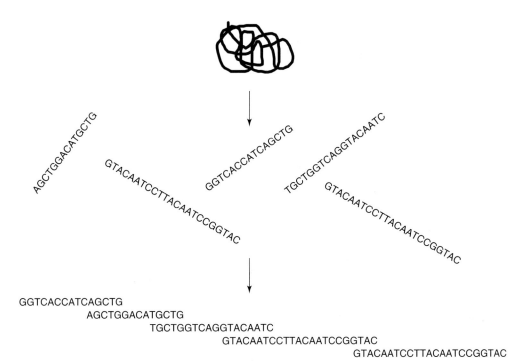

GGTCACCATCAGCTG
     AGCTGGACATGCTG
          TGCTGGTCAGGTACAATC
                GTACAATCCTTACAATCCGGTAC
                     GTACAATCCTTACAATCCGGTAC

Figure 4.22 • Shotgun sequencing. DNA is fragmented and the fragments are sequenced. These sequences are then assembled by computer analysis, recognizing overlapping regions.

At least 50% of the human genome consists of repeated sequences, which can be grouped into several classes (Figure 4.23). **Simple sequence repeats** consist of multiple copies of a short sequence, for example a di-, tri-, or tetranucleotide repeats. There are blocks of repeated sequences clustered at the centromeric region of chromosomes that we will consider further in Chapter 6. **Segmental duplications** consist of blocks of 10 to 300 kb that are copied from DNA at one site and move to another (Hot Topic 4.1). **Pseudogenes** are inactive copies of RNA, processed to remove introns that have been inserted into DNA. The final category is **transposon-derived repeats**, of which there are four major classes to consider: **long interspersed elements (LINEs)**, **short interspersed elements (SINEs)**, **LTR retroposons**, and **DNA transposons**.

LINEs range from 6 to 8 kb; they include a promoter site for RNA polymerase II and encode two proteins, one of which is a reverse transcriptase, which copies RNA into DNA. The LINE sequence is transcribed into RNA, which then moves to the cytoplasm where the two proteins are translated. These then bind to the RNA, which moves back to the nucleus, where it is reverse transcribed into DNA, which in turn may reinsert itself into the genome. In many cases, the reverse transcription does not copy the entire sequence, producing a LINE insert that remains inert. SINEs are 100 to 400 bp in length and have an RNA polymerase III promoter, mostly derived from tRNA genes. SINE sequences do not encode protein, but can use the LINE reverse transcriptase to copy their RNA into DNA and insert into the genome. LTR retroposons consist of retroviral-like elements. These include the long terminal repeat elements (LTR) required to support transcription and the two characteristic genes of the retrovirus, *gag* and *pol* (the reverse transcriptase). Reverse transcription of these elements occurs in the cytoplasm, with the DNA copy then being transported to the nucleus, where insertion occurs. Insertion of incomplete retrovirus-like elements results in many nonfunctional partial sequences in the genome. DNA transposons are similar to the transposable genetic elements found in bacteria. These encode an enzyme, transposase, which can cut the transposon out of the genome and then reinsert it at other sites. Transposable genetic elements have been viewed as parasitic sequences within the genome, although there is evidence that some may play a role in regulation of protein translation. Transposable elements also have been important in evolution, leading to creation of new genes. Most of the transposable elements in the human genome are currently inactive, but there are examples of gene mutations that have been attributed to transposition into a gene, disrupting its function.

What are the different kinds of repeated sequences?

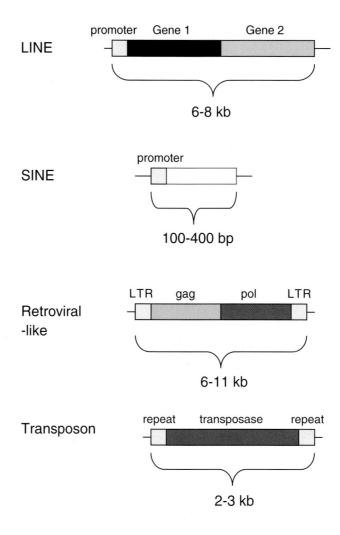

Figure 4.23 • Four classes of transposable genetic elements.

Hot Topic 4.1   SEGMENTAL DUPLICATIONS

Analysis of the human genome sequence has revealed that upwards of 5% of the genome consists of regions referred to as segmental duplications. A segmental duplication is defined as a set of sequences at least 1 kb in length with 90% or greater homology. Some segments can exceed 200 kb. Segmental duplications play a major role in driving chromosomal rearrangement. This is important in evolution, where it is responsible for chromosomal changes that drive speciation, and also in medicine, where chromosomal abnormalities lead to congenital anomalies and cancer.

Segmental duplications are not evenly distributed either along or among chromosomes. Some chromosomes are particularly rich in segmental duplications; as much as 25% of the Y chromosome consists of segmental duplication, for example. Segmental duplications are disproportionately located near centromeres and telomeres. It is not clear how segmental duplications arise. It is thought that some begin with insertion of a set of sequences into a chromosomal region (Figure 4.24), followed by unequal crossing over events that duplicate blocks of DNA.

We have already seen in Chapter 2 that unequal crossing over between repeat units can underlie deletion or duplication of chromosomal segments. This mechanism is responsible for many deletion and duplication syndromes, such as the neuropathy Charcot–Marie–Tooth disease (MIM 118200), velocardiofacial syndrome, Williams–Beuren syndrome (MIM 194050), and many others. In evolution, recombination events involving segmental duplication are thought to have led to inversions and other rearrangements that underlie speciation. For example 18 of the 23 human chromosomes are nearly identical among other primates, and pericentric inversions comprise the major differences among the remaining chromosomes. Segmental duplications may also be involved in the creation of new genes. Genes in a duplicated segment may be under less selective pressure, since they represent a "spare copy." There are many examples of duplicated gene sets in the human genome. These include the globin loci (see Chapter 13) and the opsin genes involved in color vision.

Hot Topic 4.1 SEGMENTAL DUPLICATIONS continued

Recently, it has become apparent that there is some degree of polymorphism in the number of repeat units of some large duplicated segments. This is referred to as large-scale variation. It remains to be determined whether these variants have functional consequences, for example serving as risk factors in the occurrence of common disorders.

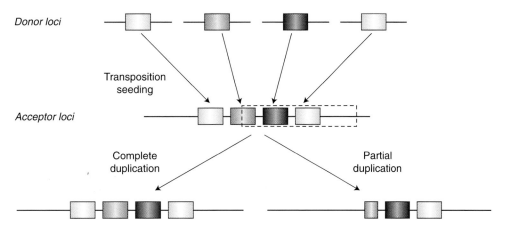

Figure 4.24 • Proposed mechanism of generation of segmental duplication. Segments of DNA are copied into a chromosomal region ("acceptor locus"). Duplication of all or part of this region leads to generation of multiple copies of the entire block, or part of the block. Adapted by permission from Macmillan Publishers Ltd: Samonte RV, Eichler EE. Segmental duplications and evolution of the primate genome. Nature Reviews Genetics 2002;3:65–72.

Genomics, Bioinformatics, and Systems Biology

The sequencing of the genome has spawned a set of new approaches to biological investigation. We will briefly consider three here: genomics, bioinformatics, and systems biology.

Genomics involves the study of large sets of genes, or gene products, up to and including the entire genome, or the entire set of transcripts ("**transcriptome**") or proteins ("**proteome**"). Genomics relies on high-throughput, automated approaches, such as the "gene chip," in which thousands to hundreds of thousands of DNA sequences can be affixed to spots on a glass chip and used to detect the presence of homologous sequences in a test sample (Methods 4.3). This approach can be used to rapidly detect sequence variants in a large number of samples or to characterize the entire set of transcribed genes in a particular tissue sample. The term "physiological genomics" has been coined to relate changes in patterns of gene expression or particular sets of genetic variants to specific physiological states in health or disease. "Chemical genomics" characterizes the alteration in behavior of genes or gene products in response to exposure to chemicals, and can be used to probe physiological responses or screen for potential new drugs.

What new disciplines have been spawned by the Human Genome Project?

Methods 4.3

Gene chips

Genetic studies have historically focused on genes one at a time, but tools are now at hand that permit wider-scale studies of the structure and function of large sets of genes simultaneously. One of the key technologies used in this effort is the "gene chip." The basic principle is that specific DNA sequences, either fragments isolated from a cell or synthetic oligonucleotides, can be fixed in place at a specific site on a glass chip. The sequences are attached using a photochemical reaction and an automated system, making it possible to create arrays with hundreds of thousands of sequences. The DNA on the chip can correspond

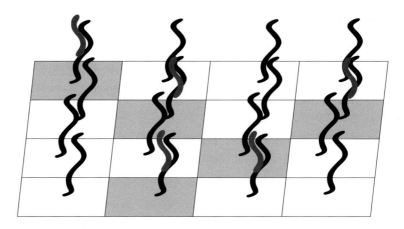

Figure 4.25 • Genomic DNA analysis using gene chips. Each cell of the grid contains single-stranded oligonucleotides with a specific DNA sequence. The test sequence will only hybridize with sequences in cells that contain an exact match. Genotype for the test sequence can be inferred from the specific cells where hybridization occurs.

with genomic sequences, or can be homologous to RNA sequences and used to probe gene expression. We will explore the use of gene expression arrays in Chapter 8. An example of genomic DNA analysis is shown in Figure 4.25. Each "cell" of the array contains an oligonucleotide that corresponds with a segment of a gene of interest. Adjacent cells contain the same sequence except for a change of one base. Every possible base change at any position in the sequence can be created and placed in a cell. The test sample of DNA is then labeled with a fluorescent marker and hybridized with DNA in the array. DNA will hybridize only with oligonucleotides in cells that contain an exact set of complementary bases. A computer system will identify the cells with hybridization signals, from which can be inferred the genotype for the test sample at any site for which oligonucleotides are present. This approach permits the simultaneous genotyping of a sample for thousands of SNPs.

Bioinformatics involves the use of computers to catalog and analyze large sets of biological data. Bioinformatic approaches have been applied to the human genome sequence to help identify genes or control elements. One particularly valuable tool is the comparison of sequences among different species. A major effort is underway to sequence the genomes of a wide variety of prokaryotic and eukaryotic organisms. Aside from providing information on the evolution of these species, such sequence comparisons help to identify functional regions that have been conserved through evolution.

Systems biology takes an integrated approach to the study of complex biological phenomena. Genes, gene products, proteins, and metabolites do not act in isolation, but interact with one another to form an integrated network. Systems biology involves an effort to understand how these networks are structured and how perturbations of a component of the network affect the whole. Much of the scientific effort of the past century, including the sequencing of the genome, can be seen as a reductionist approach aimed at identification of the individual components of biological systems. The task of systems biology is to put these pieces back together to obtain an understanding of how they function as a whole to make a living organism.

CONCLUSION

The success of the Human Genome Project has brought medical genetics, and medicine in general, to a new level. It has opened the door to the detailed study of the inner workings of the cell, as well as the ways in which cells communicate with one another and with the environment. Mysteries of development and physiology are coming to be solved at a rapid pace. There remains the daunting task of putting all this information together to unravel what might be called the "wiring diagram" of the organism. This will keep at least a generation of biologists and other scientists in fields such as computer science, physics, and chemistry, busy for a long time. Over the coming years, medical practice will be transformed as the underpinnings of health and disease increasingly come to light through this effort.

REVIEW QUESTIONS

4.1 If DNA from a genomic library were inserted into bacteria as part of a lambda phage expression vector, would you expect that a functional gene product would be obtained?

4.2 A fully penetrant autosomal dominant disorder is linked to a marker gene A, with alleles 1 and 2. Which of the following children (Figure 4.20) is recombinant (shaded symbols are affected individuals)?

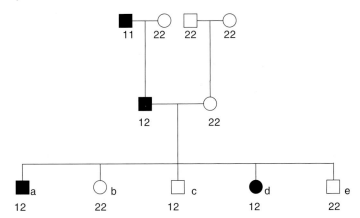

4.3 You are performing a linkage study with a marker that you think might represent the gene for a specific trait. At a $\theta = 0$ the lod score is $-\infty$. What does this tell you about your hypothesis that the marker locus is the disease gene?

4.4 How does having the complete gene sequence facilitate the process of positional cloning?

4.5 What would be the expected consequence if a LINE sequence were to insert itself into an exon of a gene?

FURTHER READING

General References
Alberts B, Johnson A, Lewis J, Raff M, Roberts K, Walter P. Molecular Biology of the Cell, 4th edn., 2002, New York: Garland Science.

Lewin B. Genes VIII, 2003, Upper Saddle River, NJ: Prentice Hall.

Lodish H, Berk A, Zipursky L, Matsudaira P, Baltimore D, Darnell J. Molecular Cell Biology, 5th edn., 2004, New York: Freeman.

Wall JD, Pritchard JK. Haplotype blocks and linkage disequilibrium in the human genome. Nat Rev Genet 2003;4:587–597.

Human Genome
Lander ES, *et al.* Initial sequencing and analysis of the human genome. Nature 2001;409:860–921.

Venter JC, *et al.* The sequence of the human genome. Science 2001;291:1304–1351.

Clinical Snapshot 4.1 Huntington Disease
Landles C, Bates GP. Huntingtin and the molecular pathogenesis of Huntington's disease. EMBO Rep 2004;5:958–963.

Clinical Snapshot 4.2 Cystic Fibrosis
Lewis MJ, Lewis EH 3rd, Amos JA, Tsongalis GJ. Cystic fibrosis. Am J Clin Pathol 2003;120:S3–S13.

Methods 4.2 DNA Sequencing
Shendure J, Mitra RD, Varma C, Church GM. Advanced sequencing technologies: Methods and goals. Nat Rev Genet 2004;5:335–344.

Ethics 4.1 Genetic Determinism
Holtzman NA. Eugenics and genetic testing. Sci Context 1998;11:397–417.

Hot Topics 4.1 Segmental Duplication
Samonte RV, Eichler EE. Segmental duplications and evolution of the primate genome. Nat Rev Genet 2002;3:65–67.

5
Multifactorial Inheritance

INTRODUCTION

The best studied genetic traits are not necessarily the ones responsible for the greatest world-wide burden of genetic disease. Single-gene disorders tend to be sharply defined traits, for which the genetic contribution lies close to the surface. These were the first disorders to be recognized as inherited and the first to be studied at the biochemical, and then the molecular, level. Genes do not function in isolation, however, nor is the human a closed system isolated from its environment. Therefore, it should be no surprise that among the most common and important of genetic traits are those that are determined by combinations of multiple genes and their interactions with the environment. This is referred to as multifactorial inheritance. In this chapter we will explore the concept of multifactorial inheritance and see how new genomic tools are being used to dissect out the genetic contributions to common disorders.

KEY POINTS

- Multifactorial traits are determined by a combination of genetic and nongenetic factors. Evidence that genes contribute to a trait includes familial clustering, monozygotic twin concordance, and studies of heritability.
- Two models of multifactorial inheritance are the additive polygenic model and the threshold model.
- Most common disorders include at least some genetic component. The identification of these genes is a major goal of current research in human genetics.
- Genes that contribute to multifactorial disorders can be identified using SNPs in association studies or transmission disequilibrium studies.

CONCEPT OF MULTIFACTORIAL INHERITANCE

The concept of multifactorial inheritance arose from the observation that there are traits that tend to cluster within families, yet are not transmitted in accordance with Mendel's laws as dominant or recessive traits. Examples include congenital anomalies, such as cleft lip or palate, spina bifida, and pyloric stenosis. They also include relatively common disorders, such as hypertension and diabetes mellitus. In this section we will look at the evidence for a genetic contribution to such traits, and at models of multifactorial inheritance.

Evidence for Multifactorial Inheritance

What kind of evidence supports multi-factorial inheritance of a trait?

There are many lines of evidence that support the contribution of genes towards the determination of multifactorial traits. The major approaches used are family analysis, twin studies, and, for quantitative traits, studies of heritability.

Geneticists measure familial clustering with a variable λ, which is the ratio of the frequency of the trait in relatives divided by its frequency in the general population. This can be easily measured by looking at the frequency of the trait among siblings as compared with the general population, in which case the variable is λ_s. For an autosomal recessive trait the frequency in

TABLE 5.1 Empirical data on recurrence risk of selected congenital anomalies in first-degree relatives

Anomaly	Population incidence	Recurrence risk (%)
Cleft lip ± cleft palate	1/1000	4.9
Congenital dislocation of hip	1/1000	3.5
Pyloric stenosis	1/500	3.2
Club foot	1/1000	2–8

siblings is expected to be 1/4, and for an autosomal dominant it will be 1/2. The value of λ_s will depend on the population frequency of the disorder. For the autosomal recessive disorder cystic fibrosis in the northern European population, λ_s will be (0.25)/(0.0004) = 625; for the dominant disorder Huntington disease λ_s will be (0.5)/(0.0001) = 5000. For the congenital anomaly pyloric stenosis (see Table 5.1) λ_s will be (0.032)/(0.002) = 16. The expected values for λ_s for dominant, recessive, and multifactorial traits are as follows:

$$\text{Autosomal dominant } \lambda_s = \frac{1/2}{x} = \frac{1}{2x}$$

$$\text{Autosomal recessive } \lambda_s = \frac{1/4}{x} = \frac{1}{4x}$$

$$\text{Multifactorial } \qquad \lambda_s = \frac{1}{\sqrt{x}}$$

where x is the population frequency of the trait.

Multifactorial traits have also been studied by analysis of the segregation of these traits through families. Computer models are generated that assume the role of one or more genes, exerting dominant or recessive inheritance, with various levels of penetrance and factoring in interactions with the environment. Data from families then are evaluated, and the relative likelihood that observed data fit with the various models is determined. This **complex segregation analysis** has been used successfully to discern the genetic contribution to a number of common phenotypic traits.

Twin studies involve comparison of the rate of concordance for a trait in monozygotic (identical) twins as compared with the concordance rate in full siblings. Monozygotic twins are formed as the result of cleavage of the early embryo into two embryos. These embryos are derived from a single fertilization event, so are genetically identical. One would expect full concordance in monozygotic twins for a trait that is entirely determined by genes. This is indeed the case for fully penetrant, monogenic traits, for example the disorders cystic fibrosis or sickle cell anemia. Monozygotic twins will not be fully concordant for a multifactorial trait, since factors other than their shared genes, such as environmental exposures, may also play a role. In general, the greater the rate of concordance among identical twins as compared with full siblings, the greater the genetic contribution to the trait (Table 5.2).

Another approach, which applies to quantitative traits such as height or blood pressure, is to estimate the **heritability** of a trait (Methods 5.1). The term was coined by geneticists who were measuring genetic and environmental contributions to measurable traits in plants and animals. The variance in such a trait can be partitioned into that which is contributed by genetic factors, environmental factors, covariance between the two, and measurement variance. Genetic factors in turn can be subdivided into those that represent additive effects of multiple genes and those that reflect interactions between genes. Environmental factors can be similarly partitioned. Heritability is defined as the proportion of variance contributed by genetic factors,

TABLE 5.2 Concordance rate for common congenital anomalies in identical and nonidentical twins

Trait	Concordance	
	Identical twins (%)	Full siblings (%)
Cleft lip and palate	40	5
Pyloric stenosis	22	4
Clubfoot	32	3
Congenital dislocation of hip	33	4

Source: Data from Smith DW, Aase JM. Polygenic inheritance of certain common malformations. J Pediatr 1970;76:653–659.

and is traditionally considered in two forms: "heritability in the broad sense" focuses only the additive genetic factors, whereas "heritability in the narrow sense" looks at all genetic factors, whether additive or interactive. For human traits we are usually interested in any genetic contribution, whether additive or interactive, and therefore focus on the latter.

Methods 5.1

Heritability concept and estimation of heritability from phenotypic correlation in family members

$$V_P = \overbrace{V_A + V_D}^{\text{genetic variance}} + \overbrace{V_E + V_I}^{\text{environmental variance}} + Cov_{GE} + \overbrace{V_M}^{\text{measurement variance}}$$

V_A = additive genetic variance
V_D = deviation due to dominance and epistasis
V_E = environmental variance
V_I = interaction variance
Cov_{GE} = covariance of genetics and environment

Heritability in broad sense $h^2 = \dfrac{V_A}{V_P}$

Heritability in narrow sense $h^2 = \dfrac{V_G}{V_P}$

Relationship	Heritability
Monozygotic twins	$h^2 = r$
Sib–sib or dizygotic twins	$h^2 = 2r$
One parent–one offspring	$h^2 = 2r$
Midparent–offspring	$h^2 = r/\sqrt{0.5} = r/0.7071$
First cousins	$h^2 = 8r$

r = correlation coefficient for quantitatively measurable trait.

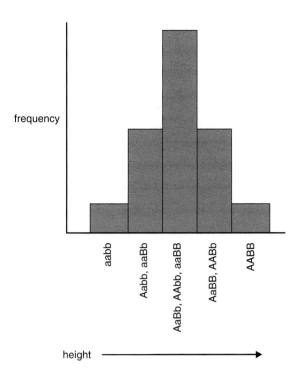

Figure 5.1 • Simple hypothetical two-locus model for inheritance of height. The dominant alleles each add 2 cm to the height and are assumed to be equally distributed in the population, with frequency of each allele being 0.5. According to this model, 1 in 16 individuals will have the genotype *aabb* and be the shortest. Likewise, 1 in 16 will be *AABB* and be tallest. One-fourth will have a single dominant allele or a single recessive allele. The majority will be of average height, having two dominant alleles. Note that, according to this model, it is the number of dominant alleles that determines height, not the specific combination (i.e., *AaBb* and *AAbb* give the same height).

Heritability can be estimated by looking at the degree of correlation of a trait in family members with different degrees of relationship. Heritability can be directly estimated from the concordance rate in monozygotic twins. Full sibs (including nonidentical, or dizygotic, twins) will share about half their genes, so heritability is estimated at twice the correlation between them. Other values for estimating heritability from the phenotypic correlation of family members are shown in Methods 5.1.

Models of Multifactorial Inheritance

What are the major models of multifactorial inheritance?

The simplest model of multifactorial inheritance assumes the action of multiple genes, but not environmental factors. This is referred to as polygenic inheritance. As an example, consider a hypothetical genetic system in which two separate loci are involved in determining final adult height (Figure 5.1). There are two alleles at each locus, one dominant, which adds 2 cm to final height, and the other recessive, which adds nothing. Suppose that a person with the genotype *aabb* would be 150 cm tall. Someone with all dominant alleles would then measure 158 cm. A person with the genotype *AaBb* would be 154 cm, as would a person with the genotype *aaBB*. The effects of these genes, then, are additive with respect to height. If alleles are equally distributed, the additive model predicts a normal distribution of the quantitative trait in the population.

Many of the traits that are subject to multifactorial inheritance are quantitative, such as height and blood pressure. It is relatively easy to see how additive effects of multiple genes or environmental factors could determine the values of such traits. Other traits, particularly congenital malformations, are less easy to explain by the additive polygenic model. Such all-or-nothing traits are better explained by the **threshold model** of multifactorial inheritance.

The threshold model assumes that there is a "liability" toward development of a disorder that is normally distributed in the general population (Figure 5.2). This liability is composed of contributions from both genetic and environmental factors that can lead to expression of the trait. Individuals will have more or less liability toward the trait, depending on how many of the predisposing genes they have inherited and the degree to which they are exposed to the relevant environmental factors. Up to a point, they will not display signs of the trait. When a threshold of liability is crossed, however, the trait appears. Some will exceed threshold because of having many genetic risk factors and little environmental risk, whereas in others the major

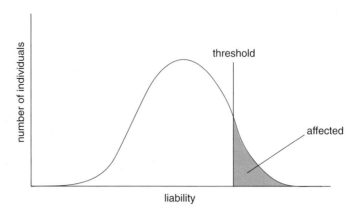

Figure 5.2 • Threshold model for multifactorial inheritance. There is a liability toward the trait that consists of a combination of genetic and nongenetic factors and is normally distributed in the population. The trait is expressed only in individuals whose liability exceeds a threshold.

contribution to liability may be environmental but, once the threshold is reached, the effect is the same.

An interesting observation has been made in some multifactorial disorders that is explained by the threshold model. Some disorders display a sex predilection, affecting either males or females more often. Neural tube defects, for example, tend to occur more often in females. Another example is pyloric stenosis (Clinical Snapshot 5.1), which is more common in males. The recurrence risk of pyloric stenosis is higher for families in which the proband is female than where the proband is male. The reason is that a female, being more rarely affected, is presumed to require a greater liability for threshold to be crossed (Figure 5.4). A couple having a daughter with pyloric stenosis is likely to transmit a greater number of genes predisposing to the disorder and therefore has a higher recurrence risk than those who have had a son with the disorder. Recurrence, by the way, is more likely to occur in a son than in a daughter, as the male would require less liability to cross the threshold.

The threshold model is based on statistical analysis of the clustering of traits in families. The notion of genetic liability may seem vague. What is really going on? The answer is mostly unknown, as there are few multifactorial traits in which the contributing genetic factors have

---

CLINICAL SNAPSHOT 5.1

▨ Pyloric stenosis

James is a 20-day-old seen in the emergency room for persistent vomiting. He was born after a full term, uncomplicated pregnancy. He has been breast-fed and seemed to have a good suck, but he has been spitting up a lot of his feeds from the first day. During the last 24 hours, however, he has been vomiting everything he has been fed, sometimes very forcefully. During this time he has become increasingly sleepy, and now shows little interest in feeding. Examination reveals a lethargic baby with a depressed anterior fontanelle and no tears when crying. A small mass is palpated in the left upper quadrant of the abdomen. Blood studies reveal low chloride and potassium and a metabolic alkalosis. A diagnosis of pyloric stenosis is confirmed by ultrasound and James is taken to surgery for a laparoscopic pyloroplasty. He is discharged from the hospital 2 days later.

Pyloric stenosis is due to hyperplasia of the muscles at the pylorus of the stomach and causes obstruction to gastric emptying (Figure 5.3). Infants present in the early weeks of life with recurrent vomiting, dehydration, and electrolyte imbalance due to loss of hydrochloric acid from the stomach and excretion of potassium and retention of hydrogen ions in the kidney. Surgical incision of the obstructing muscles is curative. Pyloric stenosis occurs in 2 to 4/1000 children with a 4:1 prevalence of affected males to affected females. It tends to cluster in families, with an increased risk among siblings or offspring of affected individuals. Inheritance is multifactorial, with no specific gene yet discovered that contributes to pathogenesis. Because of the male predominance, recurrence risk is higher in boys than girls. If the proband is female, however, the recurrence risk is higher than if the proband is male.

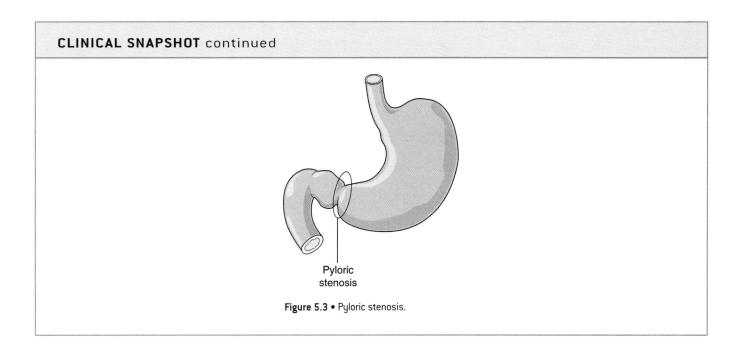

Figure 5.3 • Pyloric stenosis.

been identified. It is believed that genetic liability is accounted for by alleles at one or more loci that individually are unable to cause a distinctive phenotype. The phenotype emerges only if an individual has some critical combination of alleles at these loci. Sometimes this is sufficient to produce the phenotype, and at other times it just leads to susceptibility to an otherwise harmless environmental agent.

GENETICS OF COMMON DISEASE

Much of the progress in medical genetics during the past 50 years has applied to relatively rare, single gene or chromosomal disorders. In contrast, progress in understanding the genetic

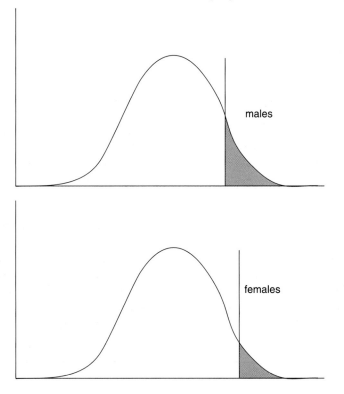

males

females

Figure 5.4 • The threshold for expression of a multifactorial trait may differ in males and females. In this example, the threshold is higher for females. A couple with an affected daughter can be assumed to have a greater overall liability and, therefore, a higher recurrence risk.

TABLE 5.3 Hypothetical case–control study testing hypothesis that allele 2 of a single nucleotide polymorphism is associated with asthma

	Asthma	No Asthma
Allele 2 present	30	10
Allele 2 not present	70	90

The polymorphism consists of a C (allele 1) or an A (allele 2) at one site in a gene of interest. Genotype is tested in 100 people with asthma and 100 controls. In this example, allele 2 is present (either homozygous or heterozygous) in cases with asthma more often than in controls. Relative risk of asthma given allele 2 is $30/70 \div 10/90 = 3.86$.

contribution to conditions that are the cause of more common diseases, such as cardiovascular disease, diabetes, and cancer, has been much slower. This is a consequence of the enormous complexity of these common disorders as compared to rarer conditions that result from mutations in single genes. Only recently have the tools of molecular genetics begun to penetrate more complex disorders.

There is substantial evidence that most, if not all, common disorders have a genetic component. The evidence is gathered from many of the approaches described earlier in this chapter – the disorders tend to cluster in families, there is increased concordance in identical twins, etc. In rare instances there are families that display single gene Mendelian inheritance of a trait such as hypertension, diabetes, or Alzheimer disease. Aside from these exceptional cases, though, it is believed that the common forms of these disorders are the combined result of both genetic and environmental factors, and that there are multiple genetic factors, each of which may contribute only modest increments of liability towards the condition. The major challenge is to define which genes these are, and how they make their contributions. We will explore the approaches currently in use to dissect the genetics of common disorders later in this book.

Genetic Association Studies

How can genetic association studies reveal the genetic factors involved in common disorders?

In spite of major success in the identification of genes involved in rare disorders, study of the genes involved in common disorders has been a much more difficult challenge. As we have seen, most common disorders have multifactorial etiology, with a combination of multiple genes interacting with the environment at the basis of pathogenesis. One approach to the study of genetic factors in common disorders relies on large population studies, looking for genetic variants that are associated with an increased risk of disease. In its simplest form this is done using the **case–control study** (Table 5.3). A set of individuals who display the phenotype under study (cases) are compared with a group who are matched as closely as possible, but who do not have the phenotype (controls) (Hot Topics 5.1). Genetic studies are then done to determine whether there is a significant difference in the frequency of a genetic trait between cases and controls. A relative risk calculation is done, comparing the frequency of the trait in cases versus controls. A relative risk greater than 1 indicates that the genetic variant is positively associated with the disorder; a value less than 1 indicates a protective association. It is important to recognize that association is not synonymous with "cause." The case–control study cannot establish a causative effect of a genetic trait with a disorder. The association could be due to an etiological contribution of the genetic trait, but not necessarily. An alternative would be that the genetic trait resides nearby another, untested marker that is truly the etiological factor.

What kinds of genetic traits can be tested in an association study? For many years, relatively few genetic markers were available. Some of the most impressive progress involved the study of association with alleles in the human lymphocyte antigen (HLA) locus on

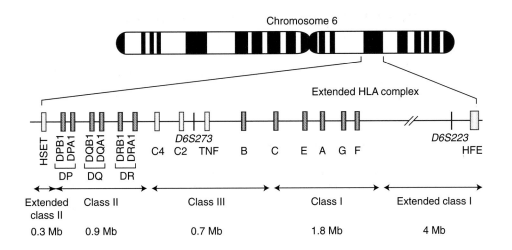

Figure 5.5 • HLA locus. Redrawn from Undlien DE, Lie BA & Thorsby E. Trends in Genetics 17:94, copyright (2001) with permission from Elsevier.

Hot Topic 5.1 LARGE COHORT STUDIES

The ability to carry out a case–control study is dependent on access to a large cohort affected with the phenotype of interest. Ideally, cases will come from a single homogeneous population, thus minimizing the likelihood that different genetic risk factors are acting in different individuals. The phenotype needs to be defined as precisely as possible. Common disorders, such as diabetes or hypertension, can be the ultimate outcome of a number of distinct pathological processes. Diabetes, for example, may result from an autoimmune process or insulin resistance due to obesity. All cases in an association study should be similar in terms of the origin of their disease. This may be aided by "subphenotyping" – identifying cases through use of a test rather than a broad phenotypic categorization. In diabetes, for example, this could be a test for β-cell antibodies, insuring that all cases have an autoimmune cause of their disease.

These various restrictions create challenges in the assembly of large groups of cases. To facilitate that process, several large, prospective cohort studies have been launched. In the United Kingdom, a project called Biobank (http://www.ukbiobank.ac.uk/) will follow a cohort of 500,000 adults for up to 30 years, tracking health status and obtaining blood and urine samples. In Iceland a private company, deCODE Genetics (www.decode.com), has established a database and DNA bank that will track the health status for over 100,000 Icelanders. The goal is to identify genes that contribute to the risk of common diseases and then to develop pharmaceuticals based on knowledge of the disease pathophysiology. Another study of 100,000 individuals has been planned in Estonia (http://www.geenivaramu.ee/). In the US, the National Human Genome Research Institute is considering plans to launch a prospective study of 500,000 individuals. Private companies in the US are establishing independent tissue banks and patient databases.

---

chromosome 6 (Figure 5.5). The HLA locus is a region that includes multiple, highly polymorphic genes that are involved in regulation of the immune response. Specific alleles have been found to be associated with a variety of disorders, most of which involve an aberration in the immune response (Table 5.4). An example is a form of arthritis called ankylosing spondylitis (MIM 106300). Individuals with the HLA-B27 allele have a 20- to 30-fold relative risk of having this disorder. Success has also been achieved in Alzheimer disease, where association has been found with one of the apolipoprotein E alleles (Clinical Snapshot 5.2).

In recent years the major focus has been on SNPs, many of which reside within the coding sequence of genes. Case–control studies using SNPs are designed to determine whether a

TABLE 5.4 HLA–disease associations

Disorder	Antigen	Relative risk
Ankylosing spondylitis	B27	69.1
Juvenile rheumatoid arthritis	B27	3.9
	DR8	3.6
Ulcerative colitis	B5	3.8
Psoriasis	Cw6	7.5
Multiple sclerosis	DR2	6.0
Narcolepsy	DR2	130.0

$$\text{Relative risk} = \frac{(\% \text{ antigen-positive patient} \times \% \text{ antigen-negative controls})}{(\% \text{ antigen-negative patient} \times \% \text{ antigen-positive controls})}$$

Source: Data from Carpenter CB. The major histocompatibility gene complex. In: Isselbacher K, Braunwald G, Wilson J, *et al.*, eds. Harrison's Principles of Internal Medicine, 13th edn.

specific genotype is found more commonly in cases or controls. Most studies are based on choosing SNPs from candidate genes that are deemed likely to be associated with disease based on a hypothesis about their physiological role in the disease process. This has produced a vast literature of reported associations, but the studies are plagued by problems of poor reproducibility from one population to the next. Such studies are also limited by the imagination of the investigator to choose an appropriate SNP for study. In addition, the case–control approach is vulnerable to an artifact referred to as population stratification by ethnicity. This is the occurrence of a spurious association due to the population being of mixed ethnicity. If

CLINICAL SNAPSHOT 5.2

▪ Alzheimer disease

Sid is 70 years old and it is clear to his family that his mental capacities have been slipping. He frequently forgets things and is constantly losing things. He has good memory for events of long ago, but does not seem to remember things said to him just hours ago. He frequently loses his way and recently had to stop driving after a minor accident. Sid denies that there is anything wrong with him, but reluctantly agrees to a visit to his doctor. His examination reveals normal physical findings, but poor recent memory. An MRI scan is done, which reveals only cortical atrophy. Blood tests are done, with mostly unrevealing findings, although he is found to have the ε3/ε4 apoE genotype. A clinical diagnosis of Alzheimer disease is made.

Alzheimer disease (AD) is a common form of progressive dementia, with over 4 million people in the US thought to be affected. It presents with memory loss and confusion and may include language problems, poor judgment, agitation, and hallucinations as it progresses. There are no distinct physical manifestations and diagnosis is established clinically. Brain atrophy is seen by MRI, though this is a nonspecific finding. Pathology includes amyloid plaques and neurofibrillary tangles (Figure 5.6).

Alzheimer disease is an example of a multifactorial trait. Rare instances of early-onset (<65 years of age) AD can be due to single gene autosomal dominant inheritance. Three genes have been identified. These encode presenilin 1 (MIM 104311) and 2 (MIM 600759) and amyloid beta A4 protein (MIM 104760). For late-onset AD there is an association with alleles at the locus for apolipoprotein E (ApoE) (MIM 107741). There are three common alleles, ε2, ε3, and ε4. The ε4 allele is found in individuals with Alzheimer disease about three times as often as in controls. The allele is nevertheless found in controls, and many with AD do not have the ε4 allele. Therefore, testing for ε4 does not diagnose AD; in an individual with a history of the disorder, however, ApoE testing can provide another bit of evidence in support of the diagnosis.

CLINICAL SNAPSHOT continued

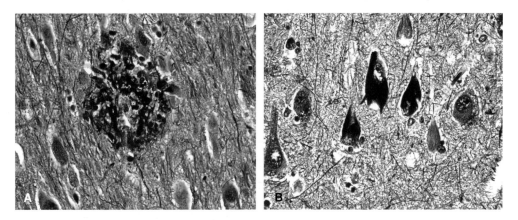

Figure 5.6 • Amyloid plaque (A) and neurofibrillary tangles (B) in a section of brain from an individual with Alzheimer disease. (Courtesy of Dr. Steven Carroll, University of Alabama at Birmingham.)

the disease is more common in a particular ethnic group and the genetic trait is incidentally more common in this same group, the study may reveal a spurious association of the trait with the disease.

Transmission Disequilibrium Testing

Various experimental approaches have been proposed to deal with these limitations. One that is designed to avoid population stratification by ethnicity is the transmission disequilibrium test (TdT). The principle of TdT is that a polymorphism is linked to a risk factor for disease, and that it is in disequilibrium with the risk factor. Disequilibrium implies not only that a pair of loci is linked, but also that specific alleles at the two loci are found as a haplotype more often than would be expected due to chance. This association of alleles most often reflects a relatively recent mutation of one of the alleles and a low rate of recombination between the loci (Figure 5.7). The TdT test is based on the idea that in a family where the disease occurs, it is more likely that the allele believed to be associated with the risk factor is transmitted to the affected individual than its counterpart allele (Figure 5.8). It is possible that the allele itself is the risk factor, but it is also possible that some other allele is the actual risk factor – all that is required is that the test allele be in linkage disequilibrium with the risk factor if it is not the factor itself. TdT testing requires collection of triads of an affected individual and both parents. The phenotype of the parents is irrelevant. What is necessary is that the transmission (or lack of transmission) of the allele under study can be scored in each triad. TdT analysis is not

How does transmission disequilibrium testing overcome errors due to population stratification?

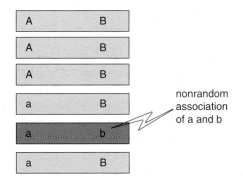

nonrandom association of a and b

Figure 5.7 • Linkage disequilibrium occurs when a mutation (in this case of B to b) occurs on a specific haplotype, in this case allele "a." Each rectangle in the figure represents a different chromosome in the population. For some period of time, "b" will be located on a haplotype with "a," until recombination occurs to create haplotypes of "b" with "A."

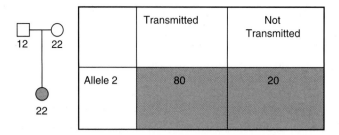

	Transmitted	Not Transmitted
Allele 2	80	20

Figure 5.8 • Hypothetical example of transmission disequilibrium study. Triads of two parents and a child, the latter affected with a disorder of interest, are genotyped, determining how frequently a parent who is heterozygous for an allele of interest transmits the allele to an offspring. In families with the pedigree structure shown, since the father is heterozygous for the alleles, there is a 50% chance that the child will inherit 2 from him, and hence be homozygous. The observed frequency of transmission (0.80) exceeds 50%, supporting the hypothesis of an association of allele 2 with the trait.

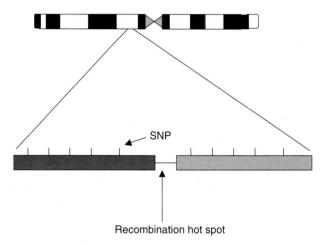

Figure 5.9 • Haplotype blocks of single nucleotide polymorphisms. The genome is organized into 10- to 20-kb blocks that are transmitted more or less intact from generation to generation, separated by "hot spots" where recombination is most likely to occur. Single nucleotide polymorphisms within a block tend to be in linkage disequilibrium with one another; therefore, a single SNP ("tag SNP") can be used as a marker for the entire group within a block.

vulnerable to population stratification by ethnicity since the association of the allele is tested family by family. It doesn't matter whether the allele is rare or common in the ethnic group from which a particular family is derived; if it is present in that family, its segregation can be tested. The major challenge with TdT analysis is the need to collect DNA from an affected individual and both parents. For adult-onset disorders, such as Alzheimer disease, it may be difficult to find affected individuals with two living parents for study.

With several million SNPs now available for analysis, it ought to be possible to find a SNP that is associated with almost any disorder. Confining the analysis to candidate SNPs means that unexpected associations will be missed. A truly comprehensive analysis would require an unbiased search of SNPs that cover the entire genome. If one were to use a SNP every 1000 bases, it would require 3 million SNPs to cover the genome. For a case–control study with 50 individuals in each group, this would require 300 million genotypes. Even with automated genotyping at pennies per genotype, the cost of such analysis would be prohibitive.

A recent discovery about the evolution of the human genome has suggested a shortcut to this analysis (Figure 5.9). It has become clear that there are blocks of human genomic DNA that have been transmitted more or less intact for most of human history, with "hot spots" for recombination separated by regions of relatively little recombination. These blocks, which have an average size of 10 to 20 kb, consist of a group of SNPs that are in linkage disequilibrum. The implication is that a single SNP, called a "tag SNP", can be used as a marker to represent an entire block, reducing genotyping task by an order of magnitude. Another approach that may help to bring the dream of a whole genome search for association within reach is analysis of allele frequencies in pools of DNA, one from cases and one from controls. Quantitative

CLINICAL SNAPSHOT 5.3

■ Diabetes mellitus

Don is a 55-year-old man who is being seen for a routine physical examination and blood pressure check. He has a history of chronic hypertension, for which he is on medication. His physical examination reveals moderate obesity and a blood pressure of 150/88. He has mild hypertensive changes in his retinal blood vessels. As part of his evaluation a urinalysis is done, which reveals the presence of glucose in his urine. A blood glucose measurement is subsequently done and is also found to be elevated. A diagnosis of type 2 diabetes mellitus is made.

Diabetes mellitus (DM) is a disorder of glucose metabolism. Ordinarily, glucose uptake into cells is mediated by insulin, a peptide hormone synthesized in β cells of the pancreas and secreted in response to a rise in blood sugar. Individuals with DM either fail to produce insulin in normal quantities or have a deficient responsiveness.

There are two major types of DM, types 1 and 2. Type 1 DM tends to have onset in childhood and is due to autoimmune destruction of β cells. It is a multifactorial trait with both genetic and environmental components. The major genetic factor is linked to the HLA locus on chromosome 6. Several specific HLA gene alleles are associated with type 1 DM in different populations. In addition, there is a VNTR polymorphism near the 5′ end of the insulin gene that also is a risk factor (Figure 5.10).

Type 2 DM is most often an adult-onset disorder and is usually associated with decreased responsiveness to insulin. Type 2 DM is also multifactorial. There are rare families with single gene inheritance of an entity referred to as maturity-onset diabetes of youth (MODY). A variety of different genes have been implicated, including genes involved in β-cell development or insulin secretion. More commonly, type 2 DM occurs sporadically. Association studies have been done to identify genes that contribute to risk. One gene, peroxisome proliferator-activated receptor-gamma (*PPARG*) (MIM 601487) has been shown in multiple studies to have an allele that is associated with type 2 DM, though having the allele conveys only a very small increase in relative risk. It is likely that multiple genes are involved in the etiology of type 2 DM, with different combinations involved in different individuals.

Insulin gene

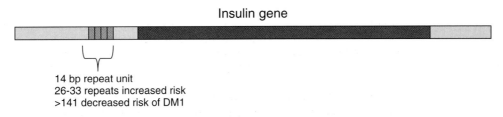

14 bp repeat unit
26-33 repeats increased risk
>141 decreased risk of DM1

Figure 5.10 • A tandem repeat polymorphism 5′ to the insulin gene that conveys risk of type 1 diabetes mellitus, with smaller repeat numbers conveying increased risk.

analysis of allele frequencies in pooled samples of DNA allows direct comparison of cases and controls for each allele, requiring only a single determination of genotype for each pool.

These approaches are beginning to bear fruit by revealing genetic variants that are associated with common disorders (Clinical Snapshot 5.3). We will explore the progress in one area later in this book when we consider risk assessment for common disorders (Ethical Implications 5.1).

CONCLUSION

Understanding the genetic contribution to common disorders is one of the major goals in genetics and medicine. It is widely anticipated that this will yield new approaches to prevention through early identification of individuals at risk. It will also produce new insights into pathophysiology that may be translated into new approaches to prevention and treatment. It is likely that insights into the genetics of common disorders will occur gradually, one disorder at a time. It is through this effort, however, that genetics will exert its maximal effect on the day-to-day practice of medicine.

ETHICAL IMPLICATIONS 5.1 • Predictive testing

Should predictive testing based on genetic association be offered as part of routine clinical care? Although it is widely antici-pated that this will be done at some point, there are few examples in current practice. There are several cautions that should be observed in the clinical application of predictive tests by genetic association.

1. Tests based on genetic association are not diagnostic tests. The test result will indicate relative risk for a disorder, not whether the disorder is currently present or someday will be present. Many individuals with the allele that is associated with disease will never become symptomatic.
2. Tests based on genetic association cannot exclude disease. Although having a specific allele may increase relative risk of a disorder, not having the allele does not mean that an individual will not develop the condition.
3. Relative risk of disease in individuals of a specified genotype can differ in different populations, as can the frequency of any specific allele. Data that are relevant to the population from which a particular patient is derived should be used to assess relative risks when possible.
4. There can be significant risks associated with predictive tests. These include stigmatization, anxiety, and the possibility of loss or denial of employment, health, disability, and/or life insurance. Laws to protect against such discrimination vary from state to state in the US and federal law has not yet been enacted.
5. There may be limited benefit associated with predictive tests, particularly if there is no means of prevention of the occur-rence of the disorder.

REVIEW QUESTIONS

5.1 A pair of identical twins is found not to be concordant for a phenotypic trait. Does this mean that the trait is not genetically determined?

5.2 A couple have a son affected with a multifactorial trait that occurs more often in females than males. For their next child, is it more likely that a son or daughter would be affected?

5.3 A case–control study shows that a particular SNP allele is associated with a 2.3-fold increased relative risk of disease. What does this imply about the relationship of the SNP to the disease?

5.4 Why is transmission disequilbrium testing not vulnerable to the effects of population stratification by ethnicity?

5.5 How will the haplotype map facilitate whole genome analysis for association of SNPs with common disorders?

FURTHER READING

General References

Newton-Cheh C, Hirschhorn JN. Genetic association studies of complex traits: design and analysis issues. Mutat Res 2005;573:54–69.

Cardon LR, Abecasis GR. Using haplotype blocks to map human complex trait loci. Trends Genet 2003;19:135–140.

Glazier AM, Nadeau JH, Aitman TJ. Finding genes that underlie complex traits. Science 2002;298:2345–2349.

Clinical Snapshot 5.1 Alzheimer Disease

St George-Hyslop PH, Petit A. Molecular biology and genetics of Alzheimer's disease. C R Biol 2005;328:119–130.

Clinical Snapshot 5.2 Diabetes

Barroso I. Genetics of type 2 diabetes. Diabet Med 2005;22:517–535.

Rewers M, Norris J, Dabelea D. Epidemiology of type 1 Diabetes Mellitus. Adv Exp Med Biol 2004;552:219–246.

Ethics 5.1 Predictive Testing

Evans JP, Skrzynia C, Burke W. The complexities of predictive genetic testing. Brit Med J 2001;522:1052–1056.

Hot Topics 5.1 Large Cohort Studies

Collins FS. The case for a US prospective cohort study of genes and environment. Nature 2004;429:475–477.

Cambon-Thomsen A. The social and ethical issues of post-genomic human biobanks. Nat Rev Genet 2004;5:866–873.

6

Cell Division and Chromosomes

INTRODUCTION

If each of the 25,000 or so genes were independently replicated and assorted to daughter cells the process of cell replication would be hopelessly chaotic. In fact the process is highly organized, with the genome packaged into 23 pairs of chromosomes which are replicated, line up in the cell, and split into strands that segregate to the daughter cells. In this chapter we will focus on this process from multiple points of view. First, we will explore the processes of mitosis and meiosis and see how the cell cycle is regulated so that DNA replication and cell division are co-ordinated. Second, we will look at the structure of chromosomes and how the genome is packaged. Finally, we will look at the techniques used to study chromosomes and at the major types of chromosomal abnormalities.

KEY POINTS

- The cell cycle is a highly regulated process that consists of four phases: G1, G2, S, and M.
- Somatic cell division is the process of mitosis, where an equal copy of the nuclear genome is distributed to each daughter cell. Germ cells are formed by the process of meiosis, which reduces chromosome number to the haploid state and also provides an opportunity for genetic recombination.
- Mitotic chromosomes are highly condensed structures, which include recognizable landmarks.
- Analysis of chromosomes can be performed by collecting dividing cells in culture, swelling the cells in hypotonic saline, fixing the chromosomes onto slides, and staining them with a variety of special stains.
- The technique of fluorescence in situ hybridization (FISH) can be used to detect small deletions or identify chromosomes involved in complex rearrangements.
- Abnormalities of chromosome number or structure underlie human developmental disorders or cancer.
- The presence of one or more extra complete chromosome sets is referred to as polyploidy, and usually is lethal.
- Aneuploidy is the presence of a nonintegral number of the haploid set. A number of trisomy syndromes have been characterized.
- Structural abnormalities include deletions, duplications, inversions, rings, and translocations.
- Individuals who are balanced translocation or inversion carriers are at risk of having offspring with chromosomal imbalance.
- Microdeletion syndromes consist of deletion of multiple, contiguous genes, and are best detected using FISH or comparative genomic hybridization.
- Uniparental disomy or deletion can underlie specific syndromes associated with deficiency in imprinted genes.

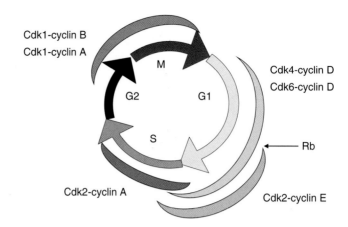

Figure 6.1 • Proteins, referred to as "cyclins" bind with specific cyclin-dependent kinases (CDKs), which phosphorylate specific proteins to initiate the events of G1, S, G2, and M.

CELL DIVISION

The process of cell division is fundamental to the growth and propagation of all living organisms. In eukaryotic cells the basic process is called **mitosis**. Mitosis consists of the replication and separation of chromosomes as well as distribution of cytoplasmic contents to two daughter cells. Germ cells undergo a specialized form of cell division called **meiosis**. Meiosis results in production of haploid gametes and also provides the opportunity for genetic recombination.

The Cell Cycle

What are the major events in the cell cycle?

Rapidly dividing cells have a relatively constant interval between successive rounds of cell division. This interval is marked by sets of events that have come to be known as the cell cycle (Figure 6.1). Following the end of mitosis, the cell enters **G1** (gap 1), which is a time when housekeeping genes and other genes are transcribed and translated. Next is **S** phase, when DNA replication occurs. Following S is **G2** (gap 2), an interval during which the cell prepares for **M** phase, mitosis. The timing of the events in the cell cycle is highly regulated by a set of proteins that include **kinases**, which activate other proteins by phosphorylation, and **cyclins**. Specific cyclin proteins are expressed or activated at specific points in the cell cycle to help move the cell to the next point. S phase requires several hours. Some regions of the genome, usually containing genes that are actively transcribed, replicate early, whereas others, particularly including inactive genes, are replicated late. S phase is also a time when the DNA repair system is invoked to repair damaged DNA. A set of proteins, referred to as **checkpoint proteins**, cause the cell to pause, assess the extent of DNA damage, and then either repair the damage or undergo **apoptosis**, programmed cell death. A major protein involved in this process is **p53**, initially discovered as the product of a gene, *TP53 (MIM 191170),* involved in many types of cancer. In fact, many other checkpoint proteins are involved in the etiology of cancer, a point that will be revisited later in this book. If the cell fails to attempt DNA repair, or proceeds through the cell cycle despite having accumulated mutations, the cell risks loss of growth control due to mutation of genes critical for the process, and may take a step towards malignancy.

Mitosis and Meiosis

What occurs during mitosis and meiosis?

The process of mitosis consists of four phases, **prophase**, **metaphase**, **anaphase**, and **telophase** (Figure 6.2). DNA replication has already occurred during S phase, so at the start of mitosis the chromosomes consist of two DNA strands, **chromatids**, joined together at the primary constriction, or **centromere** (Figure 6.3). During prophase, the chromosomes begin to condense and the nuclear membrane breaks down. The chromosomes are maximally compacted in metaphase, at which point they are lined up at the center of the cell and spindle fibers extend from **centrioles** at the two poles of the mitotic figure, connecting to the centromeres. The two chromatids separate at anaphase and move towards the poles. Mitosis is completed at **telophase** with the formation of two new nuclear membranes, and daughter cells separate by a process of **cytokinesis**.

Meiosis begins in oocytes during fetal life, whereas in males it begins for a particular spermatogonial cell sometime after puberty. Meiosis is preceded by a round of DNA replication, so

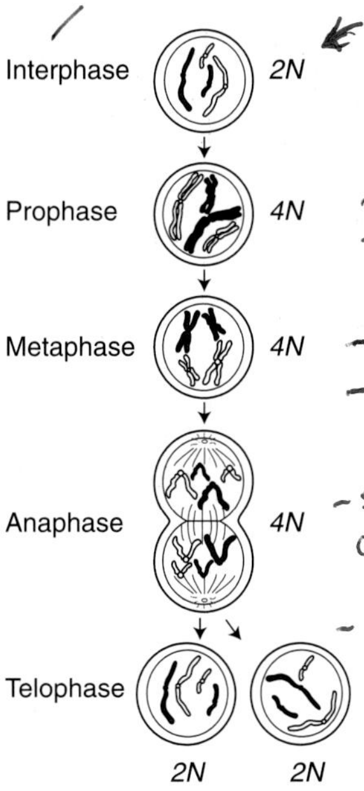

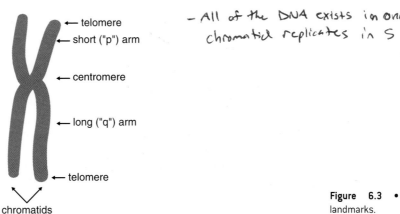

Handwritten annotations:

G1–S–G2 DNA is dispersed

DNA content

Interphase — 2N

Prophase — 4N
- Chromosomes condense (become visible @ the microscope)
- centrioles form & migrate to ends of cell

Metaphase — 4N
- chromosomes most compact & line up at equatorial plane of cell

Anaphase — 4N
- spindle fibers contract, chromosomes migrate to opposite cells
- cytokinesis

Telophase — 2N   2N

Figure 6.2 • The process of mitosis. The replicated chromosomes condense during prophase, at which time the nuclear membrane breaks down. Chromosomes line up on the spindle at metaphase and chromatids separate to the two daughter cells at anaphase. Chromosome content is indicated as diploid (2N) or tetraploid (4N) adjacent to each figure.

Handwritten: — All of the DNA exists in one chromatid, chromatid replicates in S phase

← telomere
← short ("p") arm
← centromere
← long ("q") arm
← telomere
chromatids

Figure 6.3 • Major chromosome landmarks.

at the outset there are 46 chromosomes, each of which has replicated to consist of two chromatids, just as for mitosis. There are two major rounds of cell division that occur during the process of meiosis (Figure 6.4). In the first, homologous chromosomes pair intimately and may undergo genetic recombination. The pairing is precise and involves formation of a protein structure called the **synaptonemal** complex. Recombination events always involve exchange between two DNA strands and result in a reshuffling of alleles on the recombined chromosomes (see Figure 4.7). In females, chromosome pairing begins during fetal life and continues until a particular oocyte is readied for ovulation, which is years to decades later. In males, the entire process of meiosis takes place over a period of several days. In either case, the first meiotic division is completed as the homologous chromosomes separate to either pole and two daughter cells result. In oogenesis, one of the daughter cells will become the egg, whereas the other is a smaller cell referred to as the first polar body. In either case, though, the daughter cells now contain a single copy of each chromosome, although the chromosomes each consist of two chromatids. The cells then undergo a second round of division resembling mitosis but without a preceding round of DNA replication. This produces four spermatogonia, or an egg cell and a second polar body, each with a haploid chromosome set. Meiosis thereby fulfills two crucial roles. First, it reduces the chromosome set to the haploid number, so that upon fertilization a diploid number is restored. Second, it allows for genetic recombination.

The various steps of both mitosis and meiosis are, like the cell cycle, highly regulated processes. A set of cyclins and cyclin-dependent kinases with specific activity during cell division are involved in directing the alignment of chromosomes on the spindle and the separation of sister chromatids. Spindle fibers consist of microtubules that interact with a structure at

Meiosis 1

Chiasma— pts of overlap in homologous
chromosomes during crossing over
& recombination

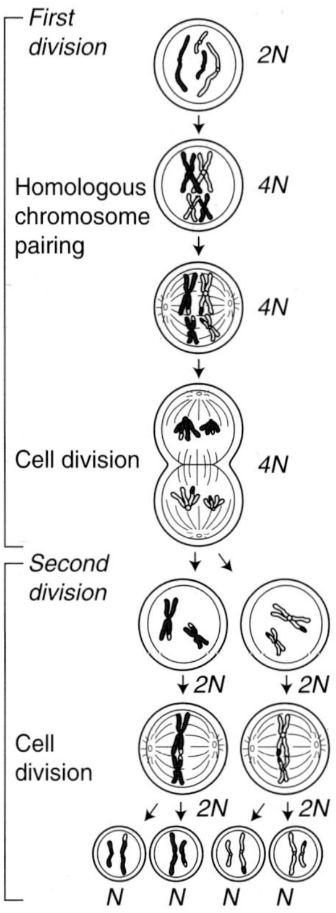

First
division   2N

Homologous   4N
chromosome
pairing

                                            4N

Cell division   4N

Second
division

                                        ↓2N   ↓2N

Cell
division

                                    ↙ ↓2N   ↙ ↓2N

                                    N   N   N   N

Figure 6.4 • Process of meiosis. Homologous chromosomes pair during the first meiotic prophase and separate in the first division. Chromatids then separate during the second meiotic division to form four haploid germ cells.

the centromere called the **kinetochore**. Proteins interact with the microtubules to function as "motors," propelling the sister chromatids (or chromosomes, in the case of meiosis) towards the spindle pole.

CHROMOSOMES

The human **karyotype** consists of 22 pairs of nonsex chromosomes (**autosomes**) and two **sex chromosomes**, XX for females and XY for males. Each chromosome consists of a single continuous DNA strand, including from a few hundred to several thousand genes. Study of both normal and abnormal chromosome structure has provided crucial tools for analysis of human developmental disorders and cancer.

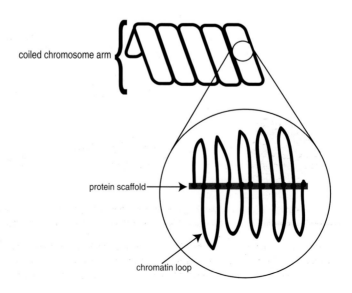

coiled chromosome arm

protein scaffold

chromatin loop

Figure 6.5 • Chromatin loops are bound to a protein scaffold to form the highly condensed mitotic chromosome.

Chromosome Structure and Analysis

Chromosomes undergo a cycle of condensation and decondensation through the cell cycle. Chromosomes are maximally decompacted during interphase, and achieve maximal compaction during the metaphase stage of mitosis, just prior to the separation of sister chromosomes to the two daughter cells. We discussed the structure of chromatin in Chapter 1. The metaphase chromosome consists of loops of chromatin bound to a protein scaffold (Figure 6.5). The overall condensation is about 10,000- to 20,000-fold relative to the "naked" DNA double helix.

Chromosomes are best visualized at or near maximum condensation in dividing cells. Chromosomal analysis is routinely performed in medical diagnostic laboratories, where it is used to detect abnormalities of chromosome number or structure. Analysis is done on rapidly dividing cells, such as bone marrow or cancer cells, or on cells grown in culture (Methods 6.1).

A number of special staining techniques are used to reveal fine structural features of chromosomes. The fluorescent dye **quinacrine** elicits a pattern of bright and dark bands that aid in chromosome identification (Figure 6.7). The same bands are also elicited by pretreatment of chromosomes (usually with the enzyme trypsin) and Giemsa staining (Figure 6.8), which obviates the need for fluorescence microscopy.

What are the major structural features of chromosomes?

Methods 6.1

Chromosomal analysis

The major source of cells used for clinical cytogenetics is peripheral blood T lymphocytes, which are stimulated to divide in culture by the lectin **phytohemagglutinin**. Cells are collected at metaphase by treatment with a spindle inhibitor such as colchicine. They are then swollen with hypotonic saline to facilitate cell membrane disruption and spread the chromosomes, fixed onto microscope slides, and stained (Figure 6.6). It was the discovery of hypotonic treatment in 1956 that ushered in the era of clinical cyto-

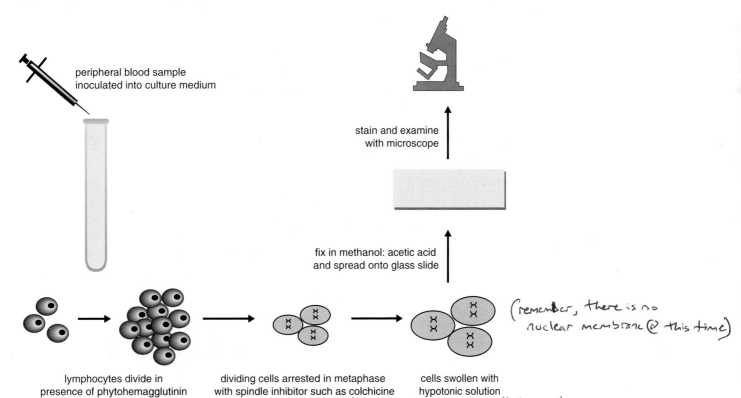

peripheral blood sample
inoculated into culture medium

stain and examine
with microscope

fix in methanol: acetic acid
and spread onto glass slide

lymphocytes divide in
presence of phytohemagglutinin

dividing cells arrested in metaphase
with spindle inhibitor such as colchicine

cells swollen with
hypotonic solution

(remember, there is no nuclear membrane @ this time)

↳ w/o spindles, chromatids are not pulled apart

Figure 6.6 • Process of analysis of mitotic chromosomes from peripheral blood. Whole blood is inoculated into a culture containing the lectin phytohemagglutinin, which stimulates the division of T cells. After 3 days in culture, the cells are swollen in hypotonic saline, fixed onto glass slides, stained, and examined through the microscope.

genetics. Prior to that, chromosomes appeared clumped within the nucleus and could not easily be distinguished from one another. The normal human chromosome number at that time was thought to be 48. Soon after the introduction of hypotonic treatment the correct number of 46 was determined. The use of peripheral blood cultures greatly simplified the collection of dividing cells for analysis. In 1959, the first human chromosome abnormality, trisomy 21, responsible for Down syndrome, was described.

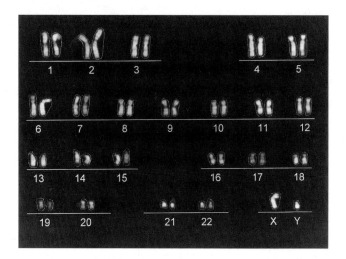

Figure 6.7 • Q-banded human chromosomes, arranged into a karyotype.

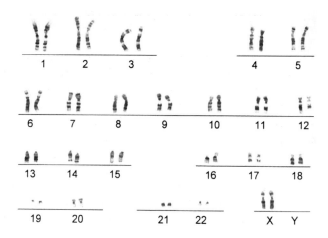

Figure 6.8 • G-banded human chromosomes, obtained with trypsin treatment followed by Giemsa staining.

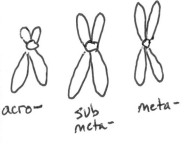

Chromosomes are classified according to size and position of the centromere into a standard array referred to as the karyotype. The centromere divides most chromosomes into long arms (designed "**q**") and short arms (designated "**p**," for petit). Chromosomes are classified as **metacentric** (centromere in the center), **submetacentric** (centromere displaced to one end), or **acrocentric** (centromere near one end of the chromosome) (Methods 6.2). The acrocentric chromosomes are 13, 14, 15, 21, and 22. The short arms of these chromosomes consist of DNA that encodes ribosomal RNA. These regions often remain decondensed, forming stalks, with small knobs at the end referred to as **satellites**.

Methods 6.2

Standard cytogenetic nomenclature

Cytogeneticists use a standardized nomenclature to describe normal and abnormal chromosomes. The nomenclature includes the chromosome number, sex chromosome constitution, extra or missing chromosomes, and chromosome rearrangements. Bands are numbered according to landmarks starting from the centromere up the short arm or down the long arm. Chromosomal rearrangements are described by noting the rearrangement and indicating the breakpoint or breakpoints. For example, a female with a deletion of the short arm of chromosome 4 with breakpoint at band p15 has the karyotype 46,XX,del(4)(p15). An abnormal chromosome generated by multiple aberrations in a single chromosome or rearrangement involving two or more chromosomes is defined as a *derivative chromosome*. An abnormal chromosome that cannot be identified is defined as a *marker chromosome*.

I.   Normal karyotype

Male: 46,XY

Female: 46,XX

II. Aneuploidy

Female with Down syndrome: 47,XX,+21

Male with trisomy 18: 47,XY,+18

Turner syndrome: 45,X

Klinefelter syndrome: 47,XXY

III. Rearrangements

Deletion: 46,XX,del(4)(p15)

Inversion: 46,XY,inv(2)(p12q12) – inversion of chromosome 2 with breakpoints at p12 and q12

Ring: 46,XY,r(13) – male with ring chromosome 13

Translocation: 46,XX,t(3;9)(p14;q21) – balanced translocation between chromosomes 3 and 9, with breakpoints at band p14 on chromosome 3 and q21 on chromosome 9. In addition to the two chromosomes involved in the translocation, there is a normal chromosome 3 and a normal chromosome 9.

Derivative chromosome: 46,XY,der(3)t(3;9)(p14;q21) – one copy of chromosome 3 is replaced by the translocation between 3 and 9, but the two chromosomes 9 are normal. This would occur due to segregation at meiosis from a balanced t(3;9) to give unbalanced products.

The centromeres are surrounded by blocks of highly repeated DNA sequences (Figure 6.9). A major component is referred to as **α satellite DNA**, which consists of thousands of copies of a 171-bp repeat. (Do not confuse this use of the term "satellite" with the acrocentric chromosome satellites described above. Satellite DNA is so-called because it consists of a highly repeated sequence that separates from the main mass of DNA by density gradient centrifugation to form a distinct band, referred to as a "satellite.") This region remains highly compacted throughout the cell cycle. The telomeres consist of 10 to 15 kb of a repeat unit GGGTTA, with repeated sequences extending for 100 to 300 kb inside of this region. **Interspersed repeated sequences** account for the banding patterns obtained with quinacrine or trypsin–Giemsa staining. Interspersed repeated sequences are short DNA segments that are scattered throughout the genome. As described in Chapter 4, two major types are called SINEs and LINEs. SINE

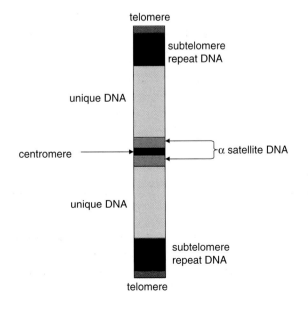

Figure 6.9 • Diagram of the major types of repeated DNA on a chromosome. Satellite DNA flanks the centromeric region. Subtelomere repeated DNA occurs just proximal to the two telomeres. Not drawn to scale.

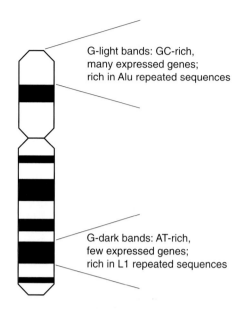

G-light bands: GC-rich,
many expressed genes;
rich in Alu repeated sequences

G-dark bands: AT-rich,
few expressed genes;
rich in L1 repeated sequences

Figure 6.10 • G-light bands are GC-rich and contain SINEs such as Alu-repeats. G-dark bands are AT-rich and contain LINE sequences, such as L1.

sequences are GC-rich and tend to be found in gene-rich areas, whereas LINEs are AT-rich and are found in gene-poor regions (Figure 6.10). Quinacrine fluorescence is enhanced by AT bases and quenched by GC, accounting for the Q-bands. G-banding reflects differences in protein binding and condensation, which is greater in AT-rich, gene-poor regions.

Chromosome banding patterns have been of critical importance in permitting fine structural analysis of chromosomal abnormalities that are responsible for congenital anomalies or malignancy. More recently, the technique of **fluorescence *in situ* hybridization (FISH)** has been used to identify particular DNA sequences on the chromosomes (Methods 6.3).

CHROMOSOME ABNORMALITIES

The ability to examine human chromosomes in readily accessible tissues, such as peripheral blood, led to the discovery of innumerable examples of abnormalities of chromosome number or structure. These abnormalities tend to occur in two settings: individuals with congenital anomalies and in somatic cells obtained from malignant tissue. We will explore cancer cytogenetics in detail in Chapter 8; here we will take a closer look at chromosomal abnormalities and their developmental consequences. Three main types of chromosomal abnormalities will be considered: **polyploidy**, **aneuploidy**, and **chromosomal rearrangements**, as well as the cytogenetic consequences of imprinting disorders.

Polyploidy

What are the clinical consequences of polyploidy?

The normal diploid number of chromosomes arises by fertilization of a haploid egg by a haploid sperm. Polyploidy represents the occurrence of one or more entire extra sets of chromosomes. **Triploidy** is the presence of 69 chromosomes, three haploid sets; **tetraploidy** is 92 chromosomes, four sets. Polyploidy is generally not compatible with survival. Most polyploid embryos spontaneously miscarry. Rare triploid fetuses survive to livebirth, though the condition is associated with severe congenital anomalies and virtually all of the infants die. Triploidy results from aberrant fertilization events, including fertilization by two sperm (**dispermy**), or fusion of a polar body with the egg cell, producing a diploid ovum that results in triploidy upon fertilization.

Aneuploidy

What happens when there is one chromosome too many or too few?

The term **aneuploidy** refers to the presence of a nonintegral multiple of the haploid number of chromosomes, usually one chromosome more or less than the diploid number due to **trisomy** (an extra chromosome) or **monosomy** (a single copy of a particular chromosome).

The first human chromosomal abnormality to be recognized was **trisomy 21**, which results in **Down syndrome**. Down syndrome is a well-recognized clinical disorder characterized by a

Methods 6.3

Fluorescence *in situ* hybridization (FISH)

The principle of FISH is illustrated in Figure 6.11. DNA on the microscope slide is separated into single strands, but the strands remain in position on the fixed chromosomes. A purified DNA sequence is labeled with a fluorescent dye and also separated into single strands. A solution of this labeled "probe" DNA is then placed on the slide. Wherever the probe DNA finds homologous chromosomal DNA a stable double helix will form. The sites of binding of probe DNA to the fixed chromosomes can be visualized by fluorescence microscopy.

FISH enables detection of the deletion of small chromosome regions (Figure 6.12). This is usually accomplished using FISH probes corresponding to specific DNA segments that are located in a

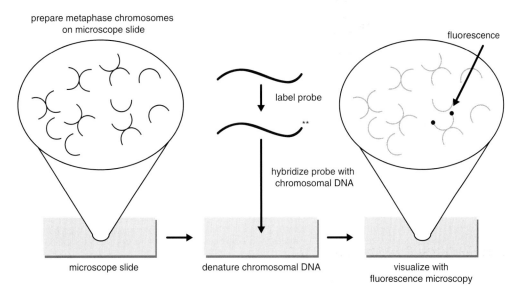

prepare metaphase chromosomes
on microscope slide

fluorescence

label probe

hybridize probe with
chromosomal DNA

microscope slide   denature chromosomal DNA   visualize with
fluorescence microscopy

Figure 6.11 • Fluorescence in situ hybridization. Metaphase chromosomes are fixed onto slides and DNA is separated into single strands. A single-stranded, fluorescently-labeled DNA "probe" binds to homologous DNA on the slide, and sites of binding visualized by fluorescence microscopy.

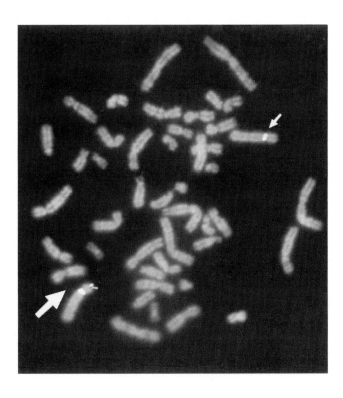

Figure 6.12 • Deletion of subtelomeric sequences from one copy of chromosome 4. Both copies are labeled at the centromere with a probe specific to chromosome 4. The normal chromosome (lower left, large arrow) has labeling of the subtelomeric region, whereas the deleted chromosome (upper right, small arrow) has no subtelomeric labeling due to a deletion.

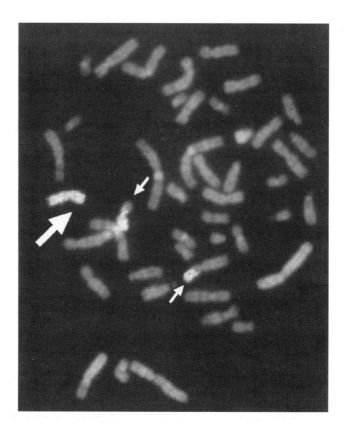

Figure 6.13 • Chromosome painting reveals a balanced translocation. The normal homolog is indicated by the large arrow at the left. The two small arrows show two parts of a reciprocal translocation.

chromosome region of interest. In addition, FISH can be used to paint individual chromosomes (Figure 6.13). This requires the use of "cocktails" of multiple FISH probes that are uniquely located on a specific chromosome. Chromosome painting is useful in identification of the origin of genetic material that contributes to rearranged chromosomes. It is now possible to use cocktails of chromosome-specific FISH probes to paint each chromosome a distinct color, an aid in the study of complex chromosomal rearrangements. We will see later how molecular approaches are now also being turned towards the detailed analysis of chromosomal abnormalities.

fairly stereotyped set of phenotypic features (Clinical Snapshot 6.1). It was relatively easy to recognize trisomy in the early days of cytogenetic testing, since it requires only a count of chromosomes, not an analysis of fine structure for subtle changes.

The recognition of trisomy 21 in 1959 stimulated a flurry of studies of other syndromes that, like Down syndrome, produced fairly consistent clinical features yet usually occur sporadically. Two other autosomal trisomy syndromes were quickly identified: Patau syndrome due to trisomy 13 and Edwards syndrome due to trisomy 18 (Table 6.1). None of the other autosomal trisomies are compatible with live birth, and no autosomal monosomy is. Chromosomal studies of early spontaneous abortions have revealed a high frequency of aneuploidy, usually trisomy, involving any of the chromosomes. Sex chromosome aneuploidy is more readily tolerated. X chromosome monosomy, designated 45,X, produces the phenotype of Turner syndrome (Clinical Snapshot 6.2). Monosomy for the Y is lethal. Having additional X or Y chromosomes is compatible with survival, though specific phenotypes result.

TABLE 6.1 Major chromosome aneuploidy syndromes compatible with live birth

Syndrome	Chromosomal abnormality	Major features
Patau syndrome	Trisomy 13	Cleft lip and palate, severe central nervous system anomaly, polydactyly
Edwards syndrome	Trisomy 18	Low birth weight, central nervous system anomalies, heart defects
Down syndrome	Trisomy 21	Hypotonia, characteristic facial features, developmental delay
Turner syndrome	Monosomy X	Short stature, amenorrhea, lack of secondary sexual development
Klinefelter syndrome	XXY	Small testes, infertility, tall stature, learning problems
Triple-X	XXX	Learning disabilities, no major physical anomalies
XYY	XYY	Learning and behavioral problems in some individuals

CLINICAL SNAPSHOT 6.1

■ Down syndrome

Ian was born after a full term, uncomplicated pregnancy. Both his parents were 30 years old. No prenatal genetic studies were done. He was noted by the obstetrician to have features of Down syndrome at birth. His neonatal course was at first uneventful, but at 48 hours of life he was found to have a congenital heart defect consisting of a common AV canal (communication between the two atria and two ventricles). This was repaired surgically within the first year of life. He has otherwise done well, although he gets frequent colds. Now, at 4 years of age, he is a happy and mostly healthy child, speaking in sentences, and getting along well with his older sister.

Children with Down syndrome are usually recognized at birth to have distinctive facial appearance (Figure 6.14) with downslanted palpebral fissures, epicanthal folds (extra skin fold at inner canthus of eye), flat nasal bridge, as well as a flat occiput, and other features such as a single transverse palmar crease, incurved fifth finger (clinodactyly), short fingers and toes, and increased space between the first and second toes. Affected children usually have muscular hypotonia, and delayed motor and cognitive development. There are often anomalies of organ system development, such as congenital heart defects and gastrointestinal defects such as duodenal atresia. Aside from developmental delay, affected individuals have frequent upper respiratory infections, an increased risk of leukemia, and develop changes similar to Alzheimer disease at a relatively young age. Although there are individual differences for any of these features, the general similarity of the constellation of signs and symptoms led to the recognition of a common underlying cause, trisomy 21 (Figure 6.15).

Continued on p. 108

CLINICAL SNAPSHOT 6.1 continued

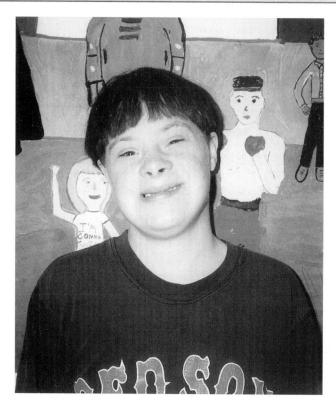

Figure 6.14 • Child with Down syndrome.

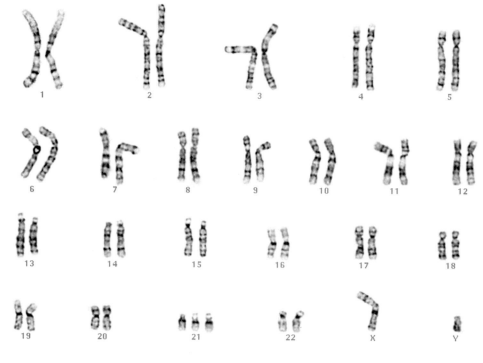

Down Syndrome   47,XY,+21

Figure 6.15 • Karyotype showing trisomy 21. (Courtesy of Dr. Andrew Carroll, University of Alabama at Birmingham.)

CLINICAL SNAPSHOT 6.2

◼ Turner syndrome

Vanessa is a 15-year-old who is referred for evaluation of delayed puberty. She has been healthy, but is increasingly frustrated that she has not begun any of the signs of puberty, including breast enlargement or menstruation. This is a significant social problem, as her friends at school are changing whereas she is not. Examination reveals that she is 4 feet 11 inches tall, which is short for members of her family. She has a webbed neck and prepubertal pattern of sexual maturation. A chromosomal analysis is sent, and she is found to have a 45,X karyotype consistent with Turner syndrome.

Turner syndrome is the chromosomal monosomy syndrome compatible with live birth. Most conceptuses with the 45,X karyotype miscarry, but some make it to term and can survive for a long period thereafter. Individuals with Turner syndrome have a female phenotype. At birth they may have swollen hands and feet due to an inadequately developed lymphatic system. *In utero* they can have massive edema, especially around the base of the neck. This stretches the skin in this region and is responsible for the webbed neck seen later in life. There may be internal malformations, especially coarctation of the aorta and renal anomalies such as horseshoe kidney. Intelligence is usually normal, but cognitive problems, including learning disabilities and difficulties with visuospatial perception, are common. Affected girls tend to be short and do not develop female secondary sex characteristics. Their ovaries degenerate into fibrous streaks and produce neither estrogen nor oocytes.

The principal karyotypic finding in Turner syndrome is a single X chromosome. Some affected girls have two Xs, including one normal and one rearranged X chromosome. The rearrangement often is a deletion, usually of the short arm, or may be an isochromosome (Figure 6.16), usually for the long arms. Some are mosaics, with one cell line having 46 chromosomes with a rearranged X and the other 45 chromosomes without the rearranged X.

Turner syndrome is only one of several sex chromosome abnormalities. Females with three or more X chromosomes tend to have developmental delay as the principal phenotype. The presence of a Y chromosome confers a male phenotype. Individuals who are mosaic for a rearranged Y and a 45,X cell line may have a testes on one side and a streak gonad on the other, referred to as "mixed gonadal dysgenesis." Males with two or more X chromosomes plus a Y have Klinefelter syndrome. This consists of atrophic testes with azoospermia, some degree of female secondary sex characteristics, and learning problems.

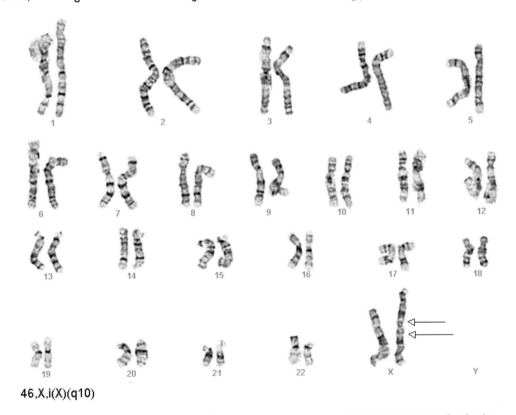

46,X,i(X)(q10)

Figure 6.16 • Karyotype from a woman with Turner syndrome showing one normal X chromosome and an isochromosome for the long arm of the X (arrows). (Courtesy of Dr. Andrew Carroll, University of Alabama at Birmingham.)

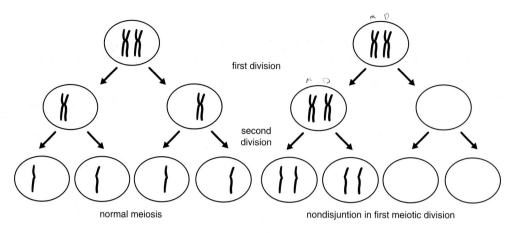

Figure 6.17 • Normal meiosis (left), and first division meiotic nondisjunction (right).

MOst common
mutational mechanism
in man

Aneuploidy results from an error in meiosis or mitosis called **nondisjunction** (Figure 6.17). Meiotic nondisjunction during the first division results in both homologous chromosomes going to the same gamete. If the nondisjunction occurs in the second meiotic division, two identical chromatids go to the same gamete. Mitotic nondisjunction must occur during somatic cell division and therefore results in mosaicism, assuming that it occurs after the first cleavage. The coexistence of a chromosomally normal cell line with an aneuploid line can ameliorate the developmental effects of trisomy. This permits survival of some fetuses with mosaic trisomy for chromosomes that would not be compatible with survival if all cells were affected. The relative proportion of trisomic and nontrisomic cells depends, in part, on when in the course of cell division the nondisjunction occurred, but also in part on the relative rate of growth and survival of the two cell lines.

Nondisjunction appears to occur most commonly in the first meiotic division in females. Hence, the vast majority of individuals with trisomy 21 have two maternal chromosomes 21 and one paternal, and the two maternal chromosomes are not identical in terms of specific alleles. Causes of nondisjunction are, for the most part, unknown. The only significant risk factor so far recognized is advanced maternal age. Risk of having a child with aneuploidy rises sharply with maternal age after about 35 years (Figure 6.18). Genetic factors may also play a role, since there are rare families with apparent clustering of instances of aneuploidy. Couples at increased risk of having a child with trisomy are now offered prenatal testing (Ethical Implications 6.1). We will explore the application of prenatal diagnosis later in this book.

The mechanisms whereby aneuploidy produces phenotypic effects are under active investigation. Increased levels of transcription have been demonstrated for chromosome 21 genes

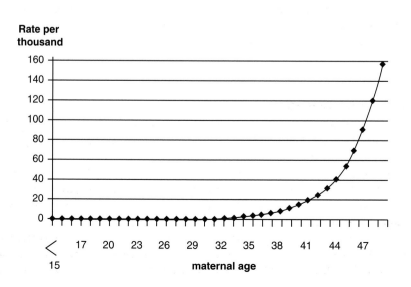

Figure 6.18 • Increase in the risk of nondisjunction resulting in trisomy 21 with advanced maternal age.

> ## ETHICAL IMPLICATIONS 6.1 • Nondirective counseling
>
> Should a couple who are at risk of having a child with a chromosomal abnormality undergo prenatal diagnosis? If they do, and a chromosomal abnormality is found, should they continue the pregnancy? These are difficult questions, and the answers are individual matters for the couple to decide. How they approach the questions depends on many factors. Have they already had a child with a chromosomal abnormality? If so, they might feel that they cannot handle the challenge of having another. But they also might experience guilt if they terminate the pregnancy, feeling that it is a refutation of the value of their previous affected child. Do they have any experience with the care of a child with a chromosomal abnormality? Do they understand the challenges – physical, emotional, and financial – of raising a child with special needs, and are they prepared? What are their personal and religious views about abortion? What about other members of their family? Moreover, there are reasons to undergo prenatal testing other than consideration of possible termination of an affected pregnancy. Some couples embark on testing in the hope of being reassured that the fetus is not affected and only begin to face the implications of an abnormal result after it has occurred. Others might wish to be tested to prepare for the care of an affected child and would not consider termination of pregnancy.
>
> The tradition in prenatal genetic counseling is to provide information and support in a nondirective manner. This means that the counselor does not advise the couple to take a specific course of action, i.e., to have prenatal testing or not, or to continue an affected pregnancy or not. Genetic counselors are trained to present all options in a neutral manner, and to support the couple whatever decision they make. The counselor tries to avoid letting his or her personal views influence the decision.
>
> Is it possible to give truly nondirective counseling? Although a counselor might try to provide information in a neutral way, subtle matters of emphasis or body language might communicate bias towards a particular course of action. Genetic counselors endeavor to recognize and minimize the impact of such bias. Nondirective counseling is not the norm in other areas of medical care. Patients usually expect a health professional to provide advice on the best course of action, for example choice of medication. As we will see later, nondirective counseling may be difficult in other areas of genetics, such as when presenting care options for a treatable disorder.

in cells from individuals with Down syndrome. It is likely that some genes will be more vulnerable to disruption of function by dosage effects than others. There are more than 200 genes on chromosome 21, so it should not be a surprise that a complex phenotype results from trisomy 21. What may be more surprising is that the phenotype is as reproducible as it is with this large degree of genetic imbalance. Recently, there has been progress in understanding the pathogenesis of the increased risk of leukemia in children with Down syndrome. The leukemias most often arise from the megakaryocyte lineage, and are associated with a mutation in the gene encoding the transcription factor *GATA1*. It is unclear why clones of cells with this mutation occur more commonly in children with Down syndrome, but one possibility is that interaction with another gene encoded on chromosome 21 confers a selective advantage on cells that acquire *GATA1* mutation. Further exploration of this mechanism, and of others involved in additional aspects of the phenotype, may be important for the prediction of individuals at risk of specific complications of trisomy, and may lead to approaches to management and even treatment.

Structural Abnormalities

Changes of chromosome structure can involve single chromosomes or an exchange of material between chromosomes (Figure 6.19). A piece of a chromosome may be lost by deletion or may be duplicated. The former results in monosomy for a group of genes, and the latter in trisomy for the genes. Chromosome segments also can be inverted – flipped 180 degrees from their normal orientation. If no material is gained or lost, the changes probably will have no phenotypic impact. Rarely, a gene may be disrupted by the chromosome breakage involved in the inversion, but there are vast regions of genetically inert material between groups of genes, so usually these breaks cause no phenotype. As will be seen below, however, such breaks can lead to unbalanced chromosomes after crossing over in meiosis. Another intrachromosomal rearrangement is formation of a **ring**. This arises from breakage of the two ends and their

What are the phenotypic consequences of structural rearrangements?

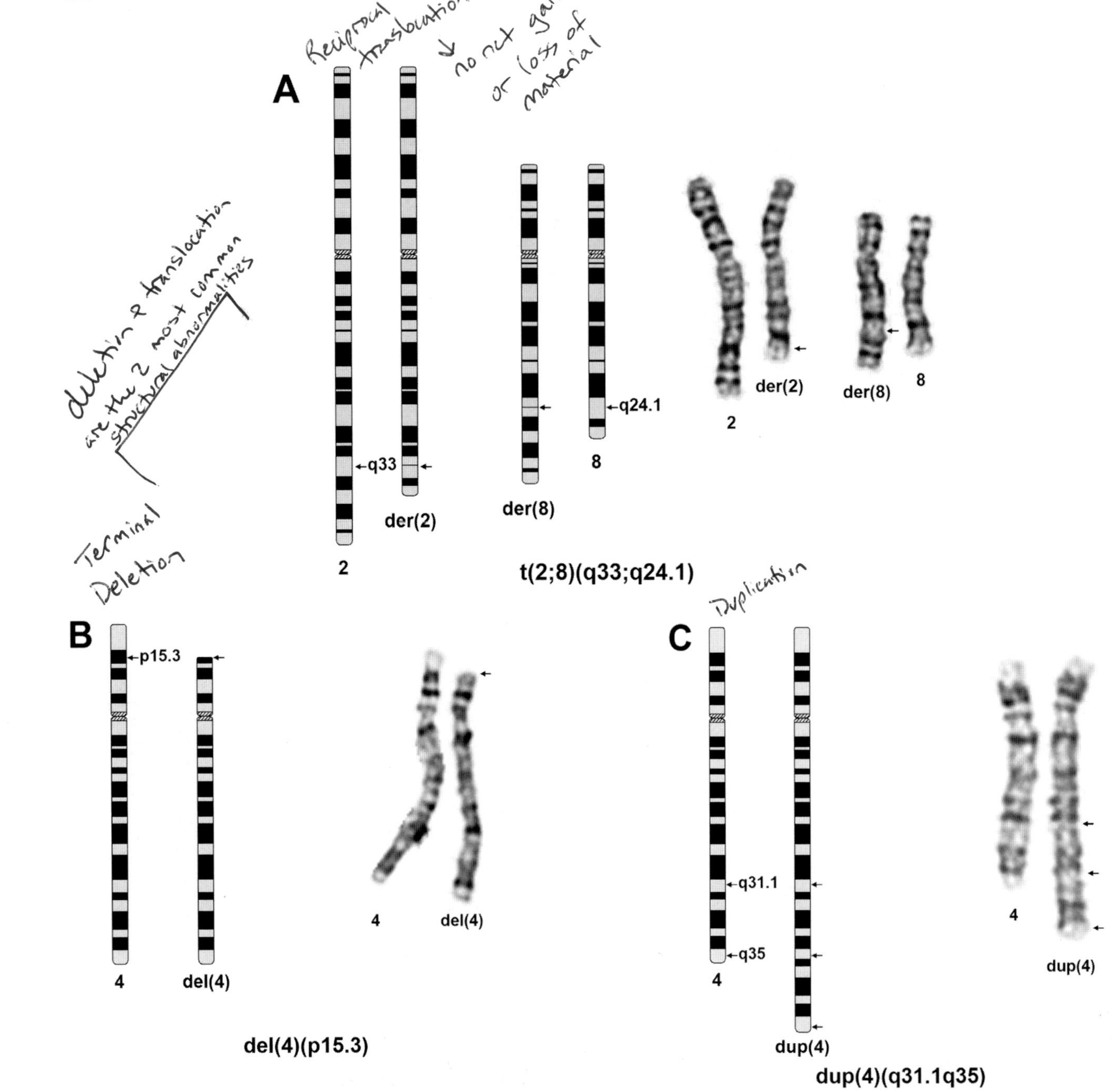

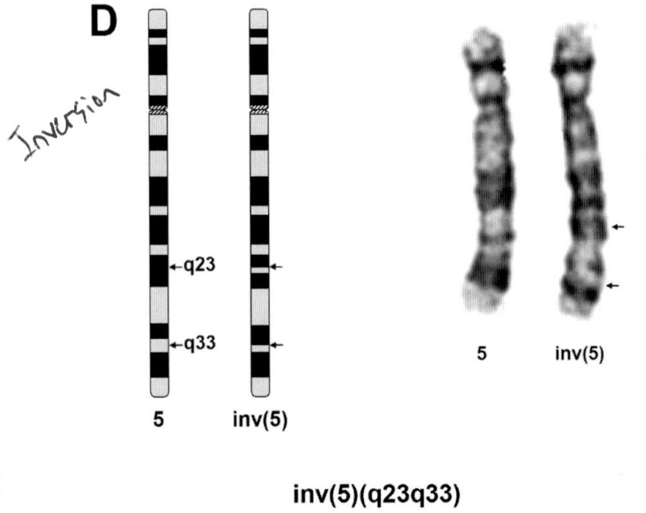

A

Reciprocal translocation

no net gain or loss of material

Deletion & translocation are the 2 most common structural abnormalities

Terminal Deletion

←q33 ←

der(2)

2

←q24.1

8

←

der(8)

der(2)   der(8)   8

2

t(2;8)(q33;q24.1)

B

←p15.3 ←

4   del(4)

del(4)

4   del(4)

del(4)(p15.3)

C

Duplication

←q31.1 ←

←q35 ←

4   dup(4)

4

dup(4)

dup(4)(q31.1q35)

D

Inversion

←q23 ←

←q33 ←

5   inv(5)

5   inv(5)

inv(5)   inv(5)

inv(5)(q23q33)

Figure 6.19 • Major types of chromosomal rearrangements; for each a photograph of the actual chromosomes is shown adjacent to an ideogram of the rearrangement. Break points are indicated by arrows. (a) Balanced reciprocal translocation between chromosomes 2 and 8, resulting in two "derivative" (der) chromosomes; (b) deletion of the tip of the long arm of chromosome 4 breaking at band p15.3; (c) duplication of part of the long arm of chromosome 4 from bands q31.1 to q35; (d) paracentric inversion of chromosome 5 involving the long arm from bands q23 to q33;

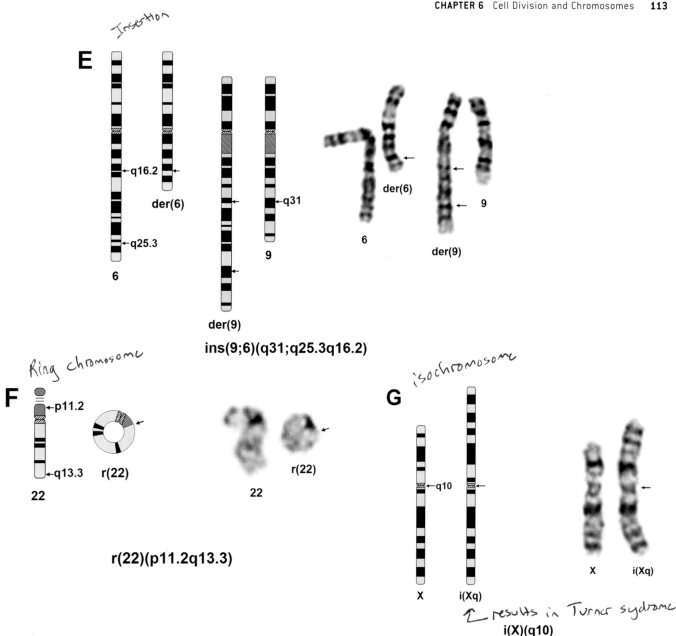

Figure 6.19 • (e) insertion of material from the long arm of chromosome 6 (from bands q16.2 to q25.3) into chromosome 9, producing a derivative chromosome 9 with extra material inserted at band q31; (f) ring chromosome 22 resulting from breaks at p11.2 on the short arm and q13.3 on the long arm, with subsequent fusion of the broken ends; (g) isochromosome for the long arm of the X chromosome, resulting in a chromosome consisting of only the long arm of the X on both sides of the centromere. (Courtesy of Drs. Andrew Carroll and Fady Mikhail, University of Alabama at Birmingham.)

subsequent fusion into a ring structure. There may be phenotypic consequences from deletion of chromatin from the two ends and also from mitotic instability of rings, resulting in trisomic or monosomic cells. **Isochromosomes** represent duplications of either the short or long arms due to misdivision of the centromere.

Translocation involves the exchange of material between chromosomes (Figure 6.20). Usually, translocations arise as apparently reciprocal exchanges. If no material is lost or gained, the translocation is said to be balanced. Balanced translocations – and inversions, for that matter – are occasionally found as variants in the general population. It is estimated that approximately 0.2% of individuals carry an asymptomatic chromosomal rearrangement. If one comes to medical attention it is usually as a consequence of the generation of unbalanced gametes during meiosis, leading to spontaneous abortion or the birth of a child with congenital anomalies. Most, if not all, translocations are reciprocal. Balanced reciprocal translocations can spawn gametes with genetic imbalance due to aberrant segregation during meiosis.

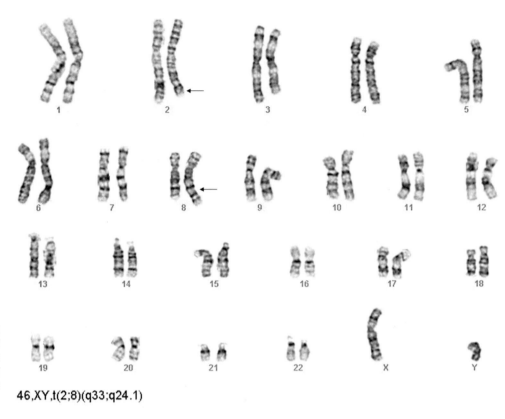

Figure 6.20 • Balanced reciprocal translocation between the long arms of chromosomes 2 and 8. Breakpoints are shown by the arrows. (Courtesy of Dr. Andrew Carroll, University of Alabama at Birmingham.)

46,XY,t(2;8)(q33;q24.1)

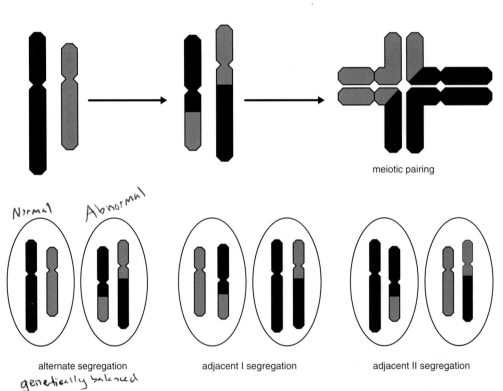

Figure 6.21 • Segregation of balanced reciprocal translocation in meiosis. Alternate segregation results in production of normal or balanced chromosomes. Separation of homologous centromeres (adjacent I) or nonhomologous centromeres (adjacent II) results in production of gametes with unbalanced chromosomes.

Meiotic pairing between chromosomes involved in a balanced translocation requires a complex association of four chromosomes – the two involved in the exchange and the two homologues (Figure 6.21). When first anaphase occurs, these chromosomes can separate in several ways. If the two normal homologues go to one cell and the two involved in the exchange go to another, the resulting gametes will be genetically balanced – either normal or both

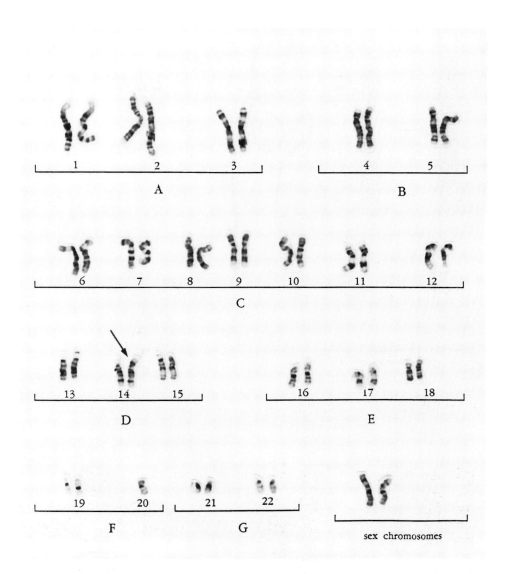

Figure 6.22 • Robertsonian translocation between chromosomes 14 and 21 (arrow) resulting in trisomy 21.

having rearranged chromosomes. Genetic imbalance will result, however, if germ cells get one normal chromosome and one rearranged chromosome. The translocation complex can also segregate so that three chromosomes go to one cell and only one to the other. Rarely, all four chromosomes can go to the same cell. Obviously, major genetic imbalance results in these instances.

Translocations account for a minority of cases of Down syndrome. Translocations between acrocentric chromosomes in which the long arms fuse at the centromeres are referred to as **Robertsonian translocations** (after the geneticist Robertson, who studied similar rearrangements in mice) (Figure 6.22). A Robertsonian translocation carrier has 45 chromosomes but is phenotypically normal. If, however, both the translocated chromosome and a normal 21 go to the same germ cell at meiosis, fertilization will result in trisomy 21. This mechanism accounts for approximately 5% of cases of Down syndrome; the phenotype is indistinguishable from Down syndrome that ensues from classic trisomy. It is important to identify translocation cases, however, because a carrier is at risk of having additional offspring with trisomy. Robertsonian translocations can be present in many members of a family, all of whom are at risk of having children with Down syndrome.

Similar rules apply to other balanced translocations, although the phenotypic consequences of imbalance are less predictable. Unbalanced offspring are trisomic for one chromosome segment and monosomic for another. Innumerable case reports describe such partial trisomies and monosomies.

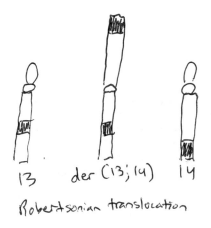

13   der (13; 14)   14

Robertsonian translocation

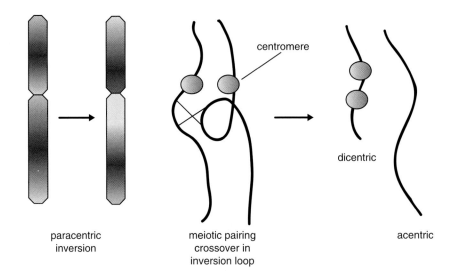

Figure 6.23 • Crossing over within an inversion loop of a paracentric inversion results in production of dicentric and acentric chromosomes. If the inversion is pericentric, deletion and deficiency chromosome products result.

Genetic imbalance can also result from meiotic segregation of inverted chromosomes (Figure 6.23). Pairing between homologues where one chromosome is inverted requires formation of a loop. Crossing over within the loop leads to duplication and deficiency of genetic material. If the inversion does not include the centromere (referred to as **paracentric inversion**), dicentric and acentric chromosomes result. These are usually unstable at mitosis and lead to nonviable phenotypes. Inversions that involve the centromere (called **pericentric inversions**) lead to partial trisomies and monosomies, some of which may be viable. Here, too, balanced rearrangement in a carrier can predispose to unbalanced products in an offspring.

Balanced chromosomal rearrangements usually come to attention through a child who has the rearrangement in an unbalanced form. Sometimes it is discovered when chromosomal analysis is done as part of an evaluation for recurrent miscarriage. Once found, other relatives may be tested to determine whether they also carry the rearrangement. Carriers are provided with genetic counseling, and prenatal diagnosis can be offered.

Chromosome deletion syndromes also affect gene dosage. Deletion of large segments or of entire chromosomes usually is poorly tolerated. Except for 45,X Turner syndrome, there are no other whole-chromosome monosomy syndromes compatible with live birth. Smaller dele-

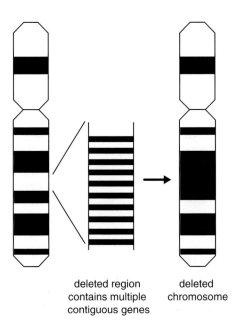

Figure 6.24 • Deletion of multiple contiguous genes results in complex microdeletion syndrome phenotypes.

TABLE 6.2 Some chromosome microdeletion syndromes

Syndrome	Major features	Chromosome region
del (1p)	MR, seizures, growth delay, dysmorphic features	1p36
Williams	Characteristic facies Supravalvar aortic stenosis Developmental impairment	7q11.23
Langer–Giedion	Exostoses, abnormal facies, developmental delay	8q24.1
WAGR	Wilms' tumor, aniridia, genitourinary dysplasia, MR	11p13
Retinoblastoma/MR	Retinoblastoma, MR	13q14
Prader–Willi	Hypotonia, developmental delay, obesity	15q12
Angelman	Seizures, abnormal movements, MR	15q12
α-thalassemia/MR	α-thalassemia, MR	16p13.3
Rubinstein–Taybi	Microcephaly, characteristic facies, MR	16p13.3
Smith–Magenis	MR, characteristic facies	17p11.2
Miller–Dieker	Lissencephaly, characteristic facies	17p13.3
Charcot–Marie–Tooth	Peripheral neuropathy	CMT: dup(17p12)
Hereditary susceptibility to pressure palsies	Peripheral neuropathy	HSPP: del(17p12)
Alagille	Intrahepatic biliary atresia, peripheral pulmonic stenosis, characteristic facies	20p11.23
DiGeorge/velocardiofacial	Palatal anomalies, conotruncal cardiac anomalies, thymic hypoplasia, parathyroid hypoplasia	22q11.2
Steroid sulfatase deficiency/Kallman syndrome	Ichthyosis, anosmia	Xp22.3

MR, mental retardation; CMT, Charcot–Marie–Tooth; HSPP, hereditary susceptibility to pressure palsies.

tions may result in recognizable syndromes, however. Some involve very small segments, sometimes so small as to not be visible with a microscope. It is believed that complex phenotypes result from simultaneous deletion of a group of genes, each of which is responsible for a specific developmental process (Figure 6.24). The exact phenotype may vary according to the extent of the deletion and which genes are lost. Although the larger chromosome deletions are readily identified by standard cytogenetic analysis, deletions of fewer than a million base pairs or so cannot be resolved with the light microscope. Cytological detection of very small deletions requires the use of FISH (Hot Topic 6.1) or comparative genomic hybridization. Many microdeletion syndromes have been defined (Table 6.2; Clinical Snapshot 6.3). Although the phenotypes of these different syndromes are distinct, the deleted regions are typically flanked by repeated sequences, suggesting that this is a common mechanism for the deletion of large chromosomal regions (see Chapter 2).

[handwritten annotations at top:] measures copy number error, not structural integrity
allows you to perform multiple FISH analysis on one platform

Hot Topics 6.1 ARRAY COMPARATIVE GENOMIC HYBRIDIZATION

The resolution of FISH is limited by the requirement of light microscopic analysis to detect hybridization and the use of relatively large probes to generate sufficient fluorescence to be visible. The smallest rearrangements that can be seen are in the range of 1 million base pairs. Another approach, comparative genomic hybridization (CGH), increases the resolution to the order of tens of thousands of base pairs.

CGH was originally developed for use on fixed chromosomes on microscope slides (metaphase CGH). It involves competitive hybridization of two sets of DNA sequences, one from a test sample and one from a control sample, to the same reference genome (Figure 6.25). The two samples are fluorescently labeled with different colors – usually the test set is labeled red and the control green. If there are equal amounts of a specific sequence in the test and control samples, both will bind equally to the reference genome, giving a yellow color from the simultaneous red and green fluorescence. If a specific sequence is represented more in the test DNA because of duplication or trisomy, red fluorescence will predominate for that sequence. If there is a deletion of the sequence from the test set, green fluorescence will predominate.

The resolution of metaphase CGH is limited to the degree of detail that can be seen with the light microscope, and therefore is no greater than FISH. Another approach that is rapidly gaining widespread use is to hybridize with cloned DNA segments bound to a glass

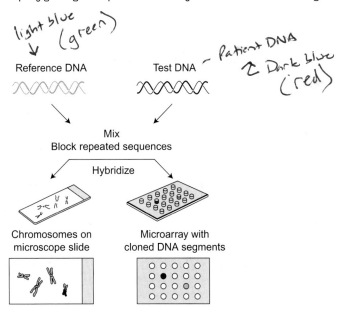

[handwritten annotations on figure:] light blue (green) → Reference DNA; Test DNA – Patient DNA ↗ Dark blue (red)

Mix
Block repeated sequences

Hybridize

Chromosomes on microscope slide

Microarray with cloned DNA segments

Figure 6.25 • Array comparative genomic hybridization. Reference DNA is labeled with a green fluorochrome (shown here as light blue), test DNA with red (shown here as dark blue). Repeated DNA sequences are blocked from hybridization by binding to purified repeated DNA. The test and reference DNAs are mixed and hybridized with human DNA sequences either on metaphase chromosomes (left) or bound in a microarray on a glass slide (right). Deletions in the test DNA appear as green (shown here as light blue) and duplications as red hybridizations (shown here as dark blue).

Hot Topics 6.1 continued

slide in a microarray, referred to as array CGH (Figure 6.26). The cloned segments currently most often consist of bacterial artificial chromosomes with specific human DNA inserts representing regions around the genome. These are often selected to cover specific chromosome regions known to be involved in deletions or duplications. Hybridization of differentially labeled control and test samples is performed, and the microarray is analyzed for evidence of disproportionate binding of either the control or test DNA to each spot in the array. Deletions or duplications of the test sample relative to the control can thereby be detected at a resolution determined by the size of the clones and their spacing in regions of interest – resolutions of tens of kb can be readily achieved with this approach. Array CGH also offers the major advantage that a large number of regions can be examined for deletion or duplication simultaneously, and at no incremental cost. Array CGH is therefore rapidly gaining acceptance as a clinical test, and will likely supplant FISH studies for detection of microdeletions or duplications in the coming years.

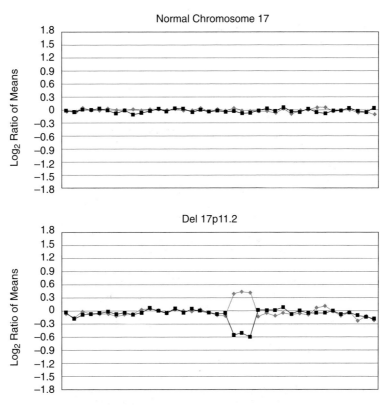

Figure 6.26 • Representative plots showing a chromosomal abnormality detected by the SignatureChip. Each clone is arranged along the x-axis according to its location on the chromosome with the most distal/telomeric p-arm clones on the left and the most distal/telomeric q-arm clones on the right. The blue line plots represent the ratios from the first slide for each patient (control Cy5/ patient Cy3) and the black plots represent the ratios obtained from the second slide for each patient in which the dyes have been reversed (patient Cy5/ control Cy3). The top panel is a normal plot for chromosome 17. The bottom panel is a plot from a patient with Smith Magenis syndrome showing a deletion of three clones from the chromosome 17p11.2 region including clones which span the *RAI* locus. (Courtesy of Signature Genomic Laboratories, LLC.)

CLINICAL SNAPSHOT 6.3

■ Velocardiofacial syndrome (VCFS)

Tess is a 4-year-old girl who is referred for a speech and language evaluation. She began to say single words well after her second birthday, and still is not speaking in full sentences. Her enunciation is also poor, and her voice is nasal. She has had many upper respiratory infections and has been followed for a heart murmur. Examination by an otolaryngologist reveals velopharyngeal incompetence (lack of complete closure of the nasopharynx by the soft palate). A chromosome study is sent and FISH reveals a deletion of the VCFS critical region on chromosome 22. A diagnosis of velocardiofacial syndrome is made.

VCFS is a congenital anomaly syndrome consisting of palatal abnormalities, congenital heart defects, and facial anomalies (Figure 6.27). The palatal anomalies can include cleft palate, submucous cleft palate, and velopharyngeal incompetence. The latter causes nasality of the voice. The cardiac anomalies tend to involve the conotrucal region, that is, the root of the aorta and pulmonary artery. These include coarctation (constriction) of the aorta, tetralogy of Fallot (pulmonic stenosis, ventricular septal defect, abnormal placement of the aortic outlet, left ventricular hypertrophy), and trucus arteriosis (common aorta and pulmonary vessel). Facial anomalies include narrow palpebral fissures and prominent nasal root. In addition, there may be decreased resistance to infection due to immunological anomalies because of underdevelopment of the thymus. The more severe instances are recognized at birth in a syndrome of congenital heart defects, hypoplasia of the parathyroids resulting in hypocalcemia, and thymic aplasia, referred to as DiGeorge syndrome. VCFS/DiGeorge syndrome is due to deletion of a region on chromosome 22q that is easily detected by FISH (Figure 6.28). In some cases, the deletion can be familial, giving rise to dominant transmission of the phenotype.

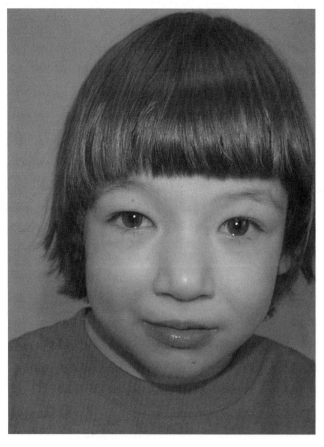

Figure 6.27 • Child with velocardiofacial syndrome. (Courtesy of Dr. Robert Shprintzen, SUNY Upstate Medical University, Syracuse, NY.)

CLINICAL SNAPSHOT 6.3 continued

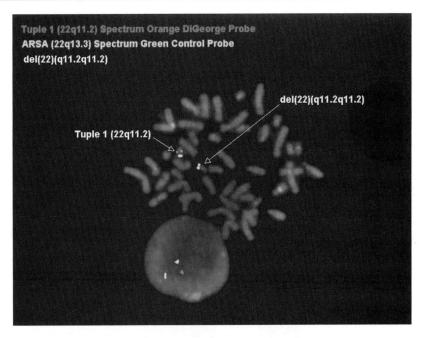

Figure 6.28 • Detection of a submicroscopic deletion of chromosome 22q11.2 by FISH with two labeled probes. The control probe (ARSA, 22q13.3, labeled green) binds to the end of chromosome 22, whereas the other probe (Tuple 1, 22q11.2, labeled red) binds to a sequence in the region that is commonly deleted in individuals with DiGeorge/ velocardiofacial syndrome. The chromosome at the right binds only with the ARSA probe, indicative of deletion of this region. (Courtesy of Dr. Andrew Carroll, University of Alabama at Birmingham.)

Imprinting and Chromosomal Abnormalities

The phenomenon of genomic imprinting has been encountered in Chapters 1 and 3. We have seen that there are certain genes that are only expressed from the maternal or paternal copy, and that this can result in complex patterns of inheritance of single gene disorders. Imprinting has also been found to have a role in determining the phenotype in individuals with certain chromosomal abnormalities.

The effects of imprinting in humans first came to light in humans through studies of rare individuals affected with the autosomal recessive disorder cystic fibrosis who had, in addition, severe growth and developmental delay. They were found to have inherited the cystic fibrosis gene mutation – along with other genes on chromosome 7 – from just one parent (Figure 6.29). This is referred to as **uniparental disomy**. Uniparental disomy is believed to be due to loss of one chromosome in a trisomic conceptus. Trisomy 7 would be nonviable, but if, early in development, one of the three copies of chromosome 7 in a trisomic embryo is lost by nondisjunction, the normal chromosome number would be restored. If the remaining copies of chromosome 7 are derived from the same parent, however, uniparental disomy results, which will have phenotypic consequences if the chromosome includes imprinted genes.

The effects of imprinting may also be detected in gene deletion syndromes. Prader–Willi (MIM 176270) and Angelman syndromes (MIM 105830) are distinct disorders that are both associated with deletions of the same region of chromosome 15 (Figure 6.30). If the deletion is of the paternal 15, however, the phenotype is Prader–Willi syndrome, whereas if maternal sequences are deleted, the result is Angelman syndrome. In some instances of Prader–Willi or Angelman syndrome, no deletion is seen, but instead there is uniparental disomy for the

How does genomic imprinting lead to distinctive phenotypes associated with chromosomal abnormalities?

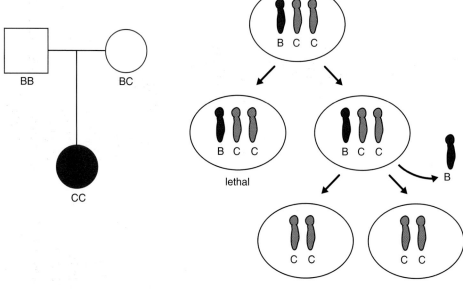

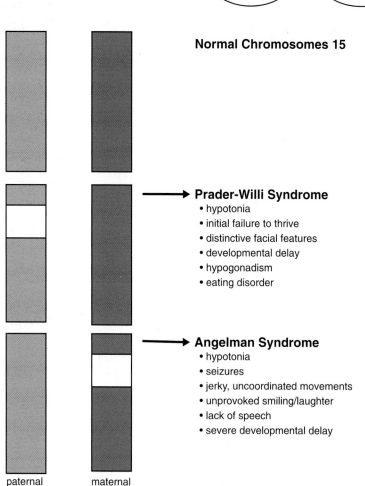

Figure 6.29 • A child is homozygous for allele c, inherited from the mother, due to phenomenon of uniparental disomy. This occurs by loss of the paternal chromosome, containing allele B, from a trisomic zygote.

Normal Chromosomes 15

Prader-Willi Syndrome
• hypotonia
• initial failure to thrive
• distinctive facial features
• developmental delay
• hypogonadism
• eating disorder

Angelman Syndrome
• hypotonia
• seizures
• jerky, uncoordinated movements
• unprovoked smiling/laughter
• lack of speech
• severe developmental delay

paternal   maternal

Figure 6.30 • Deletions of chromosome 15 result in Prader–Willi or Angelman syndrome. Deletion of paternal sequences results in Prader–Willi, whereas deletion of maternal sequences results in Angelman syndrome.

paternal (giving Angelman syndrome) or the maternal (giving Prader–Willi syndrome) copy of 15. Presumably, there are imprinted genes in this region, some of which are expressed on the paternal and some on the maternal 15. One such gene, designated *UBE3A* (MIM 601623), has been found to be mutated in some patients with Angelman syndrome.

The full range of phenotypes that result from imprinting effects has not yet been defined. Only a small number of chromosomes or chromosome regions have been implicated in clini-

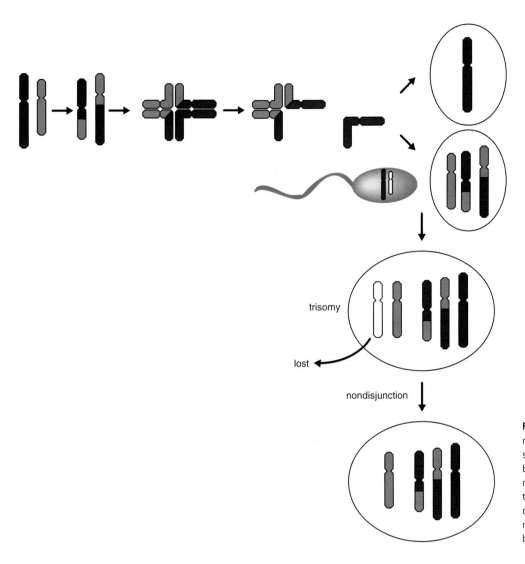

Figure 6.31 • A balanced translocation resulting in uniparental disomy. A 3:1 segregation event in meiosis results in both the balanced translocation and one normal chromosome. Upon fertilization this results in trisomy; loss of the normal chromosome from the other parent restores a normal chromosome number, but also causes uniparental disomy.

TABLE 6.3 Chromosomes implicated in clinical disorders due to uniparental disomy of the maternal or paternal chromosome or chromosome region

Chromosome	Parent	Clinical effects
15	Maternal	Prader–Willi syndrome
15	Paternal	Angelman syndrome
7	Maternal	Russell–Silver syndrome (growth delay)
6	Paternal	Transient neonatal diabetes, IUGR
11p	Paternal (duplication)	Beckwith–Wiedemann syndrome

cal disorders associated with uniparental disomy (Table 6.3). Instances have been reported wherein the offspring of a phenotypically normal, balanced translocation carrier has an abnormal phenotype in spite of having inherited the same balanced translocation (Figure 6.31). Some have been found to have inherited from the same parent both the translocation chromosome and one of the normal chromosomes involved in the translocation, resulting in uniparental disomy. Others have been found to have deletions of material not found to be deleted in the parent, suggesting instability of the rearranged chromosome. It is apparent that the full range of phenotypic consequences of chromosomal abnormalities has not yet been discovered.

CONCLUSION

The ability to study chromosome number and structure in effect launched the era of medical genetics. Since then, advances have been made in prenatal diagnosis and the resolution of cytogenetic analysis has increased to the level of thousands of base pairs. We are now seeing a convergence of cytological and molecular analysis. This will dramatically increase the power of genetic testing, improving our ability to establish diagnoses and provide counseling to families.

REVIEW QUESTIONS

6.1 What would you expect to be the effect of a complete loss of p53 function?

6.2 At what point in meiosis do homologous centromeres separate? Do all homologous segments separate at this time?

6.3 A child with Down syndrome has the genotype 1,2,3 for a polymorphism on chromosome 21 that has alleles 1, 2, 3, and 4. His mother is 1,2 and father is 3,4. In which parent did nondisjunction occur, and did it occur in the first or second meiotic division?

6.4 Are pericentric or paracentric inversions most likely to be associated with the birth of a child with congenital anomalies? Is this more likely for a large or a small inverted segment?

6.5 Uniparental disomy is a more common cause of Prader–Willi syndrome than it is of Angelman syndrome, even though both are due to loss of imprinted genes in the same region. Why is this so?

FURTHER READING

General References

Babu A, Verma RS. Human Chromosomes: Principles and Techniques, 1995, New York: McGraw-Hill.

Smeets DF. Historical perspective of human cytogenetics: from microscope to microarray. Clin Biochem 2004;37:439–446.

Sanchez I, Dynlacht BD. New insights into cyclins, CDKs, and cell cycle control. Semin Cell Dev Biol 2005;16:311–321.

Trask B. Human cytogenetics; 46 chromosomes, 46 years and counting. Nat Rev Genet 2002;3:769–778.

Marston AL, Amon A. Meiosis: cell cycle controls shuffle and deal. Nat Rev Mol Cell Biol 2004;5:983–997.

Jiang YH, Bressler J, Beaudet AL. Epigenetics and human disease. Annu Rev Genomics Hum Genet 2004;5:470–510.

Stack SM, Anderson LK. A model for chromosome structure during the mitotic and meiotic cell cycles. Chromosome Res 2001;9:175–198.

Clinical Snapshot 6.1 Down Syndrome

Patterson D, Costa ACS. Down syndrome and genetics – a case of linked histories. Nat Rev Genet 2005;6:137–147.

Antonarakis SE, Lyle R, Dermitzakis ET, Reymond A, Deutsch S. Chromosomes 21 and Down syndrome: from genomics to pathophysiology. Nat Rev Genet 2004;5:725–738

Clinical Snapshot 6.2 Turner Syndrome

Sybert VP, McCauley E. Turner's syndrome. New Engl J Med 2004;351:1227–1238.

Clinical Snapshot 6.3 VCFS

McDermid HE, Morrow BE. Genomic disorders on 22q11. Am J Hum Genet 2002;70:1077–1088.

Methods 6.1 Chromosomal Analysis

Spurbeck JL, Adams SA, Stupca PJ, Dewald GW. Primer on medical genomics. Part XI: Visualizing human chromosomes. Mayo Clin Proc. 2004;79:58–75.

Methods 6.2 Nomenclature

International System for Human Cytogenetic Nomenclature 1995. http://www.iscn1995.org/

Methods 6.3 FISH
Lee C, Lemyre E, Miron PM, Morton CC. Multicolor fluorescence in situ hybridization in clinical diagnostic cytogenetics. Curr Opin Pediatr 2001;13:550–555.

Ethics 6.1 Nondirective Counseling
Plunkett KS, Simpson JL. A general approach to genetic counseling. Obstet Gynecol Clin N Am 2002;29:265–276.

Hot Topics 6.1 Array CGH
Shaffer LG, Bejjani BA. A cytogeneticist's perspective on genomic microarrays. Hum Reprod Update 2004;10:221–226.

Mantripragada KK, Buckley PG, de Stahl TD, Dumanski JP. Genomic microarrays in the spotlight. Trends Genet 2004;20:87–94.

7

Population Genetics

INTRODUCTION

So far we have considered genetic traits from the perspective of the individual and of the family. Some, like Down syndrome, are rare traits that affect individuals throughout the world. Others, such as cystic fibrosis, are more prevalent in some populations than others. In this chapter, we will consider genetic traits from a different perspective – that of the population. Although genes act on individuals and flow through families, the forces that determine gene frequencies act at the level of populations. Study of these forces can have important implications for medicine. First, we can understand why some populations appear to be singled out for particular genetic disorders and may be relatively free of others. Second, the principles of population genetics provide tools for calculating gene frequencies to use in genetic counseling. The frequency of carriers for recessive traits cannot be determined directly but can be calculated using a simple equation that is the cornerstone of population genetics. Population genetics helps us to understand the significance of genetic variation, and has provided the basis for the intersection of genetics with public health in the form of population screening programs (Hot Topic 7.1).

KEY POINTS

- The relationship between allele frequency and gene frequency is given by the Hardy–Weinberg equilibrium. In a two-allele system if the frequency of the A allele is p and the a allele is q, then the genotype frequencies are given by p^2, $2pq$, and q^2 for AA, Aa, and aa, respectively. These frequencies will remain stable from generation to generation, provided a set of assumptions are met, including no mutation, selection, or migration, and a large population size.
- Reduction of the ability of individuals with a specific genotype to reproduce constitutes selection. This can lead to a reduction of the frequency of the allele that is selected against. Eventually, an equilibrium may be reached between loss of the allele by selection and its replacement by new mutation.
- In some instances, selection may act against homozygotes for both alleles in a two-allele system. Heterozygotes may be favored, resulting in the two alleles being retained in the population. This constitutes a balanced polymorphism, and may result in the persistence of an otherwise deleterious allele.
- If a breeding population is small there may be significant fluctuations in allele frequency from generation to generation, referred to as genetic drift.
- If a population goes through a "bottleneck" in which there are a small number of individuals, there can be major changes in allele frequency, including an increase in the frequency of a deleterious allele.

Hot Topic 7.1 PUBLIC HEALTH GENETICS

The power of genetics and genomics extends well beyond the care of individuals or families. There are profound implications for public health, with many initiatives already underway. Some of the areas of interest include:

- Programs for population screening, including carrier screening programs and newborn screening programs. The latter include screening for inborn errors of metabolism as well as conditions such as congenital deafness. Newborn screening programs have traditionally been managed at a state level, but now there is discussion about bringing consistency to programs across different states in the US.
- Quality assurance of genetic testing. As new genetic tests are developed there is a need to track the various pathogenic and non-pathogenic changes in genes. This will provide a dataset with which to judge the clinical significance of mutations found in the course of clinical testing.
- Prevention of common disorders. As genetic factors that contribute to common disorders come to light it will be important to provide public education and access to testing to insure access to tests and appropriate counseling. The public health community also has a major interest in determining which tests are appropriate for use in screening and conducting studies to determine the efficacy of screening.

Information about topics in public health genetics and genetic epidemiology are tracked on a website "HuGEnet" (www.cdc.gov/genomics/hugenet)

HARDY–WEINBERG EQUILIBRIUM

The Hardy–Weinberg equilibrium provides the cornerstone for our understanding of population genetics. The concept was established in 1908 independently by the English mathematician G. H. Hardy and the German physician W. Weinberg. Their formulation states a simple relationship between the frequency of alleles at a genetic locus and the genotypes resulting from those alleles.

What is the Hardy–Weinberg equilibrium?

Consider a gene locus with alleles A and a. Let the frequency of A be designated by the variable p and the frequency of a by the variable q. If all alleles at this locus are either A or a, then $p + q = 1$. The frequency of sperm or egg cells in the population carrying A or a will thus be p or q, respectively (Figure 7.1). If we assume that the union of germ cells carrying either A or a is entirely random, we can easily calculate the frequency of zygotes having the genotype AA, Aa, or aa. The frequency of AA will be p^2 and of aa will be q^2. The frequency of heterozygotes will be $2pq$, reflecting that Aa individuals can arise in two ways: fusion of A-bearing sperm with a-bearing eggs, or vice versa (Methods 7.1).

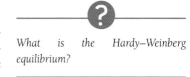

eggs

	allele	frequency	
	A	a	allele
	p	q	frequency

sperm

allele	frequency		
A	q	AA p^2	Aa pq
a	q	aA pq	aa q^2

Figure 7.1 • The frequency of A-bearing sperm or eggs is p and of a-bearing sperm or eggs is q. Assuming that mating is random with respect to genotype, that there is no mutation from A to a or vice versa, that there is no migration in or out of the population, and that mating efficiency is equal for all genotypes, the frequency of the genotype AA is p^2, of Aa is $2pq$, and of aa is q^2.

Method 7.1

Derivation of the Hardy–Weinberg Equation

The Hardy–Weinberg equation can be easily derived algebraically. Start with a population in which the frequency of $AA = x$, $Aa = y$, $aa = z$ (that is, the frequencies of the three genotypes are found to have values of x, y, and z, where $x + y + z = 1$). At this point, the frequency of $A = p = x + \frac{1}{2}y$ and the frequency of $a = q = z + \frac{1}{2}y$. We will show that, after one generation of random mating, the frequency of $AA = p^2$, $Aa = 2pq$, and $aa = q^2$.

First, let's consider all possible matings:

Mating type	Frequency	Outcome
$AA \times AA$	x^2	All AA
$AA \times Aa$	$2xy$	$\frac{1}{2}AA$, $\frac{1}{2}Aa$
$AA \times aa$	$2xz$	All Aa
$Aa \times Aa$	y^2	$\frac{1}{4}AA$, $\frac{1}{2}Aa$, $\frac{1}{4}aa$
$Aa \times aa$	$2yz$	$\frac{1}{2}Aa$, $\frac{1}{2}aa$
$aa \times aa$	z^2	All aa

A mating type such as $AA \times Aa$ can occur in two ways: The male can be AA and the female Aa, or vice versa; hence the frequency is $2xy$ (not xy).

Now let's tally the three genotypes in the next generation:

$$\begin{aligned}
AA &= x^2 + \frac{1}{2}(2xy) + \frac{1}{4}(y^2) \\
&= (x + \frac{1}{2}y)^2 = p^2 \\
Aa &= \frac{1}{2}(2xy) + 2xz + \frac{1}{2}(y^2) + \frac{1}{2}(2yz) \\
&= 2(x + \frac{1}{2}y)(z + \frac{1}{2}y) = 2pq \\
aa &= \frac{1}{4}(y^2) + \frac{1}{2}(2yz) + z^2 \\
&= (z + \frac{1}{2}y)^2 = q^2
\end{aligned}$$

The Hardy–Weinberg equilibrium depends on a number of assumptions. As already noted, mating must be random with respect to genotype. If there is preferential mating between AA and AA individuals, for example, there will be more homozygous individuals and fewer heterozygotes. Also, the population is assumed to be very large, so that statistical fluctuations will be negligible. Later we will explore the consequences of deviation from this assumption. There must be no mutation of A alleles into a, or a into A. Finally, individuals of all genotypes must be equally capable of reproduction (i.e., there must be no selection).

How is the Hardy–Weinberg equilibrium used to calculate carrier frequency of a recessive disorder? Consider the recessive condition cystic fibrosis. In this case, the A allele is the wild-type and a is the cystic fibrosis mutation. The frequency of aa – that is, of individuals affected with cystic fibrosis – is 1 in 2500 in northern European whites. Thus $q^2 = 1/2500$, and hence $q = 1/50$. Because $p + q = 1$, p must be 49/50. The carrier frequency, then, is $2pq = 2(49/50)(1/50) \approx 1/25$ in this population.

We are assuming, of course, that the cystic fibrosis gene obeys the assumptions of the Hardy–Weinberg equilibrium. The northern European population is very large, large enough to minimize random statistical fluctuation (such as the chance that only noncarriers happen to bear children in one generation). Mating may not be entirely random with respect to genotype. Some cystic fibrosis carriers may meet one another because of their affected siblings, for example, and choose either to mate or not to mate, having been brought together because of genotype. For the most part, however, cystic fibrosis carriers are not aware of their carrier status.

Two other assumptions clearly are not fulfilled. The ability of individuals with cystic fibrosis to have offspring is definitely impaired. Males with cystic fibrosis usually are infertile. Females may be fertile, but reproduction is severely limited by the medical burden of the disorder. Many cystic fibrosis homozygotes therefore do not reproduce, which should cause loss of cystic fibrosis alleles in the population from one generation to the next. The rate of change of the frequency of the cystic fibrosis allele is very slow, however, as only 1 in 2500 individuals is subject to this negative selection. Most cystic fibrosis alleles exist in heterozygous carriers who are not subject to selection.

The Hardy–Weinberg formulation also predicts that the gene frequencies will remain stable from generation to generation, provided that there is no mutation of A to a or of a to A, and no migration of individuals to or from the population, random mating, and no selection. This may seem an obvious result: Under the assumptions of an "ideal" Hardy–Weinberg population, the alleles A and a have nowhere to go; they cannot leave or enter the population by migration, be lost by infertility, change by mutation, or dwindle by chance, so their stability is assured.

The Hardy–Weinberg equilibrium applies to X-linked traits as well as to autosomal traits. For an X-linked gene, males are hemizygous; the frequency of males with the genotype A is simply the frequency of the A allele, or p. Likewise, the frequency of males with the a genotype is q. Females can be AA, Aa, or aa, with the usual frequencies of p^2, $2pq$, and q^2, respectively.

DEVIATIONS FROM THE HARDY–WEINBERG EQUILIBRIUM

The ideal Hardy–Weinberg population must fulfill several requirements that are typically not met in real populations. In this section we will explore the impact of deviators from these assumptions.

Selection

What happens if the ability to reproduce is not equal for individuals with various genotypes? To answer this, let us first consider the simple situation of a pair of alleles, A and a, with A dominant to a. Suppose that the frequency of both A and a is 0.5. If the population obeys the assumptions of the Hardy–Weinberg equation, we would expect these frequencies to remain stable over time. Approximately 25% of individuals would be AA, 50% Aa, and 25% aa.

What is the effect of selection on allele frequencies?

Now, let's change things. Suppose that aa individuals suddenly are rendered unable to reproduce. It doesn't matter how this happens: The aas might die before reproductive age or be healthy but sterile. What matters is that they do not contribute to the gene pool of the next generation. Geneticists refer to this as a **lethal trait**, but it may be only the germ cells that die.

One might expect that this change would lead to a gradual loss of a alleles and corresponding increase in the proportion of A. In the first generation after imposition of selection, 25% of individuals are aa and are lost to the gene pool. Among the survivors, the 25% AA and 50% Aa, two-thirds of the alleles are A and one-third are a, so the frequency of a diminishes from 0.5 to 0.33. In the next generation, some aa homozygotes are produced through matings between heterozygotes, and the frequency of a will decrease again due to the inability of aa individuals to produce offspring. As the frequency of a diminishes, however, the proportion of heterozygotes also diminishes, so, with each generation there are fewer and fewer aa offspring to be subjected to selection (Figure 7.2). Therefore, the rate of decrease of the frequency of a slows. A graph of the frequency of a as a function of time shows an exponential decline that approaches zero asymptotically (Figure 7.3). In an infinitely large population, a will approach, but will never reach, zero. In a real population, the day may come when there are very few Aa individuals who, by chance, happen not to produce any offspring with the a allele. At that point, the frequency of a becomes 0, and a is said to be **extinguished** and A **fixed**.

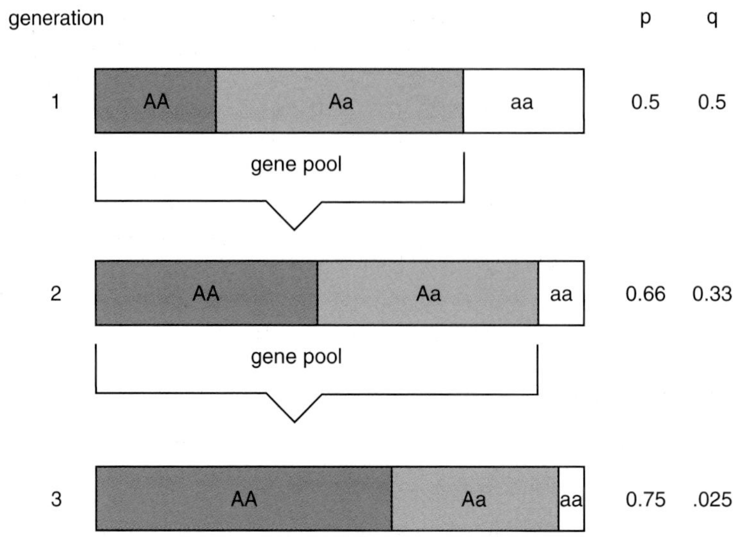

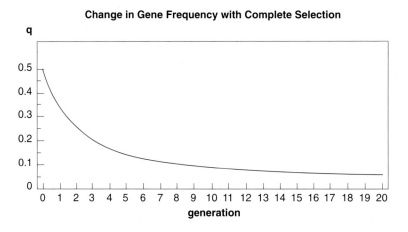

generation   p   q

1 | AA | Aa | aa | 0.5   0.5

gene pool

2 | AA | Aa | aa | 0.66   0.33

gene pool

3 | AA | Aa |aa| 0.75   .025

Figure 7.2 • Decline in gene frequency after imposition of complete selection against the homozygous recessive individuals. Only *AA* and *Aa* individuals contribute to the gene pool. The frequency of *a* diminishes in each generation owing to lack of reproduction of *aa* individuals.

Change in Gene Frequency with Complete Selection

q

0.5

0.4

0.3

0.2

0.1

0

0 1 2 3 4 5 6 7 8 9 10 11 12 13 14 15 16 17 18 19 20

generation

Figure 7.3 • Graph of *q* as a function of generations after the imposition of complete selection, assuming that, at the start, $p = q = 0.5$. Note that the frequency decreases quickly at first, as there are many *aa* individuals. As the frequency of *aa* individuals declines, however, the rate of decrease in *q* also declines.

This extreme scenario can be softened if *aa* homozygotes are able to produce some offspring but do so less efficiently than *AA* or *Aa* individuals. The *aa*s are said to be vulnerable to **selection**, or to have reduced **reproductive fitness**. The rate of decrease of the frequency of *a* will be slower, but the frequency will decrease nevertheless.

It is easy to find examples of genetic traits that are subject to selection. Consider Duchenne muscular dystrophy, an X-linked recessive trait that is lethal in males. In a given generation, the proportion of affected males is *q* and of heterozygous females is $2pq$, which is nearly equal to $2q$ because the disease gene is quite rare and thus *p* equals approximately 1. The proportion of mutant alleles lost in each generation is therefore $q/(q + 2q) = \frac{1}{3}$. The frequency of the mutant allele would dwindle gradually to near 0 unless something replenishes it, and this indeed happens in the form of new mutation. In each generation, there is a probability designated by the variable μ that a given copy of the dystrophin gene will mutate on any X chromosome. A point will be reached where this rate of new mutation exactly balances the loss of alleles in each generation, at which point the gene frequency will be stable. This can be expressed by the equation $\mu = q/3$. At equilibrium, then, the value of *q* will equal 3μ. We can measure *q*, the disease frequency, which is approximately 1 in 3000 (0.000333). This allows us to estimate that the mutation rate for this locus, or μ is 1.1×10^{-4} per gamete per generation. The wide diversity of dystrophin mutations found in different affected individuals accords with this notion that a substantial proportion (one-third) of cases arise owing to fresh mutation.

Similar arguments apply for other disorders in which new mutation counterbalances loss of alleles due to selection. In the dominant disorder neurofibromatosis type 1, which occurs with a frequency of 1 in 4000 persons, for example, approximately half of the cases in the world arise by new mutation. This predicts a gene frequency of 1 in 8000 and a mutation rate of 1 in 16,000.

Genetic disorders that have a high frequency of new mutation tend to occur throughout the world and do not display a racial, ethnic, or regional predilection. This is true for Duchenne muscular dystrophy and neurofibromatosis and reflects the fact that new mutations occur at random. Also, disorders with a high rate of new mutation tend to be genetically heterogeneous: A wide range of different mutations account for the disorder in different people. Again, this is true for Duchenne muscular dystrophy and neurofibromatosis.

Balanced Polymorphism

In contrast to Duchenne muscular dystrophy and neurofibromatosis, some genetic disorders exhibit a restricted geographical distribution (Ethical Implications 7.1). The worldwide distribution of globin disorders provides a prime example. Hemoglobin is the oxygen carrying molecule of the red blood cell. In the adult it consists of a tetramer, with two α chains and two β chains. The globin proteins each bind a porphyrin heme group which contains iron. A wide variety of genetic disorders due to globin mutations have been identified. Sickle cell anemia (Clinical Snapsot 7.1) is due to a specific β globin mutation, which results in amino acid substitution. The altered globin causes the red cells to assume a sickle shape under conditions of low oxygen tension, and these do not flow easily through small blood vessels. Thalassemia is another red cell disorder, in this case due to a deficient globin production. This results in severe chronic anemia.

What is meant by balanced polymorphism?

ETHICAL IMPLICATIONS 7.1 • Genetic variation and race

Since single nucleotide polymorphisms occur on average every 1000 bases in the genome, there should be approximately 3×10^6 base pair differences between any two persons. This represents about 0.1% of the genome, hence the commonly quoted statement that humans are about 99.9% identical from the genetic point of view. Of course, 3×10^6 single base differences is a large number in absolute terms, and accounts for phenotypic differences in traits such as physical appearance as well as differences in susceptibility to both rare and common disorders. It is also commonly pointed out that there are as many genetic differences within groups commonly identified as "races" as there are between such groups. What does this mean for the concept of "race?" Is there a biological basis for the notion?

It is indeed difficult to define in genetic terms the borders of what would constitute a "race" of people. If one looks at the distribution of allele frequencies in different populations it is apparent that the frequency of some alleles and haplotypes reflect ancestral origins. This should come as no surprise, given phenomena such as the founder effect, balanced polymorphism, and linkage disequilibrium. Members of modern populations, in many cases, bear the genetic traces of common ancestry at some point in the past. Some populations have been relatively stable for a long period, whereas in others there has been substantial migration and admixture with people of diverse origins.

"Race" is a social, political, and cultural, but not a biological concept. As we will see later in this book, there are some instances where common categorizations of race are used as surrogates for genetic traits that are prevalent in groups of individuals who share ancestral origins. For the most part, the specific genes in question are not yet known. Stratification of the population by these categorizations may have some practical utility, but also risks confusion with a long and difficult political and culture history.

CLINICAL SNAPSHOT 7.1

■ Sickle cell anemia

James is a 3-year-old African–American boy who is brought to the emergency room with leg pain and fever. He has been exhibiting symptoms of a cold for the past few days, but today woke up with a fever of 39°C, crying, and complaining that his legs hurt. His parents explain that James has sickle cell anemia. His examination shows rhinorrhea, fever of 38.5°C, and dry mucous membranes. James is exquisitely sensitive to being touched, especially in his legs. There is no visible swelling or redness to his legs, however. He is admitted to the hospital, started on i.v. fluids, pain medications, and antibiotics.

Sickle cell anemia is an autosomal recessive disorder due to an amino acid substitution (valine for glutamic acid) in the β globin gene. Adult hemoglobin consists of two α chains and two β chains (see Chapter 13). The sickle cell mutation causes the β chain to misfold, particularly under conditions of low oxygen tension. This causes the red blood cell to assume a sickle shape (Figure 7.4). Sickle cells do not pass readily through small blood vessels, which leads to tissue hypoxemia. Individuals with sickle cell anemia suffer from painful crises, due to hypoxemia of tissues such as bone. Chronic hypoxia in the spleen leads to gradual loss of splenic tissue, resulting in an increased risk of bacterial infection. For this reason, children with sickle cell anemia are treated with prophylactic antibiotics and are given intravenous antibiotics if there are signs of infection. The painful crises are treated with hydration and pain medications, and resolve over a period of days.

Sickle cell anemia is particularly prevalent among people of sub-Saharan African descent. Approximately 1 in 500 African-American births is affected. This calculates to a carrier frequency in this population of approximately 1 in 11 individuals. The mutation is also found in other parts of the world, including the Mediterranean region and the Middle East.

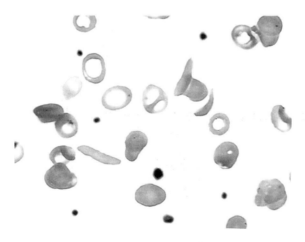

Figure 7.4 • Photomicrograph of sickle cells. (Photograph courtesy of Dr. Orah Platt, Children's Hospital, Boston.)

Globin disorders are not uniformly distributed worldwide. Sickle cell anemia is found mainly in populations from Africa (Clinical Snapshot 7.1). Thalassemia occurs in Mediterranean, Middle Eastern, and Southeast Asian populations. In 1949, the geneticist J. B. S. Haldane pointed out that the distribution of globin disorders parallels that of malaria (Figure 7.5), and proposed that malaria might constitute a selective force that could maintain globin mutant alleles in the population. Malaria is a parasitic infection of red blood cells, and at least one form, *Plasmodium falciparum*, often is fatal without treatment. How can a parasitic infection influence the worldwide distribution of a genetic trait?

The worldwide distribution of globin mutations reflects the action of two forces that mold gene frequencies. The first is referred to as **balanced polymorphism**, the second the **founder effect**. If we look back in history, and to this day in some parts of the world, most, if not all, globin

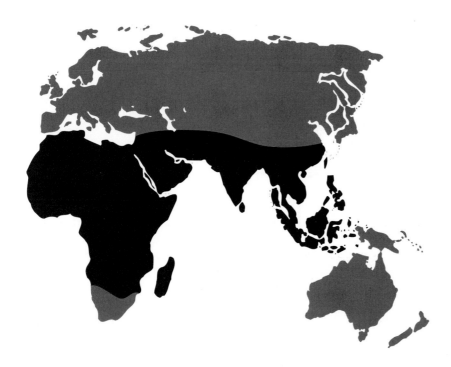

Figure 7.5 • Worldwide distribution of thalassemia, paralleling the distribution of malaria (blue area).

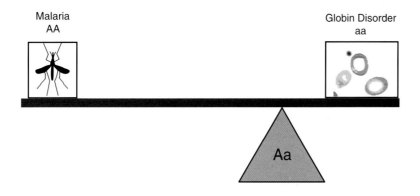

Malaria
AA

Globin Disorder
aa

Aa

Figure 7.6 • Concept of balanced polymorphism. Both the homozygous wild type and homozygous mutant individuals are subjected to selection by malaria and anemia, respectively. The *Aa* individuals have the greatest reproductive fitness and serve as a reservoir for the *a* allele.

mutations would be expected to be lethal. The rare globin mutant allele should have been gradually extinguished due to selection. At the same time, however, falciparum malaria was also often lethal. It turns out, though, that carriers of a globin mutation are relatively resistant to malaria. Homozygous normal individuals are highly susceptible to malaria, and the homozygotes for globin mutations would die of anemia. This leaves the heterozygotes as the fittest individuals in the population. Each generation, some of their offspring would die of malaria and some would die of anemia. During an outbreak of malaria in some region, large numbers might die, leaving only a few founding individuals who might be carriers for some specific globin mutation, making that mutation prevalent in their offspring. In this new population, eventually an equilibrium would be reached, such that the loss of wild-type alleles due to malaria would balance the loss of globin mutant alleles due to anemia (Figure 7.6). The globin mutation would be retained in the population for as long as the counterbalancing selective pressures are maintained.

In Chapter 2, **polymorphism** was defined as the occurrence of two or more alleles at a locus that each has a frequency of at least 1%. The case of the globin genes represents a balanced

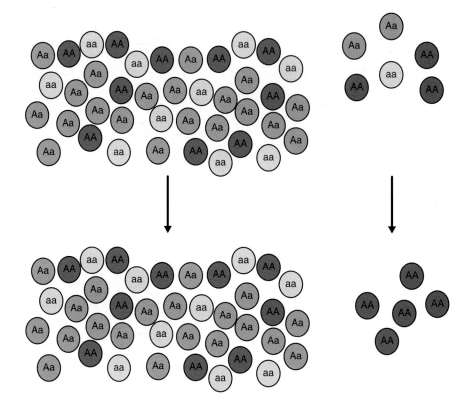

Figure 7.7 • Concept of genetic drift. In a large population with random mating, large fluctuations of gene frequency are unlikely. In a small population, however, gene frequency can change dramatically from one generation to the next, if, for example, only the *AA* individuals participate in mating by chance.

polymorphism, in which the loss of a mutant allele due to selection is balanced by the loss of the wild-type allele due to selection of a different kind. This phenomenon of **balanced polymorphism** – also known as heterozygote advantage – is well known in plants and other animals.

Founder Effect

How does the founder effect increase the frequency of an allele in a population?

The globin–malaria system is the best documented case in humans, although other examples undoubtedly exist. Heterozygote advantage may explain why globin mutations are prevalent in the malaria belt but not why different types of mutations are found in different regions. This is explained by the founder effect. The Hardy–Weinberg equation assumes that breeding in a very large population is random. Even if the frequency of an allele is low, some matings will occur that involve heterozygotes or homozygotes for the allele to maintain it in the population. If the population is very small, however, such matings might not occur, and the frequency of the allele would fall even if it were not subjected to selection (Figure 7.7). This is referred to as **genetic drift**.

The populations of Southern Italy, Greece, Central Africa, or Southeast Asia are not small, of course, but, within a region, a population may well have been subjected to a "bottleneck," perhaps due to an outbreak of malaria. If a large part of the breeding population succumbed to malaria and, among the few survivors, there was one individual with a specific globin mutation, that mutation would become more prevalent in the new population that formed in the region after the bottleneck (Figure 7.8). This illustrates the concept of founder effect.

A striking example of a founder effect has been demonstrated among French Canadians with tyrosinemia type I (MIM 276700), in which a single mutation in the enzyme fumarylacetoacetate hydrolase accounts for most cases. This disorder is an inborn error of tyrosine metabolism that leads to liver damage caused by buildup of toxic metabolites. It is rare around the world, but in the Saguenay–Lac St John region of Quebec it affects 1 of every 1846 new-

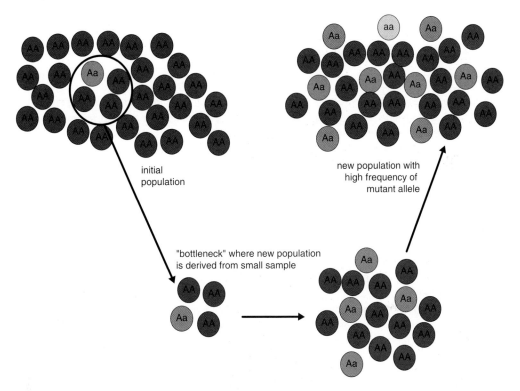

Figure 7.8 • Founder effect. The frequency of the *a* allele is low in the initial population, but a small subset, in which one individual is *Aa*, is removed from the large population and founds a new population. The frequency of *a* is markedly higher in this new population, due to its relatively high frequency in the founders.

borns, predicting a carrier frequency of 0.045, or nearly 1 in 22. DNA testing has revealed that one mutation – a splicing mutation in intron 12 – occurs in 90% of carriers in this region and therefore occurs in homozygous form in approximately 81% of affected individuals. In contrast, this mutation was found in only 28% of tyrosinemia carriers elsewhere in the world. It is presumed that the mutation was introduced into the Saguenay–Lac St John region by a founder individual sometime in the past several hundred years, and the relative isolation of the region has led to a high frequency of the allele due to the founder effect.

The founder effect has also been invoked to explain other examples of high prevalence of genetic disorders in specific populations, such as cystic fibrosis in Northern Europeans or Tay–Sachs disease (MIM 272800) (Clinical Snapsot 7.2) in Eastern European Jews, but here it cannot be the whole story. Both cystic fibrosis and Tay–Sachs disease display genetic heterogeneity, even within the populations of highest disease prevalence. The most common cystic fibrosis mutation accounts for only 70% of mutations in Europe, and at least three mutations are found among Ashkenazi carriers of Tay–Sachs disease. As for the globin mutations, it has been suggested that heterozygote advantage may, in part, explain the unusual geographic distribution of these mutations.

It is likely that selective forces have acted on other genetic traits in human history, although in most cases these forces have not been identified. Traits that are now considered deleterious may well have resulted in a selective advantage to heterozygotes at some point in history. If the same selective forces acted independently in different populations, there may be different mutations at the same locus that were subject to selection, accounting for genetic heterogeneity between populations and a founder effect within a population. These phenomena – heterozygote advantage, founder effect, and genetic heterogeneity – do not act in isolation but together represent some of the major forces that mold gene frequencies in populations.

CLINICAL SNAPSHOT 7.2

■ Tay–Sachs disease

Lewis is a 9-month-old referred for evaluation of developmental regression. He was born after a full-term, uncomplicated pregnancy and his early development was normal. He had been smiling responsively and was able to get to sitting. Over the past few months, however, he has stopped doing both. He stares blankly much of the time now, laying in his crib. He has also become quite irritable. His physical exam is normal except for the lack of interactiveness. A dilated fundoscopic exam is done, however, revealing the cherry red spot (Figure 7.9). A blood test is sent and the clinical diagnosis of Tay–Sachs disease is confirmed.

Tay–Sachs disease is an autosomal recessive disorder due to mutation in the gene that encodes the lysosomal enzyme hexosaminidase A. Hexosaminidase A is required to break down the cell membrane component GM2 ganglioside (Figure 7.10). GM2 ganglioside is found in neurons, and lack of enzyme activity leads to engorgement of lysosomes with undigested material. This is toxic and leads to neuronal loss in the brain. Children with the disorder are normal at birth and achieve normal early milestones, but after the first few months of life begin to lose abilities and regress to the point of total dependency. Most die in the first 2 years of life due to aspiration pneumonia as a consequence of swallowing inco-ordination.

Tay–Sachs disease is particularly prevalent in the Ashkenazi Jewish population, where the carrier frequency is about 1 in 30. Although this is reflective of a founder effect, there are several distinct mutations found in this population. Tay–Sachs disease is also found with increased prevalence in French Canadians, also due to a founder effect.

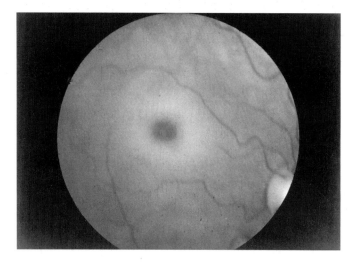

Figure 7.9 • Cherry-red spot from an infant with Tay–Sachs disease. (Courtesy of Dr. Robert Petersen, Children's Hospital, Boston.)

CLINICAL SNAPSHOT 7.2 continued

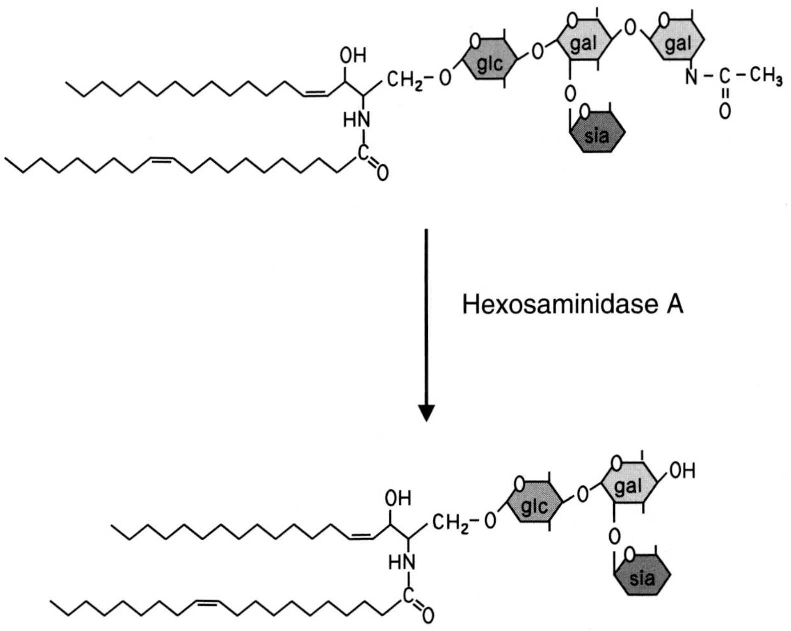

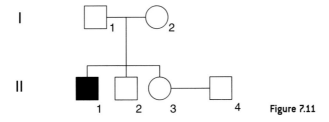

Figure 7.10 • Hexosaminidase A catalyzes the removal of *N*-acetylgalactosamine from GM2 ganglioside.

CONCLUSION

Genetic variation is the engine of evolution, and it is also a major determinate of differences in human health and vulnerability to disease. The study of population genetics has provided insights into the reasons that specific human populations bear a disproportionate burden of specific genetic disorders. The medical implications include the need to consider ancestry in assessing individual risks of disease, and the establishment of population-wide carrier screening programs. We will explore both of these applications in the second half of this book.

REVIEW QUESTIONS

7.1 Individuals II-3 and II-4 wish to know the risk of having a child with an autosomal recessive disorder that affects the brother of II-3. The population frequency of the disorder is 1 : 40,000. Calculate the risk for this couple (Figure 7.11).

Figure 7.11

7.2 Hemochromatosis is an autosomal recessive disorder in which iron accumulates in the body due to abnormal intestinal iron absorption. The prevalence of hemochromatosis is approximately 1 : 400 individuals in some Caucasian populations. Using the Hardy–Weinberg equation, what is the calculated carrier frequency? What is the risk of hemochromatosis in the child in this family

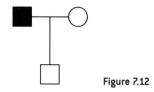

Figure 7.12

(Figure 7.12)? (Assume that both parents are from a population in which the frequency of hemochromatosis is as noted above.) It has been suggested that hemochromatosis carriers have an increased ability to absorb iron and thereby maintain adequate iron stores during times of famine. How might this explain the high prevalence of hemochromatosis?

7.3 You are asked to see a child with hereditary tyrosinemia, an autosomal recessive disorder of amino acid metabolism that causes liver failure. Both parents are of French Canadian ancestry, and come from a region of Quebec where 1:1600 newborns are affected with tyrosinemia. What is the carrier frequency of tyrosinemia in this region? You learn that 90% of mutations responsible for tyrosinemia in this population consist of the same single base change. This mutation is much less common elsewhere in the world. What is most likely to account for the high frequency of this mutation in a small region in Quebec?

7.4 A sudden wave of migration brings a large number of new individuals into a population. For an autosomal recessive trait, how long does it take for a new Hardy–Weinberg equilibrium to be reached, assuming that there is random mating between all members of the new population, including newcomers and original inhabitants?

7.5 Consider a locus with three alleles, a, b, and c, with frequencies of 0.2, 0.3, and 0.5, respectively. What is the frequency of bc heterozygotes in the population, assuming Hardy–Weinberg equilibrium?

FURTHER READING

General References

Khoury MJ, McCabe LL, McCabe ER. Population screening in the age of genomic medicine. New Engl J Med 2003;348:50–58.

Clinical Snapshot 7.1 Sickle Cell Anemia

Buchanan GR, DeBaun MR, Quinn CT, Steinberg MH. Sickle cell disease. Hematol 2004;1:35–47.

Clinical Snapshot 7.2 Tay–Sachs Disease

Desnick RJ, Kaback MM. Future perspectives for Tay–Sachs disease. Adv Genet 2001;44:349–356.

Ethical Implications 7.1 Genetic Variation and Race

Foster MW, Sharp RR. Beyond race: towards a whole-genome perspective on human populations and genetic variation. Nat Rev Genet 2004;5:790–796.

Hot Topics 7.1 Public Health Genetics

Khoury MJ, Millikan R, Little J, Gwinn M. The emergence of epidemiology in the genomics age. Int J Epidemiol 2004;33:936–944.

8

Cancer Genetics

INTRODUCTION

We have focused thus far on genetic traits present in cells throughout the body, either owing to inheritance from a parent or to new mutation. We have encountered instances in which genetic variation exists from cell to cell in an individual, owing to mosaicism for nuclear genetic traits or heteroplasmy for mitochondrial mutations. We now turn our attention to another form of somatic genetic variation, acquired genetic change leading to malignancy. Chromosomal changes in cancer cells were recognized early in the 20th century, and it was later found that environmental agents that cause cancer are also mutagenic. Families at high risk for specific cancers were recognized. All this suggested that genetic change might underlie the pathogenesis of malignancy, a hypothesis that has been overwhelmingly confirmed in recent years. It now is recognized that a tumor arises as a clonal growth, originating from genetic change in a single cell. The properties referred to as malignancy represent phenotypic features due to the accumulation of changes in multiple genes. The recognition of these genes, referred to as tumor suppressor genes and oncogenes, has led to major advances in understanding cancer biology. This, in turn, has led to improvements in diagnostic techniques and the promise of improved methods of treatment for persons with cancer. It has also shed light on the mechanisms of normal cell growth and differentiation.

KEY POINTS

- Several lines of evidence support the idea that cancer is the result of genetic changes in somatic cells.
- Two major types of genes that contribute to malignant change are tumor suppressor genes and oncogenes.
- Tumor suppressor genes contribute to transformation to cancer when both alleles are mutated. In some cases, one of the mutations is inherited, the other acquired somatically.
- Oncogenes are normal cellular genes that, when activated by mutation, convey abnormal growth properties, contributing to malignancy.
- Oncogenes encode proteins that are involved in the signal transduction pathways involved in stimulation of cell growth; tumor suppressor genes encode proteins involved in regulation of growth.
- Progression towards malignancy is a multistep process due to the gradual accumulation of genetic changes, including activation of oncogenes and loss of function of tumor suppressor genes.
- Knowledge of the molecular basis of cancer is increasingly being used to develop methods of diagnosis and new treatments.

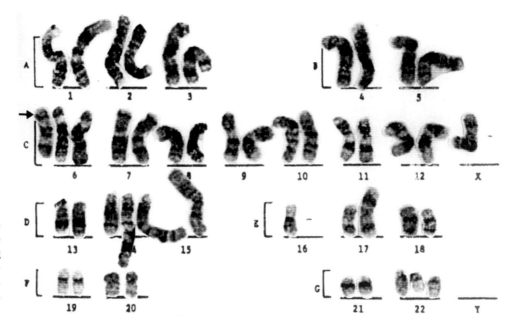

Figure 8.1 • G-banded karyotype from retinoblastoma. Numerous chromosome abnormalities are present including isochromosome for the short arm of chromosome 6 (*arrow*). (Courtesy of Dr. Brenda Gallie, Hospital for Sick Children, Toronto.)

What is the evidence that cancer is a genetic disorder?

CANCER IS A GENETIC DISORDER

A connection between cancer and genetics began to be suspected long before the existence of the gene was firmly established. The notion dates back to the early years of the 20th century, articulated by the pathologist Theordor Boveri, who noticed abnormalities of the nucleus in cancer cells. Over the ensuing decades, four lines of evidence converged to demonstrate that cancer is, in essence, a form of genetic disease. These were the observation of chromosomal anomalies in cancer, the existence of families in which cancer is transmitted as a genetic trait, the fact that carcinogens also tend to be mutagens, and the occurrence of individuals with DNA repair deficiency syndromes who are at increased risk of cancer.

The chromosomal basis of malignancy dates back to Boveri's observation, but received substantial support after it became possible to efficiently study mammalian chromosomes in the 1950s. It rapidly became clear that cancer cells often harbor multiple chromosomal rearrangements (Figure 8.1). Sometimes a particular type of cancer is associated with a specific rearrangement. This is the case in chronic myelogenous leukemia (CML), where a translocation between chromosomes 9 and 22 results in a foreshortened 22 referred to as the "Philadelphia chromosome"(Figure 8.2). The Philadelphia chromosome was used as a marker of CML long before the molecular basis for the rearrangement came to be understood (to be described later in this chapter). Many other cancers have been found to be associated with specific chromosomal markers, and others are characterized by wide-scale chromosome abnormality without a reproducible pattern. Whatever the mechanism of these chromosomal changes, it is clear that alterations of chromosome structure are common in cancer, and presumably are involved in the etiology of the disease.

Familial clustering of cancer represents the second line of evidence. Cancer is common in the general population, so virtually everyone has a family history of cancer in some relative. Some families, however, seem to be singled out for an unusually high frequency of cancer, with the disease segregating in a Mendelian pattern. An example is Li–Fraumeni syndrome (MIM 151623) (Figure 8.3), where there is autosomal dominant transmission of multiple, different forms of cancer. Other examples include various forms of colon cancer and breast and ovarian cancer. The fact that it was possible to inherit a predisposition to malignancy as the sole phenotype suggested that genes must be involved in cancer etiology.

We have seen that various types of chemicals or radiation exposure can be mutagenic. Likewise, it has been known for many years that certain chemicals and radiation can predispose to malignancy. There is very substantial overlap in the list of carcinogens and mutagens. Most, though not all, carcinogens are mutagenic, and most mutagens are capable of stimulating the growth of malignancies.

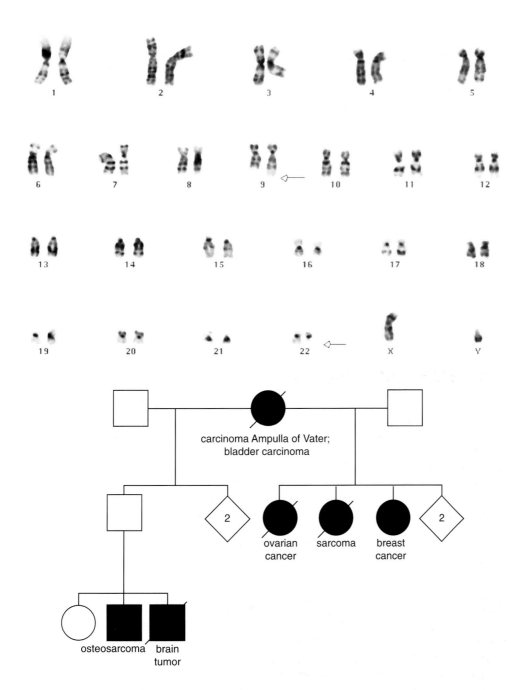

Figure 8.2 • Karyotype showing the Philadelphia chromosome, consisting of a translocation between chromosomes 9 and 22 (*arrows*).

Figure 8.3 • Pedigree of family with Li–Fraumeni syndrome. (Redrawn from Malkin D, Li FP, Strong LC, *et al.* Germ line p53 mutations in a familial syndrome of breast cancer, sarcomas, and other neoplasms. Science 1990;250:1233–1238.)

The fourth line of evidence comes from the study of individuals with disorders of DNA repair. We have seen in Chapter 2 that there is an organized system whereby the cell is able to repair DNA damage. Failure of this system causes a distinctive phenotype, which often includes a high risk of cancer. In xeroderma pigmentosum, for example, there is an inability to repair DNA damage done by UV exposure. Affected individuals are at high risk of skin cancer, resulting from sun exposure on the skin. All of the other DNA repair disorders described in Chapter 2 are associated with an increased risk of cancer, provided the affected individual lives long enough.

TUMOR SUPPRESSOR GENES

The first inroads into the molecular genetics of cancer involved the study of a rare childhood cancer, retinoblastoma (Clinical Snapshot 8.1). Retinoblastoma affects ganglion cells in the eye during early childhood. Both hereditary and nonhereditary forms exist, but both are due to disturbances in the same gene, called *Rb*, which functions as a **tumor suppressor gene**.

What are tumor suppressor genes?

CLINICAL SNAPSHOT 8.1

■ Retinoblastoma

Tom is a 2-year-old referred by his pediatrician for an ophthalmological examination. The referral was set up because the pediatrician was unable to see a red reflex in the back of Tom's right eye. A dilated fundoscopic exam is done, and a mass is seen in the retina, indicative of retinoblastoma. Tom has been in good health and his parents had not suspected a problem. There is no family history of retinoblastoma. Tom has one sibling, a 3-year-old sister.

Retinoblastoma is a malignant tumor of the retina. It occurs in young children, usually in the first few years of life. The tumor often comes to attention as an area of pallor at the back of the eye (Figure 8.4). This may be noticed during an eye examination as part of routine well-child care. Another sign of retinoblastoma is strabismus, or crossing of the eyes. Early recognition of retinoblastoma is essential for effective treatment. Retinoblastoma cells can detach from the retina and seed the vitreous of the eye. Spread also can occur back in the orbit, into the brain, and elsewhere in the body. Left untreated, the tumor is invariably fatal, but early recognition not only can be lifesaving but also can preserve vision. Treatment typically consists of radiation therapy, applied over several weeks. This usually is effective in dealing with tumors localized to the eye. Systemic chemotherapy is used if there is evidence of tumor spread. Other modes of treatment may be used for very small, intraocular tumors. These include photocoagulation (using light to burn the tumor cells through the lens of the eye), cryotherapy (freezing tumor cells through the eye), or implantation of radioactive substances into the eye. Advanced tumors that have destroyed vision may be treated by removal of the affected eye.

Prognosis in children treated for retinoblastoma has improved markedly over the years. Long-term survival now exceeds 90% for tumors recognized before systemic spread. For many, the greatest risk is posed by the development of a second, independent tumor at a different site in the same eye, in the other eye, or elsewhere in the body, especially osteosarcoma (malignant bone tumor).

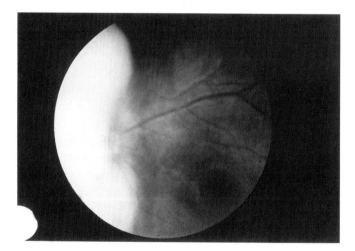

Figure 8.4 ● Photograph of retina in child with retinoblastoma. The left side of the retina is obscured by tumor. (Courtesy of Dr. Robert Petersen, Children's Hospital, Boston.)

Approximately 10% of children with retinoblastoma have a family history of the disorder (Figure 8.5). Retinoblastoma occurs in these families as an autosomal dominant trait, with approximately 90% penetrance. Among those with no family history, nearly 30% turn out to have a germinal mutation leading to familial retinoblastoma. The remainder has sporadic retinoblastoma with no genetic predisposition. The major distinguishing features of sporadic

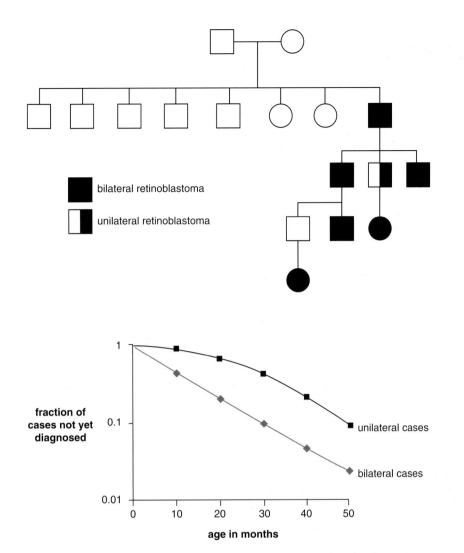

Figure 8.5 • Pedigree showing dominant transmission of retinoblastoma. Some individuals have unilateral tumors, whereas others have bilateral retinoblastoma. The father of the youngest affected female is himself unaffected, indicative of nonpenetrance. (Redrawn by permission from Vogel F. Genetics of retinoblastoma. Hum Genet 1979;52:1–54.)

Figure 8.6 • Graph of fraction of cases of retinoblastoma not yet diagnosed as function of age for individuals who developed unilateral or bilateral retinoblastomas. The rate of accumulation of cases of bilateral retinoblastoma was logarithmic, whereas the unilateral cases increased more slowly. (Data from Knudson AG Jr. Mutation and cancer: statistical study of retinoblastoma. Proc Natl Acad Sci USA 1971;68:820–823.)

versus hereditary retinoblastoma are age at onset and number of tumors. Hereditary cases often are diagnosed within the first year of life, whereas sporadic tumors may be recognized as late as age 7 to 10 years. This is not due entirely to more careful scrutiny of children in hereditary cases, especially as the majority are the result of new mutations. Hereditary cases also tend to be multifocal (occurring at several places in an eye) or in both eyes. Approximately two-thirds of those with hereditary retinoblastoma have multifocal involvement. Aside from multifocal eye involvement, there is a risk later in life of nonocular tumors, such as osteosarcoma or breast cancer.

In 1971, Alfred Knudson reviewed records of children with either unilateral or bilateral retinoblastoma. At the time retinoblastoma was first diagnosed, children who eventually developed bilateral tumors were younger than children whose tumors remained unilateral. The rate of diagnosis of bilateral cases increased exponentially with time, whereas the rate of diagnosis for unilateral cases increased much more slowly (Figure 8.6). Knudson proposed a model (Figure 8.7) in which retinoblastoma formation requires the occurrence of two separate mutation events in a retinal cell lineage. Individuals with hereditary retinoblastoma have inherited one of these mutations, and therefore all their retinal cells carry the mutation. Only one additional event needs to occur to produce a tumor. In contrast, sporadic retinoblastoma only occurs when two independent mutational events occur in the same cell lineage. This would be expected to be much rarer, and so age at onset is later and tumors are invariably unilateral. Knudson's hypothesis has come to be called the **two-hit hypothesis**. It has been the cornerstone for understanding hereditary predisposition to malignancy.

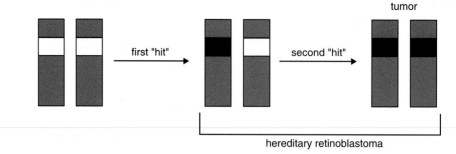

Figure 8.7 • Two-hit model. A tumor ensues when two events have occurred in the same cell lineage that knock out both copies of a gene. Two rare events must occur to produce a sporadic tumor. A person who is born with the first mutation, however, needs to acquire only one additional mutation to develop a tumor.

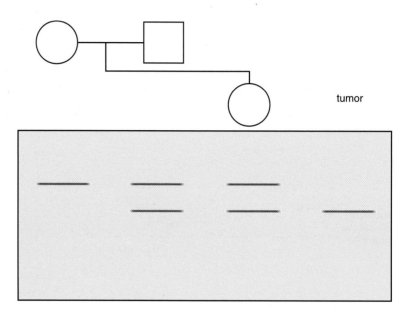

Figure 8.8 • Loss of heterozygosity for polymorphic marker on chromosome 13. DNA from the mother, father, and daughter, as well as the daughter's retinoblastoma tumor, was digested with *Hind*III and hybridized on a Southern blot with a DNA sequence from chromosome 13q14. The mother is homozygous for the upper allele and the father and affected daughter are heterozygous. DNA from the retinoblastoma, however, shows only the lower allele, indicating loss of the upper allele in the tumor.

The molecular basis for the two-hit hypothesis was established with the cloning of a gene, now referred to as *RB1*, on chromosome 13 that was found to be the first step in retinoblastoma carcinogenesis. One copy of the gene was found to be mutated in all cells of individuals with hereditary retinoblastoma. In retinoblastoma tumors, however, both copies of the gene are mutated. Sometimes, one copy is deleted in the tumor, referred to as **loss of heterozygosity** (Figure 8.8). The copy that is lost is invariably the one inherited from the nonaffected parent. Other times that copy of the gene is not deleted, but is mutated. The net effect is that both copies of the gene are nonfunctional in tumor cells.

The retinoblastoma gene was the first of a series of genes to be identified that are associated with familial predisposition to cancer. Other examples are listed in Table 8.1. These syndromes are dominantly inherited. Tumors that occur in affected persons are seen also in the general population, but those with the hereditary form develop them earlier in life and often have multiple, independent cancers. The genes have come to be referred to as **tumor suppressor genes**. They behave in a recessive manner at the cellular level, so that both copies of the gene must be inactivated in order for a tumor to occur. Within a family, however, they act as dominant traits. What is transmitted from generation to generation, though, is not the malignancy itself but rather the risk of development of malignancy. This is conveyed by transmission of one mutant allele at the tumor suppressor locus, so that only one event need occur – mutation of the remaining normal copy of the gene – for a cell to become a tumor. For these same tumors to occur in the general population requires two rare events: mutation of the first copy of the gene and then mutation of the second copy in the same cell lineage. This does occur, but only rarely.

The term tumor suppressor gene is apt, though in one sense it is misleading. It implies that the normal function of the gene is to prevent the cell from becoming a tumor. Is this truly the

TABLE 8.1 Some tumor suppressor genes, associated syndromes resulting from germ-line mutations, and characteristic tumors

Gene	Syndrome	Major tumors
APC	Familial adenomatous polyposis	Bowel carcinoma
VHL	Von Hippel–Lindau syndrome	Hemangioblastoma, pheochromocytoma, renal cell carcinoma
TP53	Li-Fraumeni syndrome	Soft-tissue sarcoma, glioma, leukemia
BRCA1/2	Familial breast and ovarian cancer	Breast and ovarian cancer
NF1	Neurofibromatosis 1	Neurofibroma, astrocytoma, sarcoma, leukemia
NF2	Neurofibromatosis 2	Schwannoma, meningioma, ependymoma
RB	Retinoblastoma	Retinoblastoma, osteosarcoma
TSC1/2	Tuberous sclerosis complex	Cortical dysplasia, renal angiomyolipoma
WT1	WAGR – Wilms' tumor, aniridia, genitourinary anomalies, growth retardation	Wilms' tumor
P16	Familial melanoma	melanoma
MSH2, MLH1, PMS1, PMS2, GTBP,	Hereditary nonpolyposis colon cancer	Colorectal carcinoma, endometrial carcinoma
PTCH	Basal cell nevus syndrome	Basal cell carcinoma, medulloblastoma
MEN1	Multiple endocrine neoplasia 1	Islet cell adenoma, pituitary adenoma, parathyroid adenoma

normal role of these genes? Understanding the function of tumor suppressor genes and the way that loss of this function results in tumor formation requires a more complete unveiling of the various genetic changes that accompany cancer.

ONCOGENES

The discovery of the first oncogene was based on work begun long before DNA was known to be the genetic material. Peyton Rous, working at the Rockefeller Institute for Medical Research in New York in 1909, began a series of experiments that started with a chicken that had a lump on its leg. The lump was a soft-tissue sarcoma. When Rous ground up some of this tumor and injected it into other chickens they, too, developed sarcomas. The active agent was identified as a virus – in fact, a retrovirus – and was called *Rous sarcoma virus*. Decades later, it was found that of the four genes in this virus, one, referred to as *src*, is responsible for the transforming properties. When *src* is lost or mutated, the virus is no longer oncogenic.

By the 1980s, approximately 20 different retroviruses, each containing a distinct oncogene, were known to be associated with cancer. These oncogenes were identified by three-letter abbreviations, usually named for tumor types they caused (e.g., *erb*-B for erythroblastosis). The breakthrough in understanding nonretroviral malignancies was recognition that viral oncogenes are homologous with normal eukaryotic genes. For example, the viral *src* gene, or v-*src*, is homologous to a eukaryotic *src* gene, referred to as c-*src* (for cellular *src*). These normal cellular genes are referred to as **proto-oncogenes**. Apparently, the overexpression of a

What are oncogenes?

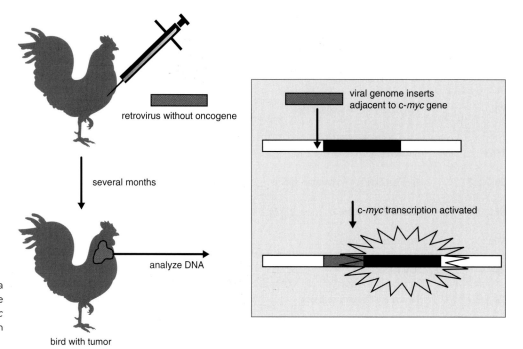

Figure 8.9 • Insertion of avian leukemia retrovirus lacking an oncogene into a site in an avian genome adjacent to c-*myc* gene. Activation of c-*myc* transcription results in tumor formation.

proto-oncogene due to regulation by the viral genome is responsible for its transforming properties.

When a retrovirus containing an oncogene infects an animal, there is usually a latent period of 2 to 3 weeks before a tumor grows. Some, however, are oncogenic with a longer latency of many months. When retroviruses infect cells, the cDNA copy of the viral genome integrates into the host cell genome. Longer-latency retroviruses do not carry oncogenes. Examination of the DNA from tumors in infected animals, however, indicates that the virus has integrated, by chance, adjacent to a cellular proto-oncogene (Figure 8.9). This places the cellular gene under the influence of the active retroviral promoter, activating the proto-oncogene and causing a tumor. Rarely, an aberrant recombination event causes the cellular proto-oncogene to incorporate into the viral genome. This is how oncogenes are "captured" from the eukaryotic genome by retroviruses.

Not all proto-oncogenes were discovered from studies with retroviruses. Oncogenes exert a dominant effect – that is, overexpression of one copy contributes some transformed properties to the cell. An assay was developed whereby DNA was isolated from tumor cells, broken into pieces, and then introduced into nontransformed cells (Figure 8.10). In the presence of calcium phosphate, the isolated DNA is taken up into the cells by a process known as **transfection**. Some DNA integrates into the recipient cell genome and is expressed. Using a mouse fibroblast cell line as recipient, it was found that transfection of tumor cell DNA resulted in isolation of fibroblast clones with some properties of transformation, such as ability to grow in soft agar. When human tumor cells were used as the donor, the transfected DNA could be identified in the mouse cells because of the presence of repeated sequences found in the human but not the mouse genome. It was found that the transforming genes corresponded in some cases with oncogenes already known to be involved in retroviral-mediated oncogenesis. Moreover, it was found that specific oncogenes tended to be involved in certain tumor types.

Oncogenes are normal cellular genes that, when their patterns of expression are changed, confer on the cell some neoplastic properties. There are many routes to oncogene activation. Some have already been mentioned – namely incorporation into a virus or insertion of a retrovirus adjacent to a proto-oncogene. Most mechanisms do not rely on viruses, though. The most direct route to proto-oncogene activation is gene amplification, wherein a block of DNA, including an oncogene and some neighboring genes, is replicated tens or hundreds of times in the cell. This probably occurs by random errors of DNA replication but, when it occurs, a

How are proto-oncogenes activated?

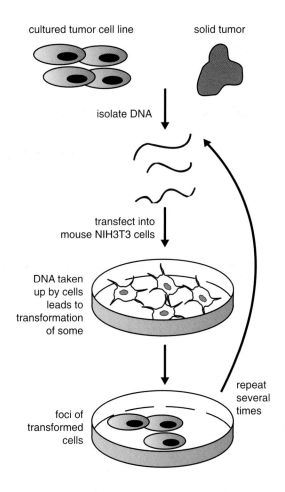

cultured tumor cell line

solid tumor

isolate DNA

transfect into
mouse NIH3T3 cells

DNA taken
up by cells
leads to
transformation
of some

foci of
transformed
cells

repeat
several
times

Figure 8.10 • Identification of transforming genes by transfection of tumor DNA into mouse fibroblasts. DNA was isolated from tumor cell lines or from solid tumors. This was added to cultures of mouse NIH 3T3 fibroblasts, which grow indefinitely in culture but otherwise do not display a transformed phenotype. Some of the human DNA is taken up by the mouse cells and, in rare instances, results in transformation of the cells. These transformed cells had abnormal appearance, grew to high density, and could be cultured in soft agar (indicating lack of requirement for a solid surface on which to grow). The process was repeated for several iterations, using DNA from the transformed cells, effectively purifying the transforming genes from the rest of the human DNA. Analysis of the human DNA in the transformed cells revealed homology with known viral oncogenes.

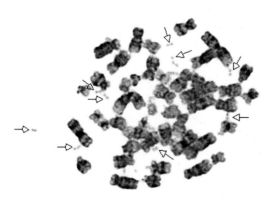

Figure 8.11 • Double minute chromatin bodies (arrows) in tumor cell metaphase. (Courtesy of Dr. Andrew Carroll, University of Alabama at Birmingham).

selective advantage is conferred on the cell, which proliferates faster than other cells in the tissue. Tumor cells with gene amplification contain tiny objects referred to as **double minute chromatin bodies**, which harbor the amplified DNA (Figure 8.11).

Another route to proto-oncogene activation is through chromosome rearrangement. This was first demonstrated in the Burkitt lymphoma tumor (Figure 8.12), which commonly includes a translocation between chromosomes 8 and 14. The breakpoint on chromosome 14 corresponds with the immunoglobulin heavy-chain locus, and that on chromosome 8 with a proto-oncogene, c-*myc*. The immunoglobulin heavy-chain gene tends to undergo rearrangement during the process of lymphocyte maturation and, on rare occasions, this

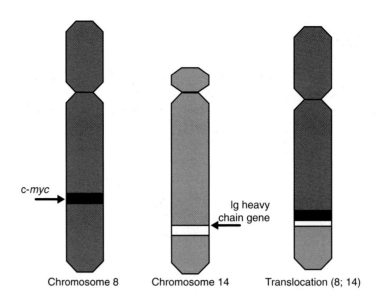

Figure 8.12 • Translocation between chromosomes 8 and 14 in Burkitt lymphoma, juxtaposing the c-*myc* proto-oncogene into the immunoglobulin (Ig) heavy-chain locus. This alters the regulation of c-*myc* expression, contributing to the malignant phenotype. (Modified from Taub R, Morton C, Lenoir G, *et al.* Translocation of the c-*myc* gene into the immunoglobulin heavy chain locus in human Burkitt lymphoma and murine plasmacytoma cells. Proc Natl Acad Sci USA 1982;79:7837–7841.)

rearrangement process goes awry. If an aberrant rearrangement juxtaposes the heavy-chain gene with the *myc* oncogene, altered expression of the oncogene ensues and contributes to tumor formation.

In most cases, activation of a proto-oncogene is not associated with a visible change in chromosome structure. The transforming gene isolated from transfection of DNA from bladder carcinoma cells is the *ras* oncogene, also a retroviral oncogene. In bladder carcinomas, the *ras* gene is found to be mutated, a single base substitution leading to an altered amino acid. The mutations tend to occur at characteristic sites in the gene and lead to an altered protein that causes transformation of the cell.

NORMAL ROLES OF TUMOR SUPPRESSOR GENES AND ONCOGENES

How do tumor suppressor genes and oncogenes function in noncancer cells?

The discovery of oncogenes and tumor suppressor genes has revealed the major cast of characters responsible for the growth of neoplastic cells. It remains for the tools of molecular biology to reveal their roles. Although this story still is unfolding, major advances have been made relatively quickly.

Dominant proto-oncogenes sort into four classes of molecules, all of which are involved in the control of cell differentiation and proliferation (Figure 8.13). The first class encodes growth factors. The prototype is the proto-oncogene c-*sis*, which encodes the beta-chain of platelet-derived growth factor. Such growth factors are able to stimulate the proliferation of certain types of cells. Overexpression, or expression of an aberrant protein, leads to enhanced cell proliferation. Tumor cells that secrete such factors and simultaneously respond to them are subject to autocrine growth control.

Growth factors must interact with membrane receptors to exert their activity, and growth factor receptors comprise the second class of proto-oncogene products. A mutation that renders a receptor active even in the absence of ligand, or that binds ligand abnormally, might render the cell independent of growth factors for control of proliferation. The proto-oncogene c-*erb-B* corresponds with the epidermal growth factor receptor. The viral v-*erb-B* is a truncated form of this receptor with abnormal activity. Binding of a growth factor leads to dimerization of the receptor and activation of tyrosine kinase domains, which leads to phosphorylation of tyrosine residues on the receptor as well as other membrane proteins. Phosphorylation serves as an activating signal that leads the proteins to interact with others. Some of these other proteins also have tyrosine kinase activity and transmit an activation signal to target proteins by phosphorylation. An example of such a downstream target is the *src* gene product.

The third class of membrane-associated proteins has the ability to phosphorylate serine or threonine residues. These include the product of the *raf* proto-oncogene. Another group consists of proteins that bind guanosine triphosphate (GTP), of which *ras* is the prototype. *Ras* is

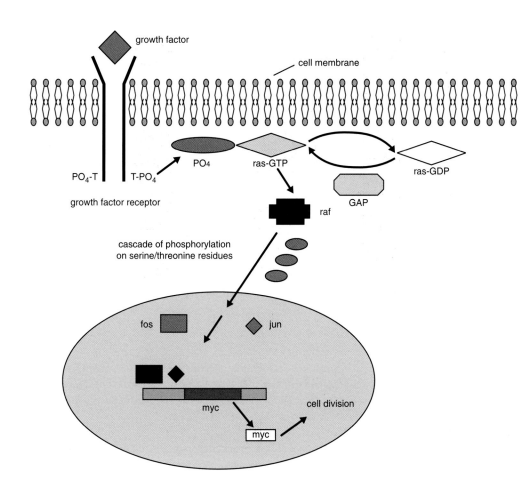

Figure 8.13 • Cascade pathway of activation of cell division involving oncogene products. A growth factor binds to a specific membrane receptor, which dimerizes and activates tyrosine kinase activity. This leads to autophosphorylation of the receptor, as well as phosphorylation of other membrane proteins at tyrosine (*T*) residues. The oncogene product *ras* then is activated by binding to guanosine triphosphate (*GTP*), which in turn leads to activation of the product of the *raf* oncogene. GTPase-activating proteins (*GAP*) convert the active *ras*-GTP into an inactive *ras*-GDP complex, limiting the duration of *ras* activation. The raf protein sets into motion a series of phosphorylation events involving other proteins, which then enter the nucleus and activate the transcription factors *fos* and *jun*. These then bind to the promoter of the *myc* gene, activating transcription. The *myc* gene product, in turn, activates other genes involved in stimulation of cell division. (*GDP* = guanosine diphosphate.)

activated by signals transmitted from membrane receptors and, in turn, transmits a signal by modification of other proteins. Oncogenic *ras* mutations lead to overexpression of the activated form of the protein or insensitivity to other proteins that regulate *ras* activity.

The final class of oncogenes is the group that controls transcription in the nucleus. These include *myc*, *jun*, and *fos*. Direct activation of these factors can lead to abnormal cell proliferation or differentiation in the absence of appropriate signals transmitted across the cell membrane and through the cytoplasm. It is here that the Rb gene product is active. The Rb protein is phosphorylated as the cell transits from G1 to S phase and plays a role in the transit of the cell from interphase to DNA synthesis. Loss of Rb activity removes this control point. The Rb protein binds to three proteins that were identified initially as oncogenes from three DNA-containing tumor viruses. These oncogenes are referred to as *E1A* (an adenovirus oncogene), *SV40 large T antigen*, and *papillomavirus E7 protein*. It has been hypothesized that overexpression of these proteins in virally transformed cells binds the Rb protein and thus inhibits it, effecting the same outcome as if Rb were homozygously mutated. In fact, expression of SV40 large T antigen in the retina of transgenic mice results in retinoblastoma formation.

The mechanism of action of other tumor suppressor genes is also gradually coming to light. The *NF1* gene product, which is mutated in individuals with neurofibromatosis type 1, is a GTPase-activating protein (GAP), which regulates *ras* activity by stimulating GTPase activity. Loss of the *NF1* gene product is believed to lead to unimpeded *ras* activity. The *TP53* gene is mutated in a wide variety of tumor types and is involved in a familial cancer syndrome, Li–Fraumeni syndrome, in which sarcomas, brain tumors, and leukemias occur with high frequency. Like Rb, the *TP53* gene appears to be involved in the regulation of the cell cycle, causing the cell to pause before DNA synthesis to repair DNA damage, or to undergo **apoptosis** (programmed cell death) if the damage is irreparable. Loss of p53 activity would allow cells to proceed through division without repairing DNA damage, and thus increase the likelihood of survival of cells with genetic alterations that may contribute to malignancy. The *APC* gene, involved in familial adenomatous polyposis (MIM 175100) (Clinical Snapshot 8.2), regulates transmission of a signal from the cell surface to the nucleus that leads to c-*myc* expression. These tumor suppressor genes have been described as having a "gatekeeper" function; that is, they regulate basic cell functions such as the initiation of proliferation, differentiation, or apoptosis.

A different type of genetic defect has been found to underlie the syndrome of hereditary nonpolyposis colon cancer (HNPCC) (MIM 114500). A hallmark of these tumors is the occurrence of a phenomenon of "**microsatellite instability**," meaning that simple sequence repetitive DNA elements show excessive size variability due to inaccurate replication (Figure 8.15). This has been attributed to loss of activity of any of six genes involved in repair of mismatched bases in DNA: *MSH2, MLH1, PMS1, PMS2,* and *GTBP* (also called *MSH6*). These function as tumor suppressor genes, in that individuals with HNPCC are heterozygous for a mutation in any one of these genes, but the tumor cells will be found to be homozygous for a mutation in one of the genes. Loss of activity leads to a hypermutable state, in which mutations will accumulate in other dominant or recessive oncogenes, leading to tumor progression. A similar

CLINICAL SNAPSHOT 8.2

■ Hereditary colon cancer

Alice is a 40-year-old who is referred for counseling following a recent diagnosis of colon cancer. She had presented with rectal bleeding and was found to have an adenocarcinoma of the rectum. A colonoscopy had then revealed multiple adenomatous polyps throughout the colon. Alice is an only child, but her mother had died of colon cancer at age 50. She has no further information about her family history.

Colorectal cancer is the second most common form of cancer in the US. Although most cases occur sporadically, there are two major syndromes associated with autosomal dominant inheritance: familial adenomatous polyposis (FAP) and hereditary nonpolyposis colon cancer (HNPCC). Individuals with FAP develop multiple adenomatous polyps in the colon and rectum (Figure 8.14), as well as the stomach and duodenum. Polyps may begin in childhood and continue throughout life, and cancer occurs in almost all affected individuals, most commonly in the third or fourth decades. Other manifestations include congenital hypertrophy of the retinal pigment epithelium, dental anomalies, and soft tissue tumors. FAP is due to mutations in the tumor suppressor gene *APC*.

Individuals with HNPCC have about an 80% lifetime risk of colon cancer but do not develop adenomatous polyps. Women with HNPCC are also at risk of endometrial carcinoma. Other cancers associated with the disorder include small bowel carcinoma, urinary tract tumors, and glioblastoma. HNPCC is due to mutation in one of several DNA mismatch repair genes. These behave as tumor suppressors in that heterozygous mutation in the germline puts the individual at risk of loss of both alleles in the tumor, leading to defective DNA repair, an accumulation of mutations, and malignant change.

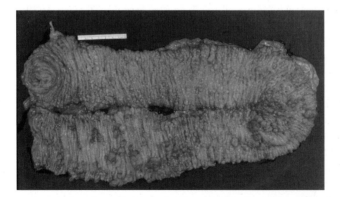

Figure 8.14 • Multiple polyps of the colon in a patient with familial adenomatous polyposis. (Photo courtesy of Dr. Ernesto Drelichman, University of Alabama at Birmingham.)

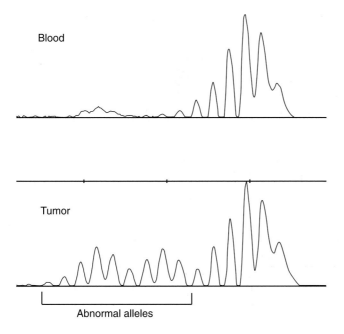

Blood

Tumor

Abnormal alleles

Figure 8.15 • Microsatellite instability. A microsatellite repeat is amplified by PCR and the length of amplified DNA analyzed by electrophoresis. The traces indicate band intensity along the electrophoresis gel. In blood DNA a set of bands is seen corresponding with two alleles of slightly different size. Multiple bands are seen due to inaccuracies of PCR amplification of the repeated sequence. In the tumor sample many additional bands are seen due to instability of the repeat during DNA replication. (Courtesy of Dr. Ludwine Messiaen, University of Alabama at Birmingham.)

mechanism underlies an increased risk of malignancy associated with a group of DNA repair disorders (see Chapter 2). These are recessively inherited, and increased risk of malignancy is due to an accelerated rate of accumulation of mutations, some of which activate dominant oncogenes or inactivate tumor suppressor genes. The genes involved in HNPCC and DNA repair disorders have been referred to as "**caretaker genes**."

A third class of genes that predispose to tumor formation is typified by *PTEN* and *SMAD4*. These genes are involved in juvenile polyposis (MIM 174900), in which benign polyps that have an increased risk of malignancy occur. Here it appears that the heterozygous mutation leads to abnormal proliferation of the stromal cells surrounding colonic epithelial cells. This is believed to result in an altered microenvironment and consequent aberrant cell growth, leading to malignant transformation. These genes have been described as having functions as "**landscapers**."

The products of oncogenes and tumor suppressor genes are part of a network of proteins that control cell growth. They represent steps in the pathway from the cell surface to the nucleus. A defect anywhere along the chain can render the cell incapable of responding to signals to stop dividing and differentiate or can trick the cell into a cycle of unstoppable proliferation.

THE MOLECULAR BASIS OF ONCOGENESIS

The path from a normal to a malignant cell comprises a series of genetic changes involving both dominant oncogenes and tumor suppressor genes. In the familial cancer syndromes, and perhaps in sporadic cancers as well, loss of a tumor suppressor gene appears to be rate-limiting: It is the change that sets into motion a cascade of events wherein genetic damage accumulates, leading to a complex set of abnormal properties. Moreover, there can be a snowballing of genetic change. As the tumor cells experience genetic damage and cell division becomes more rapid and disordered, additional damage occurs. Other tumor suppressor genes may be mutated or lost. Dominant oncogenes are activated. Novel genes may be created by translocation of two genes into one. The fusion proteins encoded by these new genes may confer new, abnormal properties to the cell. Some changes are deleterious and lead to cell death. If, however, a change occurs that causes the cell to grow faster or to be freed from dependence on a growth factor, that cell will have an advantage over others and may become the predominant cell type in the tumor. Tumor growth, then, is a process of natural selection. When the tumor finally is diagnosed, the tumor cells are highly evolved products of hundreds of generations of mutation and selection (Figure 8.16).

What are the molecular genetic changes that lead to initiation and progression of malignancy?

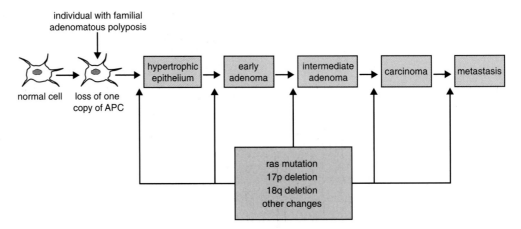

Figure 8.16 • Multistep pathway from normal cell to metastatic colon carcinoma. The rate-limiting step is postulated to be loss of the APC gene on chromosome 5. Individuals with familial adenomatous polyposis (FAP) inherit the first mutation (*APC* gene) and need to acquire only a second mutation. Other individuals need to acquire both mutations in the same cell lineage. This leads to a hypertrophic epithelium, however. Additional genetic damage is accumulated, including loss of sequences on chromosomes 17p and 18q as well as other changes. These can occur in any order but lead to progressively abnormal cells including, eventually, cells capable of metastasis. (Redrawn from Fearon ER, Vogelstein B. A genetic model for colorectal tumorigenesis. Cell 1990;61:759–767.)

Knowledge of genetic changes in malignancy has significantly improved the approach to cancer diagnosis and management. In the leukemias, cytogenetic analysis has long been used for diagnostic purposes. The first tumor-specific chromosome change to be identified was the Philadelphia chromosome in chronic myelogenous leukemia. Although originally believed to be a deleted chromosome 22, this eventually was found to represent a translocation of chromosomes 9 and 22, juxtaposing the proto-oncogene *abl* to a gene called *bcr* to generate a novel fusion gene. Detection of the Philadelphia chromosome is used in the diagnosis of leukemia and in following response to treatment. The first appearance of Philadelphia chromosome-positive cells in the bone marrow of patients after treatment is often the first sign of relapse. Sensitive detection methods based on PCR now provide early detection of such relapse, allowing treatment to be reinitiated before the tumor burden becomes substantial. The importance of the Philadelphia chromosome in developing a new treatment for chronic myelogenous leukemia will become apparent in the next section.

Diagnosis of cancer has been further refined using new approaches based on the analysis of patterns of gene expression. Tumor cells that look alike through the microscope may have very different clinical behavior and response to therapy. These differences may be reflected in expression of different sets of genes, which can now be analyzed using cDNA microarrays (Methods 8.1). Expression analysis is showing promise as a means of subclassifying tumors that may eventually guide choice of treatment and help determine prognosis.

Methods 8.1

Expression array analysis

Microarray analysis has enabled rapid analysis of the complement of genes expressed in a tissue. This provides a profile of gene expression that may be specific to the tissue in a particular physiological state. It also opens the door to searching for cancer-specific expression profiles that can be used to identify specific types of cancer and to predict response to therapy.

We have already considered the use of "gene chips" in Chapter 4. For expression analysis, the chip features contain either cDNAs or oligonucleotides that correspond with cDNA sequences. A prototypical experiment is illustrated in Figure 8.17. RNA is isolated from the tumor to be tested and labeled with a red fluorochrome. RNA isolated from a reference sample, such as a nontumor cell, is labeled in green. Both

Test RNA   Reference RNA

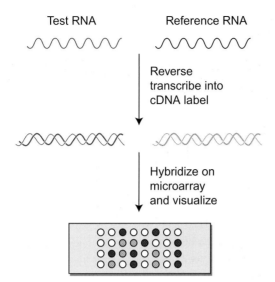

Reverse
transcribe into
cDNA label

Hybridize on
microarray
and visualize

Figure 8.17 • Microarray expression analysis. Thousands of different cDNAs are bound to a glass "chip", creating a grid with a different cDNA in each cell. RNA is isolated from a test and a control sample and made into two batches of cDNA. The test cDNA is labeled with a red fluorescent tag (shown here as dark blue) and the control is labeled with a green tag (shown here as light blue). Equal amounts of both are hybridized with cDNA bound to the chip. If an RNA species is more abundant in the test sample, the cell will show red fluorescence, whereas if the RNA is more abundant in the control, the cell will show green fluorescence. Computer analysis of the patterns of red and green fluorescence can be used to establish a profile of differences in gene expression between the two tissues.

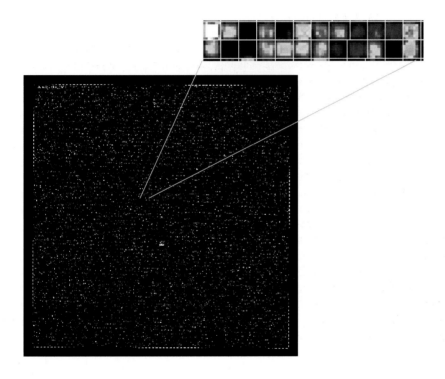

Figure 8.18 • Expression microarray of a tumor sample, with inset showing a close-up of individual cells. (Courtesy of Dr. Lihong Teng, University of Alabama at Birmingham.)

RNA samples are then hybridized with the DNA in the chip. If a particular RNA is represented more in the tumor than in the reference sample a feature will fluoresce in red; if the expression level is lower it will appear green.

Thousands of cDNAs can be included on a single chip, providing a massive amount of data on the profile of genes expressed in the test sample. Various analysis systems have been devised to make sense of this vast dataset. One approach is to perform cluster analysis, grouping samples that have in common high or low levels of expression of particular genes (Figure 8.18). This approach has been used to separate tumors that look the same pathologically into groups that have different biological behavior or response to treatment.

ETHICAL IMPLICATIONS 8.1 • Genetic testing of children

Should children be tested for risk of genetic disorders? It is common to offer genetic testing to children who display signs of symptoms of an inherited disorder. Achieving an accurate diagnosis can provide the basis for institution of treatment and providing anticipatory guidance to the family. Genetic testing can also provide a basis for accurate genetic counseling of the family.

What about testing of children for adult-onset disorders? Should a child at risk be tested for disorders such as Huntington disease, breast and ovarian cancer, or colon cancer? The consensus in the genetic community is that testing should be offered only in instances where the child will directly benefit from the outcome of testing. This may be the case for familial adenomatous polyposis, since polyps begin in childhood. A child at risk will begin to have sigmoidoscopy at around 10 years of age. If the child is found to not have inherited an *APC* mutation he or she can be spared from this uncomfortable procedure (at least until an age is reached where testing would be recommended regardless of family history). Disorders such as Huntington disease or breast and ovarian cancer usually do not present in childhood. For such disorders genetic testing is not recommended. Rather, it is suggested that testing be deferred until the child is old enough to understand the implications of testing and make an informed decision. The rationale is that the child will not immediately benefit from the results of testing, yet would be vulnerable to risks such as discrimination or stigmatization.

Genetic testing can be used not only to diagnose and monitor cancer in affected persons but also to identify some individuals at risk of developing malignancy in the first place. At present, this can be done for members of families with one of the syndromes listed in Table 8.1. Those who inherit a *TP53* mutation are at risk of developing sarcoma, brain tumor, or leukemia, characteristic of Li–Fraumeni syndrome. If the pathogenic mutation in the family is known, then any family member can be offered testing. As is increasingly true in genetics, however, knowing *how* is easier than knowing *why*. Early diagnosis of cancer usually is assumed to lead to a better outcome of treatment, but effective treatments do not exist for some of the cancers of Li–Fraumeni syndrome. The problem is especially difficult for young children (Ethical implications 8.1). Is it justified to submit children who cannot give informed consent to a lifetime of cancer surveillance, the benefit of which is unknown? Will persons found to have a *TP53* mutation be denied health insurance or employment? What are the psychological effects of being discovered to carry a mutation, and what is the impact of being found not to carry the mutation when other relatives are not as fortunate?

How can knowledge of the molecular basis of oncogenesis lead to new approaches to treatment?

NEW TREATMENTS FOR CANCER

Cancer is indeed a genetic disease, sometimes inherited but always showing somatically acquired genetic damage. The discovery of genes that underlie the transformation and progression of malignant cells is one of the great achievements in biology during the 20th century. Cancer diagnosis has been revolutionized, yet therapy still depends on the use of surgery or nonspecific killing of dividing cells with toxic drugs or radiation.

There is hope that new knowledge of the genetic mechanisms that underlie cancer may lead to novel approaches. A step in this direction has already occurred through the development of more precise means of genetic diagnosis (Hot Topics 8.1). Early diagnosis of relapsing chronic myelogenous leukemia by detection of the Philadelphia chromosome is an example. Genetic markers have also been used to distinguish histologically similar tumors that may respond differently to different means of therapy. An example is the distinction of Ewing sarcoma from neuroblastoma. These are histologically similar, small-cell, soft-tissue tumors, yet they are treated differently. Although classic pathologic markers may not distinguish these tumors, Ewing sarcomas typically have an 11;22 translocation, whereas neuroblastomas are characterized by deletion of chromosome 1p.

Hot Topics 8.1 EGFR MUTATIONS PREDICT LUNG CANCER TREATMENT RESPONSE

Non-small-cell lung cancer (NSCLC) is the most common form of malignancy in the US. Chemotherapy may prolong survival but the tumor is almost inevitably lethal in spite of treatment. Recently, a drug called gefitinib has been developed that inhibits the epidermal growth factor receptor (EGFR) tyrosine kinase activity. EGFR overexpression occurs commonly in NSCLC. Clinical trials have shown encouraging responses, but only in approximately 10 to 20% of treated patients.

Two papers have reported results that may indicate the reason for this low rate of response. Both groups examined the *EGFR* gene in patients with NSCLC who either did or did not respond to gefitinib. *EGFR* mutations were found in the majority of patients who responded to the drug, whereas few of those who did not. The mutations consisted of in-frame deletions or amino acid substitutions around the kinase domain. These mutations are gain of function changes that enhance kinase activity. Tumors with such mutations may be more dependent on EGFR activation, and therefore more sensitive to EGFR kinase inhibition by gefitinib.

This study is important because it provides a basis for stratification of the population of patients with NSCLC for further clinical trials. Those without *EGFR* mutations might be more appropriate candidates for other experimental treatments. It also provides a basis for prediction of response, although it should be noted that not all mutation-negative patients were nonresponders. Finally, it provides evidence in support of the notion that genetic testing can provide a basis for individualization of drug therapy to achieve optimal response.

Advances in therapy, though, are at a more primitive stage. Conventional modes of treatment are designed to kill all dividing cells. Side-effects result from killing of nontumor cells, and treatment failures are due to failure to kill all tumor cells. Sometimes, in fact, the tumor cells that survive develop drug resistance and may be more virulent than their predecessors. Research in cancer therapy therefore is directed toward the development of agents that are more selective for tumor cells. Approaches include inhibition of tumor blood supply, taking advantage of cell surface markers that are unique to tumor cells, or developing means of altering the activity of genes involved in oncogenesis.

The latter has taken advantage of new knowledge of the molecular genetics of cancer. The same complexity of the system that regulates cell growth, which makes the cell vulnerable to genetic changes that lead to malignancy, also offers many possible sites of intervention. Drugs are being developed that interact either with oncogenes or with other cellular proteins that interact with oncogenes. A dramatic example is a drug developed to treat CML. The *bcr–abl* gene fusion encodes a novel hybrid protein, which has the kinase activity of *abl*, but is expressed in the cytoplasm rather than the nucleus, where *abl* is normally expressed. A small molecule was developed that binds to the ATP binding site of this fusion protein, preventing binding of ATP to the site and thereby inhibiting the kinase activity (Figure 8.19). This drug, called imatinib, has produced dramatic remissions of CML, which had been largely refractory to conventional chemotherapy. The drug has also been used with success in some other tumors with mutation of oncogenes that have kinase activity. Imatinib does not cure the tumors, which

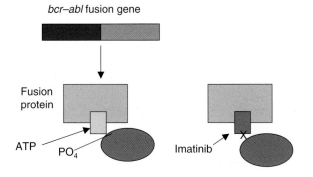

Figure 8.19 • Mechanism of action of imatinib. The *bcr–abl* fusion gene encodes a fusion protein that binds ATP and phosphorylates other cytoplasmic proteins. Imatinib competitively binds the ATP binding site and thereby prevents the fusion protein from phosphorylating other proteins.

develop resistance as mutations occur within the drug/ATP binding site. It is likely, however, that it will have a major role in treatment of CML and other cancers, along with either conventional or other mechanism-based therapies that will be used in combination.

CONCLUSION

A century of research has overwhelmingly verified the hypothesis that genetic change is the major driver of initiation and progression of malignancy. This is producing major new approaches to prevention, diagnosis, and management. Individuals at risk on the basis of family history can be identified and offered programs of surveillance and prevention, a point we will explore further in the second half of this book. Genetic approaches are gradually supplementing classical histology as a basis for diagnosis of specific cancer and choice of therapy. Ultimately, the greatest hope is the development of new treatments based on understanding the mechanisms of cancer.

REVIEW QUESTIONS

8.1 The nevoid basal cell carcinoma syndrome is characterized by the development of basal cell tumors in the skin, medulloblastoma of the cerebellum, and a number of congenital anomalies. It is transmitted as a autosomal dominant trait. The gene responsible for this disorder is found to be linked to a locus on chromosome 9. Analysis of a polymorphic marker in the linked region in a tumor and nontumor sample from an affected individual reveals heterozygosity in the patient's blood cells but absence of one allele in the tumor. What does this imply about the mechanism of action of the responsible gene regarding tumor formation? If the disorder was inherited from the father of the patient referred to above, would you predict that the allele lost in the tumor would be the one inherited from mother or father? Why might radiation therapy be a poor choice of treatment for cerebellar medulloblastomas in individuals with this syndrome?

8.2 Tumor suppressor gene mutations are often seen as constitutional mutations but oncogene mutations generally occur sporadically. What would you expect to be the consequence of germline inheritance of an activating oncogene mutation?

8.3 Why is familial predisposition to cancer associated with an earlier age of onset of tumors than occurs sporadically?

8.4 What is a mechanism by which chromosome translocation can activate a proto-oncogene? Is it possible that a translation could inactivate a tumor suppressor gene?

8.5 What is the significance of microsatellite instability when found in a colon carcinoma?

FURTHER READING

General References
Frank SA. Genetic predisposition to cancer – insights from population genetics. Nat Rev Genet 2004;5:764–772.

Garber JE, Offit K. Hereditary cancer predisposition syndromes. J Clin Oncol 2005;10:276–292.

Clinical Snapshot 8.1 Retinoblastoma
Abramson DH, Schefler AC. Update on retinoblastoma. Retina 2004;24:828–848.

Clinical Snapshot 8.2 Hereditary Colon Cancer
Jo WS, Chung DC. Genetics of hereditary colorectal cancer. Semin Oncol 2005;32:11–23.

Methods 8.1 Expression Array Analysis
Brentani RR, Carraro DM, Verjovski-Almeida S, Reis EM, Neves EJ, de Souza SJ, Carvalho AF, Brentani H, Reis LF. Gene expression arrays in cancer research: methods and applications. Crit Rev Oncol Hematol 2005;54:95–105.

Ethical Implications 8.1 Genetic Testing Of Children
Genetic Testing in Children and Adolescents, Points to Consider: Ethical Legal and Psychosocial Implications (ACMG/ASHG). Am J Hum Genet 1995;57:1233–1241.

Hot Topics 8.1 Lung Cancer Treatment

Lynch TJ, Bell DW, Sordella R, *et al.* Activating mutations in the epidermal growth factor receptor underlying responsiveness of non-small-cell lung cancer to gefitinib. New Eng J Med 2004;350:2129–2139.

Paez JG, Janne PA, Lee JC, *et al. EGFR* mutations in lung cancer: Correlation with clinical response to gefitinib therapy. Science 2004;304:1497–1500.

Genetics in Medical Practice

9
Chromosome Translocation

INTRODUCTION

Chromosomal analysis may be thought of as the first true genetic test, introduced in 1959 when trisomy 21 was found to be the cause of Down syndrome. A set of chromosomal aneuploidy syndromes was quickly discovered, making chromosomal analysis a standard part of the evaluation of an infant with congenital anomalies. Prenatal diagnosis by amniocentesis was introduced in the early 1960s. The ensuing decades have seen a progressive refinement of the approach to cytogenetic analysis, permitting precise characterization of chromosomal abnormalities at the submicroscopic and molecular levels. In this chapter we will explore the application of cytogenetic testing to diagnosis of an infant with multiple congenital anomalies. We will see how detection of the chromosomal basis for the child's problems leads to the ability to provide recurrence risk counseling and prenatal diagnosis. A variety of different approaches to prenatal diagnosis have been introduced, and pregnancies are now screened for the risk of Down syndrome. We will also look at advances in molecular cytogenetics that are rapidly changing the approach to cytogenetic analysis.

KEY POINTS

- Congenital anomalies occur in approximately 3% of pregnancies and are due to a wide variety of both genetic and nongenetic causes. Some multiple congenital anomaly syndromes are due to chromosomal abnormalities.
- Prenatal diagnosis by amniocentesis is commonly offered to women over 35 years of age due to an increased risk of trisomy, especially trisomy 21. Biochemical screening is being used to screen pregnancies for risk of trisomy.
- Chromosomal imbalance in a child can occur as a result of segregation of a balanced translocation in a parent. This leads to a risk of recurrence of the chromosomal abnormality in future pregnancies.
- The two most common approaches to obtaining fetal cells for prenatal diagnosis are amniocetesis, performed between 16 and 18 weeks' gestation and chorionic villus biopsy between 10 and 12 weeks' gestation.
- Cytogenetic analysis of fetal specimens may reveal a mixture of cells with or without a chromosomal abnormality, referred to as mosaicism. This may be indicative of true fetal mosaicism, or may arise during culture of the fetal cells.
- Molecular cytogenetic analysis, including fluorescence *in situ* hybridization and array comparative genomic hybridization are now being used to provide molecular characterization of submicroscopic chromosomal anomalies.

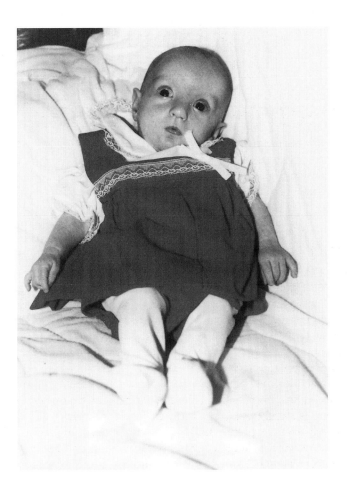

Figure 9.1 • Child with Wolf–Hirschhorn syndrome.

PART I

> *Karen was born after a full-term pregnancy. There were no medical problems during the pregnancy, but there was concern toward the end of term because her mother, Deborah, was not gaining weight as fast as expected. No prenatal testing had been done, as Deborah was 27 years old and there is no known family history of genetic problems. Deborah did have a blood test done during the second trimester, which she understood was to check that the baby was "developing normally," and she was told only that everything was "fine." An ultrasound examination done in the 8th month, though, showed the fetus to be small for gestational age. At birth, Karen weighs 4 pounds, 10 ounces. She is noted to have a number of unusual features (Figure 9.1), including widely spaced eyes, prominent nose, large ears, and bilateral iris colobomas. She is brought to the special care nursery where, on day two of life, she is found to have a heart murmur due to a ventricular septal defect. Karen is examined by a geneticist, who suggests that she might have Wolf–Hirschhorn syndrome.*

Approximately 3% of all babies are born with a congenital anomaly. In most cases, these anomalies involve a single part of the body – for example, cleft lip or a heart defect. Usually the problems are compatible with survival and can be surgically repaired. The body is formed normally beyond the one area that is malformed. There are some infants, however, who have multiple congenital anomalies, indicative of a more generalized disruption of embryonic development. Some of the malformations may be obvious (e.g., facial or limb defects). Internal organs such as the brain, heart, and kidneys often are involved as well. Surgical treatment may be possible for specific malformations, but most defects of the central nervous system, which lead to neurologic problems and developmental impairment, cannot be corrected.

Multiple congenital anomalies can occur due to many causes, such as infections acquired *in utero*, exposure to toxic agents (teratogens), and genetic factors. Genetic problems include single gene defects, chromosomal abnormalities, and multifactorial disorders.

Determining the etiology of multiple congenital anomalies can be challenging but is important both for care of the infant and for counseling of the family. Recognition of a pattern of anomalies can lead to the diagnosis of a syndrome – a constellation of distinctive features that is fairly consistent from individual to individual. Knowledge of features associated with a syndrome can alert the clinician to examine the child for internal anomalies that are not otherwise apparent. Some congenital infections can be treated with antibiotics to prevent further damage. The parents can be informed about future prospects for their child, both medically and developmentally. Finally, if a genetic disorder is identified, the family can be counseled about risks of recurrence.

Wolf–Hirschhorn syndrome consists of a set of multiple anomalies with a very distinctive facial appearance. The eyes are set widely apart and the nose is prominent. A coloboma is a defect in the formation of the iris or retina. There is often a cleft lip and palate. Cardiac defects are common and may cause heart failure in the early days of life. Usually, the brain is severely malformed, resulting in profound developmental impairment. Wolf–Hirschhorn syndrome is due to a chromosomal anomaly, specifically deletion of material from the short arm of chromosome 4.

A chromosome deletion could have been detected by prenatal analysis, but there was no indication for such testing with this pregnancy. Amniocentesis is generally offered if the mother will be 35 years of age or older at the time of delivery, due to the increased frequency of nondisjunction with advanced maternal age. Although the risk of having a child with trisomy increases with maternal age, most pregnancies occur in younger women, and hence most births of children with trisomy occur to younger women. Efforts have been made to identify those at risk of carrying affected fetuses by means other than assessment of age.

Several approaches have been developed to provide early prenatal screening for Down syndrome. The first to be widely used involves biochemical testing of analytes in the mother's blood in the second trimester. Alpha-fetoprotein is a serum protein produced by the fetus. A small quantity is excreted through the urine into amniotic fluid, and some crosses the placenta into the maternal circulation. Congenital malformations that create defects in the fetal body wall lead to large increases in amniotic fluid and maternal serum alpha-fetoprotein levels. During the course of screening for such defects, it was noticed that low amniotic fluid levels tend to occur more often if the fetus has a chromosomal abnormality, particularly trisomy 21. It was later found that addition of two other measurements – unconjugated estriol and human chorionic gonadotropin (βhCG) – increased the sensitivity of the screen. Fetuses with Down syndrome are associated with low alpha-fetoprotein and estriol levels but a high βhCG level in maternal serum. Low values for the three substances indicate a risk of trisomy 18. It is estimated that applying this "triple test" will detect 70% of fetuses with Down syndrome at a false positive rate of 5%. Addition of another analyte, inhibin-A, increases sensitivity to around 80%. Use of ultrasound to identify physical features consistent with Down syndrome, such as shortened humerus or femur or echogenic focus in the heart can increase sensitivity, but it is difficult to quantify this because of variation in the ultrasound approach used in different centers.

Although second-trimester screening is now routinely offered in most centers, approaches to first-trimester screening have been introduced and validated. The test involves measurement of nuchal translucency by ultrasound, as well as measurement of βhCG and pregnancy-associated plasma protein-A (PAPP-A) at 11 to 13 weeks. This provides a detection rate around 84% at a 5% false positive rate. Some centers combine first- and second-trimester screening, using a variety of approaches to calculate a final risk. Integrative testing provides a single risk figure based on the combined results of first- and second-trimester tests. Sequential testing involves first performing first-trimester screening and disclosure of results. If no prenatal test is done on the basis of these results, second-trimester screening is then done, with various approaches to risk assessment based on the first-trimester results.

A truly universal prenatal test for trisomy will require a risk-free and inexpensive means of fetal testing. Experiments are in progress with an approach based on analysis of fetal cells in the maternal circulation. Some fetal cells (trophoblast or blood cells) leak across the placenta just as does alpha-fetoprotein. Genetic analysis of these cells may someday actualize the dream of a risk-free test.

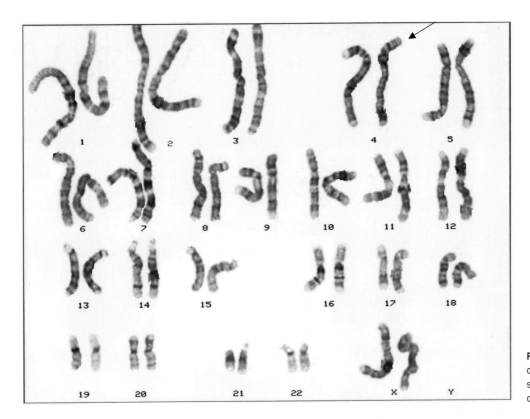

Figure 9.2 • Karyotype showing evidence of deletion of the short arm of chromosome 4, with abnormal material present on 4p (*arrow*).

PART II

Because Wolf–Hirschhorn syndrome is suspected, blood is sent to the laboratory for chromosomal analysis. Deborah and her husband Steven are told of the possible diagnosis. They are very anxious about Karen's future. They understand that the chromosomal analysis may take 2 weeks to be completed. Clinically, Karen is doing fairly well; her heart disease does not require treatment. She is being kept in the hospital mainly for nutritional support, until she gains some weight. Two weeks after Karen's blood sample is drawn, the laboratory reports that she does have a deletion involving material on the short arm of chromosome 4, with abnormal extra material attached to the end of 4 (Figure 9.2). FISH studies are done, and reveal that the extra material is derived from chromosome 8. This confirms the clinical diagnosis of Wolf–Hirschhorn syndrome, though in addition she has partial trisomy for the short arm of chromosome 8. Deborah and Steven discuss the finding with Karen's pediatrician and with the geneticist who was asked to see her. They are told that Karen has no life-threatening problems but that she will likely have significant developmental impairment. They are not really surprised at this by now, having had several weeks to adjust to Karen's condition. After nearly 3 weeks in the hospital, Karen is now gaining weight, and she is ready to be taken home.

Wolf–Hirschhorn syndrome was described in the early days of clinical cytogenetics, before chromosome banding. It is associated with deletion of material from the tip of the short arm of chromosome 4. The congenital anomalies are thought to result from loss of multiple genes in the region. The paradigm of a complex set of developmental anomalies resulting from deletion of multiple contiguous genes has been invoked for many chromosomal deletion syndromes (see Chapter 6). Efforts have been made to map the extent of deletion with specific phenotypic features in affected individuals but, the specific genes that are responsible for various aspects of the phenotype are not known.

More refined methods of chromosomal analysis have revealed that some apparent deletions are actually the result of translocations between two or more chromosomes. Sometimes these are visible with chromosome banding, but some require FISH to be detected. The

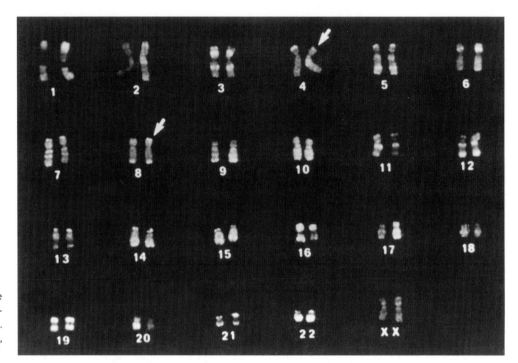

Figure 9.3 • R-banded karyotype showing balanced translocation between chromosomes 4 and 8 (*arrows*). (Courtesy of Cytogenetics Laboratory, Brigham and Women's Hospital, Boston.)

translocation in this child involves loss of material from the short arm of chromosome 4 and gain of material from the short arm of chromosome 8. The phenotype would be expected to reflect genetic imbalance of both chromosomal regions. The fact that the child has features of Wolf–Hirschhorn syndrome suggests that the chromosome 4 deletion has the predominant effect, perhaps because a larger region of chromosome 4 was lost than was gained for chromosome 8.

Most likely, the unbalanced translocation was the result of segregation of a balanced translocation in one of the parents. Chromosomal analysis of both parents should be carried out, since if one carries a balanced rearrangement there is a risk of having additional children with chromosomal imbalance.

PART III

Karen is now 2 years old. She did not require surgery for the ventricular septal defect, which closed on its own. She has had innumerable ear infections and has been hospitalized several times for pneumonia. Her parents are now interested in having other children, and speak with the geneticist to review the risk of recurrence of similar problems. It had been recommended that they have chromosomal analysis after Karen's deletion was identified, but they had put this off. Now, both parents have blood drawn. Deborah is found to have an apparently balanced translocation between chromosomes 4 and 8 (Figure 9.3). Deborah and Steven are counseled that there is a risk – in the range of 15% – for an abnormality in a subsequent pregnancy. Deborah's parents are tested, and her mother is found to carry the same translocation as Deborah. Her mother has a history of three miscarriages but no children born with congenital anomalies. Deborah is an only child. Deborah's mother had two sisters, both of whom are deceased, but each had several children. Deborah's mother is urged to inform these nieces and nephews of their potential for carrying the translocation (Figure 9.4).

We have seen in Chapter 6 how meiotic segregation of a balanced translocation can give rise to gametes with gains or losses of chromosomal segments. Alternate segregation will produce either normal chromosomes, or gametes with the balanced translocation. The unbalanced products, however, will likely result in some perturbation of development. Often, the developmental effects are of sufficient magnitude that spontaneous abortion occurs. This is

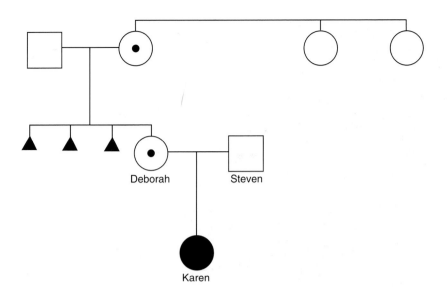

Figure 9.4 • Pedigree for Deborah and Steven.

probably the fate of most chromosomally abnormal embryos, and may occur so early that the pregnancy goes unrecognized. Only the more subtle imbalances are likely to be compatible with development to later stages of pregnancy, or development to term. These subtle imbalances, however, may be of sufficient magnitude to produce major congenital anomalies.

The risk of production of unbalanced gametes is difficult to predict. It depends on many factors, including the size of the translocated segment. Also, the risk is often different depending on whether the mother or the father is the carrier, for unknown reasons. Recurrence risks are derived empirically, but in many cases a particular translocation is unique to a particular family, making it difficult to provide accurate risk assessment.

Finding a balanced translocation in an individual warrants counseling of other family members who may also be at risk. There may be a family history of congenital anomalies, or, more commonly, of recurrent miscarriage. Chromosomal analysis should be offered to couples who have a history of recurrent miscarriage, especially first-trimester miscarriage, since most chromosomally abnormal embryos miscarry at this time in pregnancy.

PART IV

Deborah is now pregnant. Amniocentesis is done at 16 weeks and, 2 weeks later, a normal male karyotype is reported: 46,XY. Deborah and Steven are delighted when, 5 months later, a healthy baby boy is born.

For the prenatal diagnosis of genetic disorders, fetal tissue has to be obtained. There are two major ways of obtaining this tissue. At 10 to 12 weeks of gestation, a sample of the fetal placenta can be obtained with a biopsy catheter inserted either through the cervix or transabdominally – in either case, under ultrasonographic guidance (Figure 9.5). This is referred to as **chorionic villus sampling** (CVS). The tissue can be used to isolate DNA or can be grown in culture. At 16 to 18 weeks of pregnancy (and, in some centers, at 11 to 12 weeks), a sample of amniotic fluid can be withdrawn with a needle inserted transabdominally (**amniocentesis**) (Figure 9.6). This fluid contains fetal cells, mainly derived from skin and bladder (amniotic fluid is largely derived from fetal urine), that can be grown in culture.

Visualization of the chromosome structure requires access to dividing cells. Amniotic fluid cells must be grown in culture for several days, after which dividing cells are harvested and studied. Some cytotrophoblast cells obtained with chorionic villus tissue divide so rapidly that they can be harvested immediately for chromosomal analysis. Extraembryonic mesoderm can also be obtained from this tissue and grown in culture.

When a parent is known to carry a balanced rearrangement, it is relatively simple to analyze fetal chromosomes to look for evidence of imbalance. FISH probes have been developed to

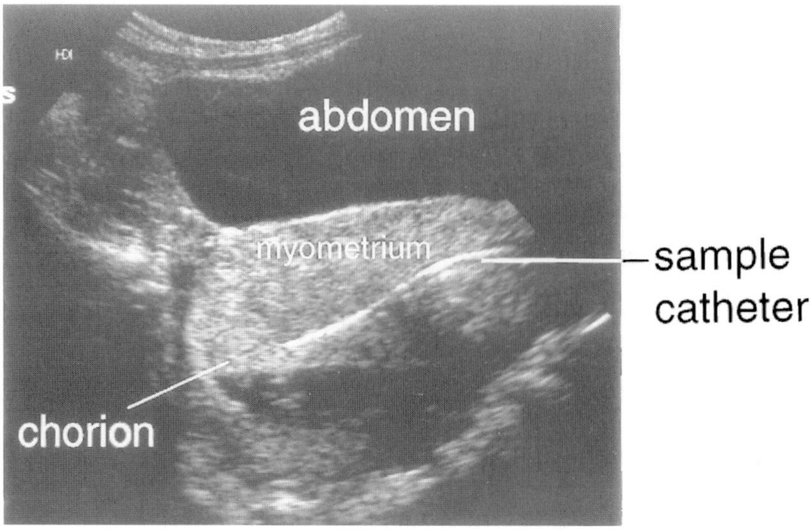

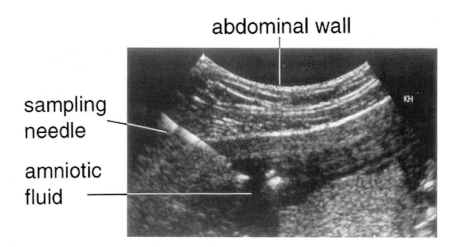

Figure 9.5 • Ultrasound illustrating tran-scervical chorionic villus sampling. In this case, a biopsy catheter is inserted through the mother's cervix, reaching the fetal chorion where a sample is taken. In other cases, a needle is inserted through the mother's abdomen to sample the fetal tissue. (Courtesy of Drs. Jodi Abbott and Deborah Levine, Beth Israel Deaconess Medical Center, Boston.)

Figure 9.6 • Ultrasound illustrating amniocentesis. A needle is inserted through the mother's abdomen into the amniotic cavity, where fluid is with-drawn for study. (Courtesy of Drs. Jodi Abbott and Deborah Levine, Beth Israel Deaconess Medical Center, Boston.)

permit rapid diagnosis of aneuploidy for the major chromosomes involved in liveborn aneuploidy syndromes (13, 18, 21, X). These probes bind to chromosome-specific DNA in uncultured interphase cells, permitting the presence of monosomy (for X) or trisomy to be detected rapidly. The approach does not detect structural rearrangements of chromosomes, or aneuploidy involving other chromosomes or chromosomal segments.

PART V

Karen is now 5 years old, and her brother Daniel is 3. Deborah is pregnant again, and this time chorionic villus sampling is done. Analysis of the direct preparation reveals three cells with trisomy 16. No trisomy 16 cells are found in the cultured preparation from the chorionic villi. Deborah and Steven are counseled that trisomy 16 cells probably are not present in the fetus but represent confined placental mosaicism. The fetus does carry the balanced translocation, but Deborah and Steven understand that this is likely to cause no problems. Five months later a healthy girl, Christine, is born.

When nondisjunction occurs during mitosis rather than meiosis, the result is chromosomal mosaicism. Detection of mosaicism by prenatal diagnosis can result in situations in which the phenotypic consequences are hard to predict. Not only is it difficult to know whether the fetus has physical abnormalities, but also the abnormal cells may not be derived from the embryo.

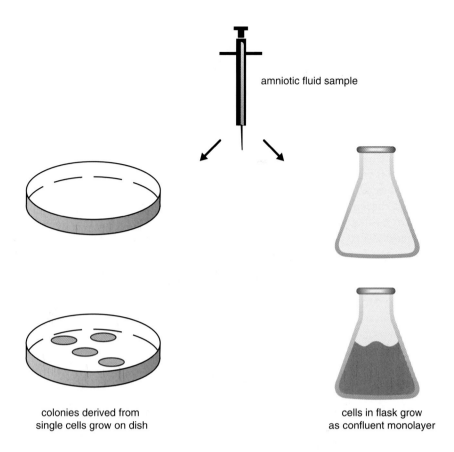

amniotic fluid sample

colonies derived from
single cells grow on dish

cells in flask grow
as confluent monolayer

Figure 9.7 • Amniotic fluid may be inoculated into culture dishes or flasks. In the dishes, single cells grow into discrete colonies. If cells are grown on cover glasses in dishes, they may be harvested *in situ* and directly examined with the microscope. In this way, cells within individual colonies may be directly examined. Cells that are inoculated into flasks grow as a confluent monolayer. These cells are enzymatically removed from the flask and harvested for chromosomal analysis.

Chorionic villus biopsy samples two cell types, neither of which is embryonic. Rapidly dividing cytotrophoblast cells are particularly prone to mitotic nondisjunction, and the mosaic chromosomal abnormalities often are not represented in the fetus. Cultured chorionic villus tissue is derived from extraembryonic mesoderm. Amniotic fluid cells originate from fetal skin and bladder, as well as from the lining of the amnion. The latter, again, are not embryonic.

This has created a dilemma in genetic counseling for many families. Mosaicism noted in uncultured chorionic villus material should be confirmed with cultured material. Mosaicism that is confined to the cytotrophoblast is much less likely to be clinically significant. For amniotic fluid analysis, it is common to grow samples in multiple culture flasks or on coverslips in multiple culture dishes (Figure 9.7), permitting analysis of colonies derived from individual cells. Sometimes chromosomal mosaicism will arise by nondisjunction in culture. This is referred to as **pseudomosaicism**. If the chromosomal anomaly is not seen in multiple cultures it is presumed to be pseudomosaic and probably is not clinically significant. On the other hand, if the abnormal cells occur in multiple cultures, true mosaicism is present. This is more likely to have phenotypic impact, although in some cases the proportion of affected cells may be low, and the exact phenotypic consequences may be difficult to predict. Many families who undergo prenatal diagnosis are not well prepared for the possibility of receiving results that are of uncertain clinical significance. This underscores the importance of genetic counseling as a component of the prenatal diagnosis process.

CLINICAL CYTOGENETICS

Chromosomal analysis was the first routine medical genetic test. In the early years of cytogenetics several distinctive syndromes were discovered (see Chapter 6) that are due to changes in chromosome number. Several disorders due to large deletions or other rearrangements were described, but it was not until the advent of chromosome banding in the late 1960s that more subtle chromosome structural changes could be routinely detected. Over the years since then the precision of chromosomal analysis has gradually improved, to the point now where molecular cytogenetic tools such as FISH and CGH arrays (see Chapter 6) permit detection of deletions or duplications with several thousand nucleotide resolution.

Standard chromosomal analysis includes a count of 20 or more metaphases to exclude mosaicism and banding, usually with Giemsa staining. Chromosomes are extended as much as possible to elicit fine structure and facilitate detection of small rearrangements. There is a wide range of indications for standard chromosomal analysis. It is performed to confirm a suspected diagnosis of a chromosomal aneuploidy syndrome such as Down syndrome, trisomy 13, Turner syndrome, etc. In some cases, such as in a child with multiple, severe congenital anomalies, the analysis may be performed emergently. Since the survival of children with trisomy 13 or 18 is very limited, it may be decided to withhold major surgical treatments if a diagnosis is confirmed.

Standard chromosomal analysis is the first-line genetic study performed for children with multiple congenital anomalies. The yield on chromosomal testing is low if there is only a single anomaly, such as isolated cleft palate, but increases if there are two or more anomalies or if the anomalies are accompanied by impaired cognitive development. High resolution analysis may reveal very small rearrangements, such as small deletions, insertions, or duplications.

Another indication for standard chromosomal analysis is for couples in which there have been recurrent first-trimester miscarriages, or with a history of infertility. The goal is to search for a balanced rearrangement, such as translocation or inversion, that predisposes to the production of chromosomally unbalanced gametes. There are many other causes of recurrent miscarriage or infertility, so cytogenetic analysis is but one component of the evaluation. The yield on chromosomal analysis tends to be higher in couples who have had previous pregnancies that have come to term, since if one carries a balanced rearrangement it is expected that some normal gametes will be produced.

Molecular cytogenetics provides additional tools for special study. Individuals suspected of having a microdeletion syndrome can be tested using specific FISH probes. In most cases these microdeletions are overlooked with standard cytogenetic analysis. FISH can also be used with subtelomeric probes to search for small deletions in the subtelomeric region. The phenotype associated with these deletions is often a nondescript one, with developmental delay, intrauterine growth retardation, and sometimes a family history of similar problems or miscarriage.

FISH can also be helpful in the identification of chromosomes involved in rearrangements. Derivative chromosomes, that is chromosomes that form as a result of segregation of a balanced rearrangement, can be difficult to identify with standard banding. Sometimes the constituent chromosomal segments can be identified by performing cytogenetic studies on both parents, looking for one with a balanced rearrangement. Otherwise, cocktails of chromosome-specific FISH probes can be used to paint specific chromosome regions, permitting identification of the abnormal material. Other techniques, such as comparative genomic hybridization or spectral karyotyping, can also be used. These require more complex technologies that are not always available within clinical laboratories. Moreover, there is limited clinical utility to identification of the exact origin of abnormal chromosomal segments, as it can be difficult to predict phenotype from this information.

CGH microarray analysis is beginning to be used for clinical cytogenetics. It offers the advantage that deletions or duplications as small as just a few thousand bases can be detected without prior knowledge of the specific chromosomal region that is involved. It can therefore be used as a general screen for diagnosis of an individual with a disorder that does not fit a specific syndrome. The major disadvantage to this approach is that it is insensitive to balanced rearrangement.

Any of these approaches can be used with prenatal samples obtained by chorionic villus biopsy or amniocentesis. In addition, blood can be obtained from the fetus by **percutaneous umbilical blood sampling** (PUBS). This is done after 18 weeks' gestation and is associated with a miscarriage rate as high as 2%. It is used to establish a diagnosis in cases where clinical suspicion of a chromosomal abnormality occurs too late for amniocentesis. This might be the case, for example, where abnormal ultrasound findings occur in the second trimester.

A new approach to prenatal testing involves **preimplantation diagnosis** (Figure 9.8). The most common approach is to perform testing on single blastomeres derived from an early embryo. Multiple oocytes are obtained by hormonal induction of ovulation and are harvested using a

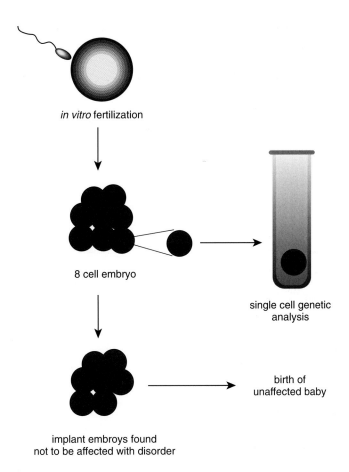

in vitro fertilization

8 cell embryo

single cell genetic
analysis

birth of
unaffected baby

implant embroys found
not to be affected with disorder

Figure 9.8 • Scheme of preimplantation diagnosis. Egg cells are obtained from the mother by insertion of a collecting catheter into the abdominal cavity, following hormone treatment to stimulate ovulation of multiple eggs. Fertilization of several egg cells is carried out *in vitro*. The embryos are brought to the eight-cell stage *in vitro*, and one or two cells from each embryo are biopsied using micromanipulation. DNA is extracted from the cells, and a sensitive assay, capable of detecting a single cell's DNA, is used to determine the genotypes of the biopsied cells. Only embryos found to be unaffected are implanted into mother's uterus and brought to term.

laprascopic procedure. These are fertilized *in vitro* and the embryos allowed to divide to the eight-cell stage. A single blastomere is removed using a micropipette. This cell can be used for FISH studies to detect a chromosome rearrangement or trisomy for which the embryo is known to be at risk. DNA can also be isolated from the cell and tested for specific mutations known to be in the family. Embryos that are found not to have the genetic abnormality in question are then implanted into the mother's uterus and brought to term. (The loss of a single cell does not impair viability.) Preimplantation diagnosis offers testing at the earliest possible stage, and is, in effect, a form of embryo selection. Most of the technology was developed as an approach to treatment of infertility, and diagnostic testing is often used for couples with a history of inability to become pregnant, sometimes because of a familial genetic disorder.

REVIEW QUESTIONS

9.1 An amniocentesis is done because of advanced maternal age and interphase FISH studies are done looking for evidence of trisomy 13, 18, and 21, as well as sex chromosome aneuploidy. Three signals are seen representing chromosome 21, indicating that the fetus will be affected with Down syndrome. Why is it important to still perform chromosomal analysis for counseling the couple?

9.2 A couple has a child with Down syndrome following a prenatal biochemical screen that did not indicate increased risk of Down syndrome in the pregnancy. They ask how the diagnosis could have been missed on the screen. What would you tell them?

9.3 A chromosomal analysis done on chorionic villus cells indicates trisomy 15, but follow-up amniocentesis shows normal chromosomes. Should the parents be reassured that the fetus will be normal, and that the initial result represents confined placental mosaicism? Are there other tests that should be done?

9.4 A child with multiple congenital anomalies has an apparently balanced translocation between chromosomes 2 and 11. Is it possible that the translocation is responsible for the child's problems? What would you do to further explore this possibility?

9.5 You are providing counseling to an adult with cleft palate and a history of congenital heart disease that was repaired as a child. He wants to know if there is risk of transmission of similar problems to the next generation. What kind of cytogenetic test would be appropriate in this setting, and if the result is positive, how would you counsel him?

FURTHER READING

Bahado-Singh RO, Choi SJ, Cheng CC. First- and mid-trimester Down syndrome screening and detection. Clin Perinatol 2004;31:677–694.

Bergemann AD, Cole F, Hirschhorn K. The etiology of Wolf–Hirschhorn syndrome. Trends Genet 2005;21:188–195.

Brambati B, Tului L. Chorionic villus sampling and amniocentesis. Curr Opin Obstet Gynecol 2005;17:197–201.

Eiben B, Glaubitz R. First-trimester screening: an overview. J Histochem Cytochem 2005;53:281–283.

Kuliev A, Verlinsky Y. Preimplantation diagnosis: a realistic option for assisted reproduction and genetic practice. Curr Opin Obstet Gynecol 2005;17:179–183.

Lau TK, Leung TN. Genetic screening and diagnosis. Curr Opin Obstet Gynecol 2005;17:163–169.

Reddy UM, Mennuti, MT. Incorporating first-trimester Down syndrome studies into prenatal screening. Obstet Gynecol 2006;107:167–173.

10
Molecular Diagnosis

INTRODUCTION

The diagnosis of genetic disorders was historically based on clinical assessment and use of various laboratory tests, including imaging, physiological tests, tests of blood, urine, or other body fluids, and biopsy of affected tissue. In some cases tests were expensive and could be invasive, even requiring hospitalization and surgery. Results were often ambiguous, sometimes requiring years before a definitive diagnosis could be achieved. Prenatal testing or testing in advance of symptoms for an individual at risk was impossible. All of this has changed with the advent of molecular diagnosis. If the gene for a genetic disorder is known and mutations can be detected, it can be possible to establish a diagnosis on the basis of testing DNA from any tissue, such as blood. In some cases, diagnosis can be definitive, rapid, inexpensive, and can be established in advance of clinical symptoms or even prenatally. Molecular diagnosis is rapidly transforming the medical practice of genetic disorders, and is beginning to have an impact on medical decision-making in the care of common disorders. In spite of its power, however, there are many pitfalls in the use of molecular diagnostic tests, both technical and ethical. In this chapter we will explore the evolution of a molecular test for one of the first disorders for which testing was available: Duchenne muscular dystrophy. We will see how the testing evolved from a linkage-based analysis to direct detection of mutations and how this has permitted prenatal diagnosis to be offered to families. We will then look at some of the challenges faced in the development and interpretation of molecular tests.

KEY POINTS

- Linkage-based testing can be offered to track a gene mutation through a family, providing molecular diagnosis even if direct mutation testing is not yet possible. Pitfalls include genetic recombination, genetic heterogeneity, incorrect clinical diagnosis in an index case, and misattributed parentage.
- Identification of the gene for a disorder permits diagnostic testing by direct mutation analysis. It can also provide a basis for the development of protein-based testing for the gene product.
- Some genetic disorders are associated with a wide range of allelic heterogeneity. In some cases, specific mutations correlate with specific clinical outcomes.
- Molecular genetic tests are often first developed in research laboratories, but clinical testing requires transfer of the test to a certified clinical laboratory.
- Clinical validity refers to the likelihood that a test result correctly diagnoses presence or absence of mutation. Clinical utility refers to the degree to which a test result guides clinical management.

Normal

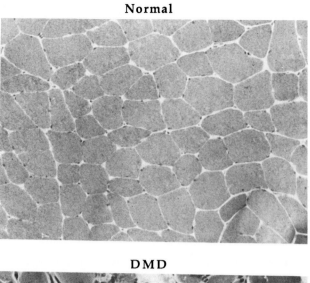

DMD

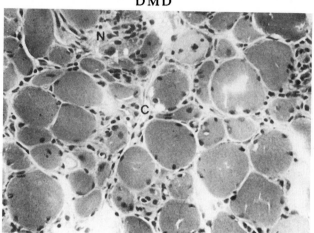

Figure 10.1 • Normal muscle (top) and muscle from a boy with Duchenne muscular dystrophy (*DMD*; bottom). The dystrophic muscle contains muscle cells of various sizes with connective tissue (*C*) and a necrotic cell (*N*).

PART I   1982

> *James and Brenda, who are both in their midtwenties, are referred to the genetics clinic. They are considering starting a family but are concerned because Brenda has a half-brother, Charles (same mother, different father), who has Duchenne muscular dystrophy. This diagnosis was made at age 4, when Charles was evaluated for delayed language development. At that time, it was noted that he had achieved motor milestones normally in the first year of life but had difficulty climbing stairs and was considered to be clumsy in preschool. A serum creatine phosphokinase assay revealed a level of 11,000 mU/ml (normal less than 30), and a muscle biopsy showed a pattern typical for Duchenne muscular dystrophy (DMD) (Figure 10.1). Charles is now 18 years old. He has been wheelchair-bound since age 11 and has profound weakness of all proximal muscles (Figure 10.2). He has experienced several bouts of respiratory infections, the most recent of which required prolonged hospitalization. His cognitive function is impaired as well, his IQ having been measured as being in the 80s a few years ago, when his muscle strength was better. James and Brenda are concerned that they are at risk of having a child with DMD. Having read literature from the Muscular Dystrophy Association, they are also interested in knowing whether they could have a child with a milder disorder, Becker dystrophy.*

Duchenne muscular dystrophy (DMD) is characterized by progressive loss of muscle strength. Because it is inherited as an X-linked recessive trait, it occurs mostly in males. The symptoms are usually noticed in the early years of life. A child with the disorder will learn to walk but develops clumsiness and may not get to running. The large muscles of the pelvic

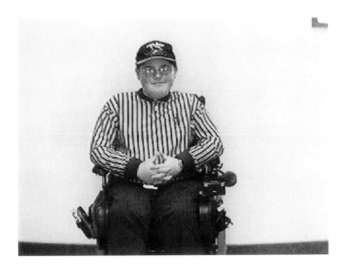

Figure 10.2 • Boy with Duchenne muscular dystrophy.

girdle usually are the first to display weakness. This is most obvious when the child is asked to stand quickly from a lying position. Weakness of the hip muscles causes the child to use the hands to help support the body as he rises (Gower sign). The calf muscles are enlarged, although muscle mass is not increased (pseudohypertrophy) and he may walk on tiptoe. Gradually, strength diminishes in muscles throughout the body. Most boys with DMD become wheelchair-bound by late childhood or their early teen years. They develop weakness in the shoulder girdle and, eventually, in the arms and even the hands. Ultimately, they may be essentially paralyzed, except for finger and toe movements. Movements of the eyes, however, are not affected. The heart muscle is also involved, causing a dilated cardiomyopathy and leading to cardiac failure, which is exacerbated by severe scoliosis that limits breathing. There is an accompanying cognitive impairment found in many. Boys with DMD die in their late teens or early twenties. No medical treatment has been determined to be effective.

Increased levels of serum creatine phosphokinase (CPK) can be an indicator of muscle disease. CPK is an enzyme found in skeletal muscle, heart, and brain. When muscle cells are damaged, CPK leaks into the serum. Boys with muscular dystrophy have extremely high CPK levels. This is true even at birth, before muscle weakness is apparent. The definitive diagnostic test for muscular dystrophy is muscle biopsy. A small piece of muscle is removed and examined with the microscope. Dystrophic muscle is characterized by degenerating muscle cells and increased connective tissue and fat.

Becker dystrophy is a related disorder, in which the same muscle groups are affected as in DMD but the age of onset is later and the rate of progression slower. It is also transmitted as an X-linked recessive trait. At the time when Charles's disease was diagnosed, there were no tests to distinguish Duchenne from Becker dystrophy, and it was unclear whether these disorders were due to mutations at the same or at different genes.

PART II

Further investigation of the family history reveals that Brenda's mother had a brother who also received a diagnosis of DMD. He had died at age 17 of pneumonia. Brenda's mother has a healthy brother as well. No other family members are known to have muscle disease (Figure 10.3). The genetic counselor explains to James and Brenda that Brenda's mother is an obligate carrier of DMD and therefore that Brenda is at 50% risk of being a carrier. The only means of carrier testing is blood CPK analysis. CPK testing is done on Brenda and on her mother and is repeated three times. The CPK tests confirm that Brenda's mother is a DMD carrier, as was known from the family history. Brenda's results indicate that she is not a carrier, but she is told that these results do not definitively rule out carrier status.

Duchenne muscular dystrophy is transmitted as an X-linked recessive trait. A carrier female may have affected brothers, and has a 50% risk of transmitting the trait to any of her sons.

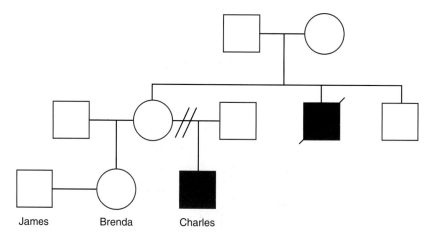

Figure 10.3 • Pedigree of Brenda and James's family.

James   Brenda   Charles

Sometimes one will encounter a family in which there are no affected male relatives. If the mother has few or no brothers or maternal uncles this may be due to chance. The mutant gene may not have been passed to any male relatives in recent generations, and therefore the phenotype may not have been encountered in the family. Usually, it is difficult to obtain reliable medical information for more than one or two generations in the past so, if males were affected in earlier generations, this information may not be known to current members of the family.

Alternatively, just as was the case for autosomal dominant traits, X-linked recessive traits may arise by new mutation. In this case, the mutation may have occurred in the egg cell that produced the affected boy or may have arisen in the sperm or egg that produced his mother. The distinction is important, because in the latter case the mother is at risk of having additional affected sons, whereas in the former case her risk is low. Germ-line mosaicism has also been seen for X-linked traits. We will explore options for carrier testing in the next section.

Serum levels of CPK can be elevated in females who carry the DMD gene mutation. Muscle cells actually are a syncytium containing multiple nuclei derived from the fusion of immature myoblasts. Any individual myoblast in a carrier has a 50% likelihood of having an active mutant or normal X chromosome and therefore a 50% chance of expressing the muscular dystrophy mutation. Muscle cells with a chance preponderance of mutant-expressing nuclei will be prone to destruction and will release CPK. Muscle is capable of regeneration, though, so over time, damaged cells may be replaced by healthier muscle, causing the CPK values to decrease and thereby accounting for false negative tests. CPK can also be released from muscle cells damaged by simple trauma, including the trauma of vigorous exercise, thereby accounting for false positive tests. These testing problems are ameliorated somewhat by performing tests on several separate occasions, which allows the clinician to discount a single, aberrantly elevated value. Clearly, CPK testing is an imperfect carrier test. Approximately two-thirds of DMD carriers have elevated CPK values, and approximately 5% of women in the general population have elevated values.

PART III   1983

> *Based on the information they received in the genetics clinic, James and Brenda decide to try to become pregnant. In 1983, they telephone a genetic counselor at the clinic, who informs them that prenatal diagnosis of DMD has been done in a few families using RFLPs for a number of nearby loci. Blood is drawn from Brenda, her mother, her father, Charles (who has DMD), Brenda's healthy maternal uncle, and both her mother's parents. Brenda turns out to be heterozygous at two loci that flank DMD, namely D2 and L128 (Figure 10.4). D2 recognizes two alleles in PvuII-cut DNA (6.0-kb and 6.6-kb); L128 recognizes two alleles in TaqI-cut DNA (12-kb and 16-kb). Brenda is found to be "informative" for these flanking markers, so prenatal diagnosis is offered. The fetus from this pregnancy is determined, by karyotype analysis from*

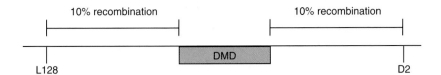

Figure 10.4 • Map of region surrounding DMD gene, indicating flanking markers L128 and D2.

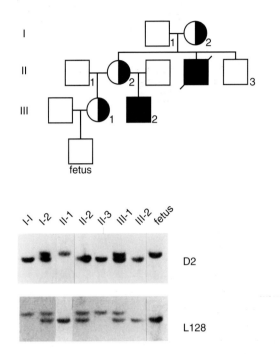

Figure 10.5 • Results of Southern analysis with D2 and L128 probes. The pedigree is shown at the top and the Southern blot results at the bottom.

an amniocentesis specimen, to be male, and DNA studies are performed on cells from the fetus (Figure 10.5).

The probable haplotypes with respect to DMD, D2, and L128 are shown in the pedigree. The DMD mutation is in coupling with the 6.0-kb D2 allele and the 12-kb L128 allele in II-2. This can be determined because II-2 had to receive the 6.0- and 16-kb haplotype with the normal DMD allele from her father. A recombination must have occurred in I-2, leading to either II-2 or II-3, because in II-3 the maternal 6.0-kb D2 allele is in coupling with the wild-type allele of the DMD locus. Because we do not know whether the crossover occurred in the meiosis leading to II-2 or II-3, the coupling phase of I-2 is uncertain, as indicated. The consultand, III-1, received the 6.6-kb D2 allele and the 12-kb L128 allele from her father. She therefore must have received the 6.0- and 16-kb alleles from her mother. Barring recombination between the DMD mutation and L128 in II-2, III-1 is likely not to be a carrier (actual risk of being a carrier is approximately 20% based on DNA analysis, less if negative CPK testing is taken into consideration).

The male fetus received the grandpaternal 6.6-kb and 12-kb alleles from III-1. He is therefore unaffected, unless his mother was a carrier and a double crossover occurred between L128 and DMD on one side and D2 and DMD on the other [probability of (0.20)(0.20)(0.20) = 0.008]. He therefore has a greater than 99% chance of being unaffected (Figure 10.6).

The power of genetic linkage to map the DMD gene was recognized soon after the development of mapping strategies involving RFLPs. The DMD gene was known to reside on the X chromosome, and experience with rare individuals with chromosome translocations who had DMD indicated that the gene might reside at a specific site on the short arm. Gene mapping studies were undertaken using the then newly discovered restriction fragment length polymorphisms to study extended families with DMD. By 1983, the DMD locus was mapped to a precise region on the short arm of the X chromosome and a linkage map of the region was available.

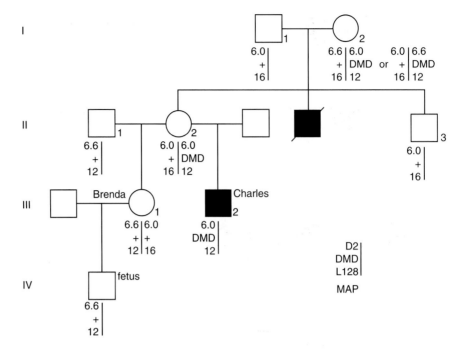

Figure 10.6 • Pedigree indicating alleles for L128 and D2.

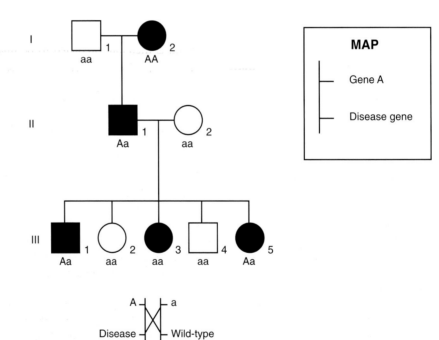

Figure 10.7 • Linkage-based diagnosis in a family with an autosomal dominant disorder. Father II-1 is heterozygous for a closely linked marker with alleles *A* and *a*. *A* is in coupling with the disease gene in him, as he inherited both *A* and the disease allele from his mother, I-2. Children III-1 and III-5 inherit both *A* and the disease, and children III-2 and III-4 inherit both *a* and the nondisease allele. Child III-3 is a recombinant, as shown.

This knowledge permitted carrier testing and prenatal diagnosis in some families, based on tracking the affected gene through the family. The basic strategy is shown in Figure 10.7. Here an individual (II-1) has an autosomal dominant disorder for which no laboratory diagnostic test exists. He is heterozygous for a marker gene closely linked to the disease gene that has two alleles, *A* and *a*. His partner is homozygous *aa*. In this family, we know that *A* is in coupling with the disease because II-1 inherited both the disease and the *A* allele from his mother, I-2. There are five children. III-1 and III-5 both have inherited the *A* allele from father and, of course, *a* from mother. Because they received the marker allele in coupling with the disease, they would be predicted to be affected and, indeed, they are. III-2 and III-4 got *a* from both parents and are predicted to be unaffected, as they are. Child III-3 would seem to be prob-

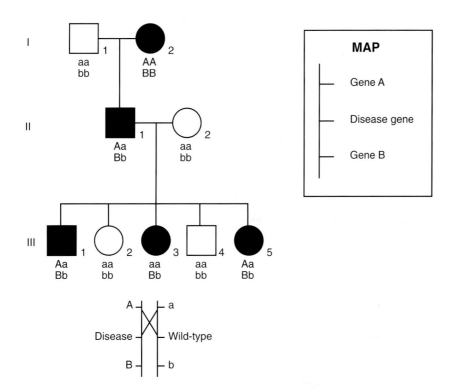

lematic, however. She got the *a* allele from her father and is therefore predicted to be unaffected, yet she has the disorder. This illustrates an important pitfall of linkage-based diagnosis, which is genetic recombination.

We have already seen how genetic recombination can change the association of particular alleles on a chromosome without changing the order of gene loci. Recombination between a marker gene and a disease gene can lead to a diagnostic error in a family linkage study. There are a number of ways to deal with this possibility.

First, the probability of recombination between the marker and disease should be known from the studies that established linkage in the first place. This allows an estimate to be made of the accuracy of a genetic linkage study. In Figure 10.7, if the recombination frequency between the marker and the disease is a value θ, then the accuracy of a diagnosis in the third generation is $1 - \theta$. For example, if the marker is 3 cM from the disease gene, then the risk of disease in individuals III-1 and III-5 is $(1 - 0.03) = 0.97$; likewise, the risk of disease in individuals III-2, III-3, and III-4 would be 0.03 (or the likelihood of being unaffected is $[1 - 0.03] = 0.97$). Obviously, it is advantageous to use very tightly linked markers for diagnostic testing whenever possible.

Another strategy for dealing with recombination is to use flanking markers. This is illustrated in Figure 10.8. Here genetic recombination can be readily detected because the combination of flanking markers in an individual changes as a consequence of recombination. In this case, individual III-3 inherited *a* and *B* from father, whereas we know that in II-1 *A* and *B* were in coupling. Therefore, a crossover must have occurred somewhere between *A* and *B*. If *A* and *B* are approximately equidistant from the disease locus, we would have no way of knowing whether it is more likely that the crossover occurred between *A* and the disease or between *B* and the disease. The diagnosis in III-3 would therefore be indeterminate. If the markers are not equidistant from the disease gene, their relative distance from this gene can be used to estimate the likelihood that the crossover occurred on one side or the other, and hence whether or not the child is likely to be affected. In practice, though, markers are likely to be more or less equally separated from the disease gene. The use of flanking markers at least alerts one to the fact that recombination has occurred.

There are a number of other limitations of the use of genetic linkage data for diagnostic purposes. First, unlike most diagnostic tests, this approach requires study of a family, not just an individual. Relatives in two or more generations must be available and willing to participate in the study. Some may be deceased, or it may be difficult to motivate some to provide a blood sample, perhaps because of poor relations in the family or because of fear of what the test will show. Linkage studies have revealed, for example, a fairly high incidence of **misattributed parentage**. Most often this involves a situation in which the stated father of a child is not the biologic father (inferred from the fact that the child has an allele that could not have been inherited from the father). Often in such cases, the stated father is not aware that the biologic father of a child is different, setting up a sensitive and awkward situation in genetic counseling.

Second, linkage testing is not informative for all families. The parent who carries a mutant gene must be heterozygous for the linked marker or markers, and the alleles in this parent must be distinguishable from those of the partner. These criteria are more likely to be met if there are many markers available that are linked to a disease gene of interest and that flank the disease gene. It also is helpful to have markers that are highly polymorphic, which means that there are multiple alleles at the locus and heterozygosity is common in the population.

Third, and most important, is the issue of genetic heterogeneity. Because we are not determining directly the gene mutation, linkage-based testing relies on the assumption that the disease gene in the family is indeed linked to the marker gene. If diagnosis of the disease in the proband is incorrect, any inference of diagnosis based on linkage in another member of the family will also be incorrect. Even if the diagnosis in the proband is correct, however, genetic heterogeneity can provide misleading results. This would occur if there are many genes at different locations that can account for a given phenotype. If the wrong gene is tracked through the family, the results of linkage analysis will not indicate inheritance of the true disease-causing gene. Therefore, if genetic heterogeneity is known to exist, linkage studies must be used with great caution.

Despite these limitations, linkage analysis can be a very powerful approach to providing genetic diagnosis in a number of settings. It can be used for prenatal diagnosis, as fetal DNA can be obtained from chorionic villus biopsy or amniocentesis. Also linkage analysis can provide presymptomatic diagnosis. In many disorders, signs and symptoms of disease may not be apparent early in life, yet linkage analysis can indicate who is likely to be affected in a family at any time. This can be useful in identifying those who need to be followed medically for potentially treatable complications and for providing genetic counseling. Such use, however, can also open Pandora's box, possibly creating major psychological and adjustment problems for a person in whom a diagnosis of being affected is made years or even decades in advance of the appearance of symptoms.

PART V   1986

> James and Brenda read in the newspaper that the DMD gene has been cloned. They call the genetic counselor who informs them that, for some families, direct detection of deletions, representing the gene mutation, is possible. This offers a chance for more precise prenatal diagnosis. Shortly afterward, Brenda becomes pregnant for the second time. A piece of frozen muscle from Charles's biopsy (obtained 15 years earlier) was found and tested for expression of dystrophin. The absence of dystrophin in Charles is interpreted as consistent with Duchenne, as opposed to Becker, muscular dystrophy, which in turn is consistent with the clinical history. DNA from Charles is still available in the laboratory and, after digestion with BglII, this is hybridized with cDNA probes from the DMD locus. On the basis of the findings from this study, prenatal diagnosis is undertaken, this time using material obtained at 10 weeks' gestation from a chorionic villus biopsy (Figure 10.9).

The DMD gene was cloned in 1985, one of the first to be identified using the positional cloning approach. The gene product consists of a membrane protein more than 400 kDa in size. It is expressed in muscle cells, including skeletal muscle, smooth muscle, and cardiac muscle. It is also found in brain tissue but nowhere else in appreciable abundance. Even in muscle, the protein is a minor species, comprising less than 0.002% of the total muscle protein. Antibodies were raised to the protein and used to effect immunofluorescent staining of tissue sections. Fluorescent staining was found to outline each muscle cell in cross-section, con-

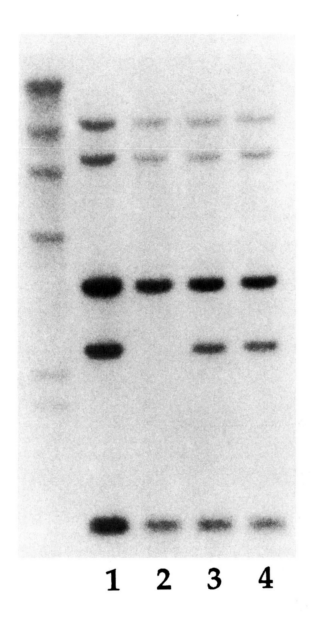

Figure 10.9 • Identification of a dystrophin deletion by Southern analysis. Lane 2 contains DNA from Charles, in which one band is missing. This corresponds with exon 51 of the dystrophin gene. His mother's DNA is in lane 1. Lanes 3 and 4 contain DNA samples from the previous pregnancy and the current prenatal sample, respectively.

1 2 3 4

firming cell membrane localization (Figure 10.10). This new protein had not been known to exist prior to its discovery through positional cloning of the muscular dystrophy locus. It was therefore dubbed **dystrophin**, though its function was still unknown.

Studies of DNA from males with both Duchenne and Becker dystrophy revealed a high frequency of deletions in each disorder (Figure 10.11). This demonstrated that the disorders are allelic but, as the deletions were mapped, no simple pattern emerged to distinguish Duchenne patients from Becker patients. Deletions were widely distributed over the length of the gene, with no clustering of deletions in Duchenne or Becker dystrophy. The size of deletion also did not correlate with phenotype: large deletions were found in some with the milder Becker dystrophy, whereas some with severe Duchenne dystrophy had small deletions.

Phenotypic correlations were more successful at the protein level. Western blot studies revealed a total absence of dystrophin in muscle biopsies from males with DMD (Figure 10.12). Immunofluorescence studies of DMD biopsies revealed muscle cells lacking the characteristic membrane-associated staining. Males with Becker dystrophy, in contrast, were found to have dystrophin in their muscle, but this dystrophin was aberrant in quantity or quality (or both). Some were found to have deficient amounts of a more or less normal-sized dystrophin. Others had dystrophin of lower or, rarely, higher molecular weight than normal. Correlation of the presence or absence of dystrophin with the Duchenne or Becker phenotype was found to be so good that the protein test came to be incorporated into the diagnostic evaluation of boys

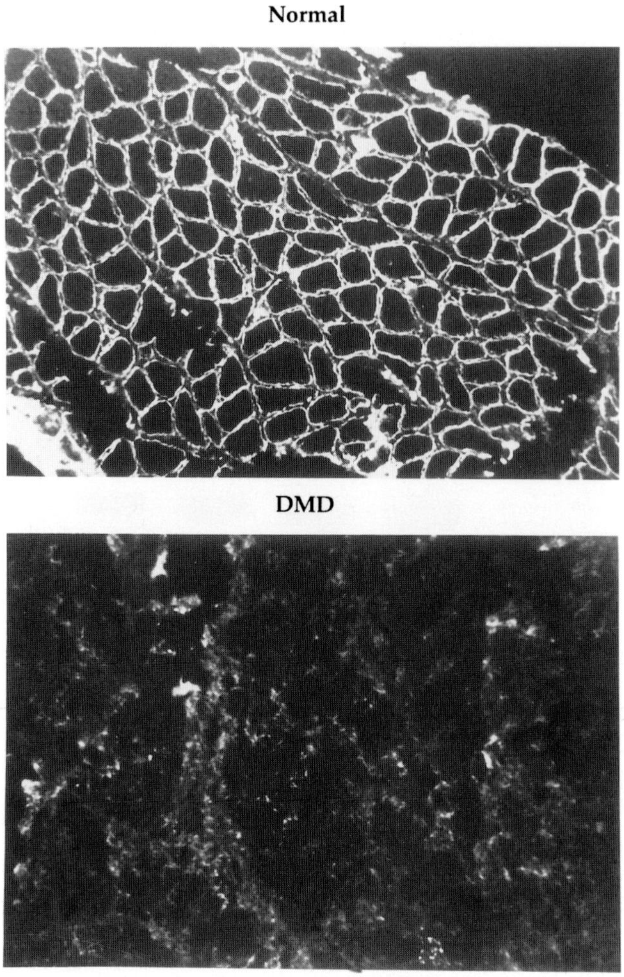

Normal

DMD

Figure 10.10 • Immunofluorescent staining of dystrophin in normal muscle (top) and in muscle from a boy with Duchenne muscular dystrophy (bottom). In the normal muscle, bright staining outlines each muscle cell in cross-section, indicating that dystrophin is located near the cell membrane. No dystrophin staining is found in the dystrophic muscle. (Courtesy of Dr. Louis Kunkel, Children's Hospital, Boston.)

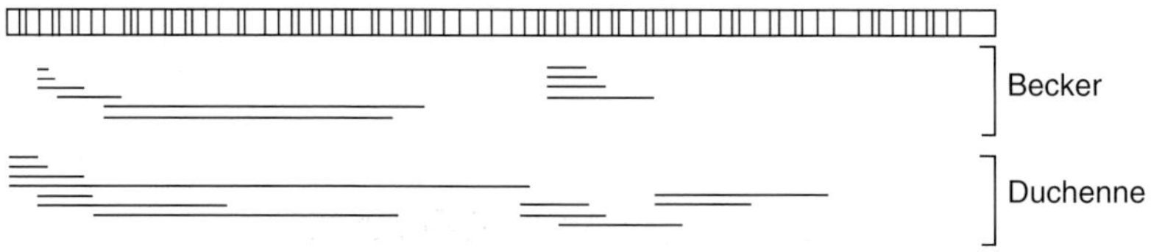

Figure 10.11 • Map of dystrophin gene, with vertical lines indicating exons (not drawn to scale). Below the map, the extent of some deletions responsible for Duchenne or Becker dystrophy are indicated. The sizes of deletions are indicated approximately. (Data based on the work of Koenig M, Beggs AH, Moyer M, *et al.* The molecular basis for Duchenne versus Becker muscular dystrophy: correlation of severity with type of deletion. Am J Hum Genet 1989;45:498–506.)

with muscular dystrophy. Absence of dystrophin predicts DMD, the presence of abnormal dystrophin predicts Becker dystrophy, and normal dystrophin means that some other diagnosis should be considered. This greatly improved the precision of pathologic diagnosis and the ability to predict disease progression.

The basis for genotype–phenotype correlations was found by analysis of the codons at the beginnings and ends of exons (Figure 10.13). Exons do not necessarily end at the third position of a triplet, completing the codon for an amino acid. Often the last base of an exon is the first or second base of a codon. As long as the first base of the next exon picks up where the previous exon left off to complete the codon, the reading frame of the protein is preserved. The protein will be shorter by whatever was lost in the deleted region but otherwise will be translated from end to end. If, however, two "noncompatible" exons are juxtaposed in the spliced message, a frameshift will occur. This inevitably leads to a stop codon after a short distance. The protein product will be severely truncated and probably degraded in the cell. Most

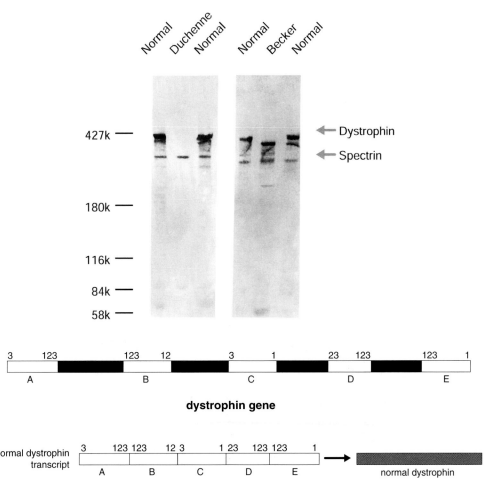

Figure 10.12 • Western blot of Duchenne and Becker dystrophy muscle biopsies. The muscle protein spectrin also is stained, to serve as a control. (Courtesy of Dr. Louis Kunkel, Children's Hospital, Boston.)

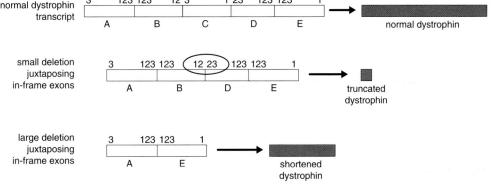

Figure 10.13 • Reading-frame hypothesis. The reading frame at the beginnings and ends of exons (exons indicated by *white boxes* in gene) are shown at the top. The numbers *1, 2,* and *3* correspond with the first, second, and third bases of a triplet codon, respectively. Hence, exon A, which ends with *123,* includes the complete codon for an amino acid at its end; exon C, in contrast, ends with *1,* with exon D supplying the second and third bases to complete a codon. The normal dystrophin transcript is spliced together to provide a complete code for the dystrophin protein. A small deletion that removes exon C results in production of an out-of-frame transcript (see *circle*), producing a truncated protein. A larger deletion of exons B through D results in an in-frame transcript, which produces an intact, although shorter-than-normal, transcript. (Modified with permission from Monaco AP, Bertelson CJ, Liechti-Gallati S, Moser H, Kunkel LM. An explanation for the phenotypic differences between patients bearing partial deletions of the DMD locus. Genomics 1988;2:90–95.)

cases of DMD are thus caused by deletions that create frameshifts resulting in complete absence of dystrophin. Becker dystrophy usually is associated with in-frame deletions that allow production of an internally deleted, but partially functional, protein product.

The **reading-frame hypothesis** explains most, but not all, cases of Duchenne or Becker dystrophy due to deletion. Some very large in-frame deletions can produce DMD. Also, some out-of-frame deletions can produce a Becker phenotype, probably due to exon-skipping events.

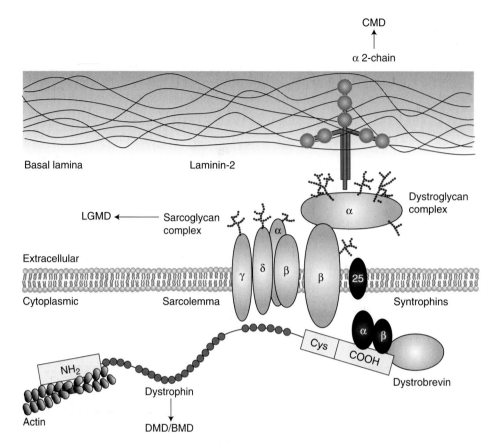

Figure 10.14 • Diagram of muscle cell membrane (sarcolemma), dystrophin, and the dystrophin-associated protein complex. Dystrophin is located inside the cell and binds actin at its N-terminus and the syntrophins, sarcoglycans, and dystrobrevin at the C-terminus. Mutations in dystrophin are responsible for Duchenne muscular dystrophy/ Becker muscular dystrophy (DMD/BMD). Mutations in the various sarcoglycans give rise to limb-girdle muscular dystrophy (LGMD), and laminin mutations result in congenital muscular dystrophy (CMD). (Redrawn from Bonnemann C, McNally E, Kunkel LM. Beyond dystrophin: current progress in the muscular dystrophies. Curr Opin Pediatr 1996;8:569–582.)

When the dystrophin message is spliced, sometimes one or more exons are spliced out of the final message. Such alternative splicing events generate slightly different proteins and can occur as normal events in some tissues. Alternative splicing can result in juxtaposition of compatible exons despite the presence of a deletion, preserving the reading frame. In such instances, the protein will be of reduced size but will otherwise be intact, resulting in Becker dystrophy.

In addition to Duchenne and Becker dystrophy, there are a number of additional forms of muscular dystrophy, most of which display autosomal recessive rather than X-linked inheritance. In many cases these have been found to be due to mutations in genes encoding proteins that interact with dystrophin. Dystrophin binds to a number of other proteins, including a set at the C-terminal end that link dystrophin with the extracellular matrix (Figure 10.14). Loss of function of any of these proteins by mutation leads to a muscular dystrophy more or less similar to Duchenne dystrophy, but with autosomal recessive transmission.

Although dystrophin analysis of muscle provides an accurate diagnostic test, it is invasive, with attendant high costs and risks. Also, dystrophin is not expressed in amniotic fluid cells or in chorionic villus tissue. Protein testing therefore does not provide a useful basis for prenatal diagnosis. The finding of a high frequency of gene deletion in affected individuals opened the way to direct mutation testing. At first, deletions were identified by Southern analysis. A set of subclones of the cDNA were used as hybridization probes, producing a complex set of bands when genomic DNA was cut with a restriction enzyme, because each clone recognizes many (10 or more) exons. A male with a deletion lacks the bands that correspond with deleted

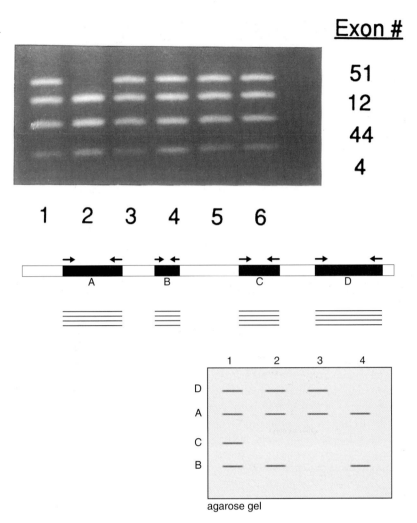

Figure 10.15 • Multiplex polymerase chain reaction analysis of exons 51, 12, 44, and 4 of the dystrophin gene. Bands corresponding with each exon are indicated at the right. Charles's sample is in lane 2, showing an exon 51 deletion. DNA from the current pregnancy is in lane 3. Lane 1 is a control, showing all four bands. Other lanes contain samples for other males.

Figure 10.16 • Multiplex PCR analysis of dystrophin gene deletions. Exons A, B, C, and D are amplified in a single PCR reaction (*arrows* indicate PCR primers). The products (shown below each exon) are separated by size on an agarose gel and are visualized by DNA staining. The order of exons in the gel is related to size, not position in the gene. Lane 1 shows all four exons. Exon C is deleted in the sample tested in lane 2, exons B and C are deleted in lane 3, and exons C and D in lane 4. Note that exons that are adjacent in the gene are not necessarily adjacent in the gel. (Based on technique of Chamberlain JS, Gibbs RA, Ranier JE, Nguyen PN, Caskey CT. Deletion screening of the Duchenne muscular dystrophy locus via multiplex DNA amplification. Nucleic Acids Res 1988;16:11141–11156; and from Beggs AH, Koenig M, Boyce FM, Kunkel LM. Detection of 98% of DMD/BMD deletions by PCR. Hum Genet 1990;86:45–48.)

DNA. A complete search of the dystrophin gene requires hybridization with 10 cDNA probes and scanning of dozens of bands for deletion. This is an expensive and laborious process, but it allows molecular diagnosis or prenatal diagnosis in two-thirds of cases.

PART VI   1989

Brenda's pregnancy in 1986 resulted in the birth of a healthy son. A third prenatal diagnosis is undertaken in 1989. This time the polymerase chain reaction is used to detect the mutation in Charles and to study the fetal DNA obtained by chorionic villus biopsy (Figure 10.15). The testing reveals that the fetus, a male, has not inherited the DMD mutation.

The invention of the polymerase chain reaction (PCR) led to the development of an efficient, accurate, and inexpensive test for deletions. Oligonucleotide primers were made that were homologous either with intron sequences that immediately flank specific exons or with sequences at the beginning and end of certain exons. This allowed PCR amplification of individual exons. The products could be visualized by separation in an agarose gel and staining with ethidium bromide (Figure 10.16). It was found that several exons could be

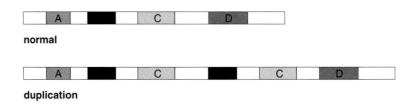

Figure 10.17 • Diagram of duplication in the dystrophin gene. The duplication juxtaposes exons C and B, which can result in an in-frame or an out-of frame transcript.

simultaneously amplified in the same reaction, producing one band per exon. This is referred to as **multiplex PCR**. The order of bands in the gel is related to the exon size of the PCR product and not to the location of the exon in the gene. A male with a deletion would be missing bands corresponding with deleted exons.

A combination of 18 sets of PCR primers can identify 98% of all known dystrophin deletions. Diagnostic errors are very rare. The PCR test can be performed very rapidly – even within 1 day – and at much lower cost than muscle biopsy. It can be done with very small quantities of DNA, including prenatal samples. Often both the 5′ and 3′ borders of a deletion can be inferred from the PCR analysis, allowing a distinction of Duchenne from Becker dystrophy by the reading-frame hypothesis. Many clinicians now rely on DNA testing before proceeding to muscle biopsy to diagnose Duchenne or Becker dystrophy, resorting to muscle biopsy only if the deletion test is negative.

Approximately two-thirds of affected males have a dystrophin gene deletion. What about the others? Among the remaining one-third, nearly 15% have been found to have duplications of the dystrophin gene (Figure 10.17). Duplications have been identified by quantitative analysis of band intensity on Southern blots hybridized with cDNA probes. The analysis is difficult and time-consuming, as relatively small differences in hybridization intensity must be discerned among dozens of bands. The pathogenesis of dystrophin abnormalities due to duplication is similar to that of deletion: production of abnormal dystrophin in Becker dystrophy or juxtaposition of out-of-frame exons leading to lack of dystrophin expression in Duchenne dystrophy.

The remaining dystrophin mutations are gradually coming to light. Generally, they consist of mutations of one or a small number of base pairs, including small deletions, insertions, and single base changes. Direct sequencing of the dystrophin coding sequence and flanking intron–exon borders can reveal such mutations, though the testing is expensive and laborious.

PART VII   1992

> *It has long seemed likely that Brenda was not a DMD carrier, although prenatal testing was offered because it was difficult to be certain. Recently, an assay has been developed that provides more definitive carrier testing for dystrophin deletions. Quantitative PCR is performed on a sample of DNA from Brenda. It is concluded that she is not a DMD carrier.*

The advent of a simple and reliable test for dystrophin deletions was a great help for diagnosis in affected individuals and for prenatal diagnosis. One of the difficult challenges in genetic counseling in muscular dystrophy is identification of carriers. The daughters of a carrier are at 50% risk of being carriers and often are interested in having their carrier status determined (Figure 10.18). Also, Duchenne or Becker dystrophy often arises as a sporadic event in a family. Approximately one-third of the time this is due to new mutations, but two-thirds of the time the mother of a sporadically affected male is found to be a carrier.

We have already seen that CPK testing provides a crude carrier test but is subject to both false positive and false negative results. Linkage analysis sometimes helps to resolve carrier status but not if the proband is the only affected member of the family. For those families in which a deletion is found in the proband, direct analysis for carrier status should be possible.

Detection of heterozygous deletions is far more challenging than detection of hemizygous deletions. Quantitative analysis of band intensity on a Southern blot is technically difficult. Band intensity may vary from band to band on a blot, reflecting differences either in amount of DNA loaded on the electrophoresis gel or in efficiency of transfer of DNA fragments from

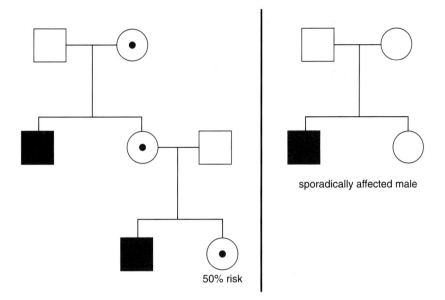

sporadically affected male

50% risk

Figure 10.18 • Two types of pedigrees encountered in families with Duchenne or Becker dystrophy. The family on the left includes two obligate carrier females and a woman at 50% risk based on family history. In the family on the right, there is one affected male. His mother has a 66% risk of being a carrier, and his sister, therefore, a 33% risk.

gel to membrane. To carry out quantitative analysis, it is necessary to compare corresponding bands from a test subject and a normal control, using bands outside the deleted region to correct for differences in the amount of DNA present in the blot. Quantitative analysis of PCR products is also challenging, but techniques have been developed that permit measurement of PCR products with sufficient precision to distinguish individuals with one or two copies of a sequence. These can now be used to determine carrier status in women at risk of carrying a DMD deletion.

For females with sporadically affected sons, carrier testing, however it is done, can give deceptive results. Approximately 10% of such females have gone on to have a second affected son despite negative carrier testing. These women are presumed to represent mosaics, in whom either the mutation is confined to cells in the germline or somatic cells with the mutation cannot be detected against the background of normal cells. The practitioner must bear this possibility of germ-line mosaicism in mind when counseling a family with one affected son.

MOLECULAR DIAGNOSIS OF GENETIC DISORDERS

This case illustrates the evolution of molecular diagnosis of genetic disorders due to mutation in single genes. Beginning in the 1980s it became possible to map genes using linkage-based approaches, but for the most part the genes themselves were unknown at that time. The linkage approach could be used, however, to track the gene mutation through the family and provide diagnostic testing, with the limitations of genetic recombination, genetic heterogeneity, etc., discussed above. Over the years, the process of gene identification has become easier, so the gap between gene mapping and gene identification may be brief. This enables direct analysis of a gene mutation, avoiding many of the caveats of a linkage-based test. Linkage is still used, however, in some instances. Some disorders are associated with a wide range of genetic heterogeneity, that is, a wide range of different mutations in different individuals. It may be impractical to identify all possible mutations in affected individuals. The gene map is very dense now, with simple sequence repeat markers available flanking most genes and very closely linked, vastly improving the likelihood of informative linkage markers that provide very accurate testing.

Molecular diagnostics are rapidly being incorporated into medical practice, as genes responsible for disease are increasingly being identified. Direct mutation tests must be developed and validated for each gene. In some cases, such as sickle cell anemia, a single mutation accounts for virtually all affected individuals. In others, there may be a larger, but limited, repertoire of mutations known to be associated with disease. The diagnostic challenge can be substantial due to both allelic and locus heterogeneity. The entire coding sequence, as well as intron–exon borders, may need to be sequenced in order to detect mutations.

Most genetic tests begin life in a research laboratory where the gene is identified, but use of the test for clinical decision making involves validation and performance in a clinical diagnostic laboratory. In the United States, clinical laboratories are certified under the Clinical Laboratory Improvement Amendments (CLIA). A laboratory that provides a genetic test for diagnostic purposes and charges a fee for that service must be certified under CLIA. Aside from developing and validating a new test, the clinical laboratory must insure that there are no patents that are violated by offering testing on a fee-for-service basis. Many gene sequences are patented by the laboratories that first identified the sequence. In some cases, patent-holders exercise rights to restrict the license to offer testing, and may force testing to be performed in specific, designated laboratories.

There are a wide variety of technologies now in use to detect mutations. The specific approach depends, in part, on the types of mutations to be detected and the volume of tests that need to be done. Automated approaches to sequence-based analysis are increasingly being used, and the technology is evolving rapidly. In general, the analytical validity of DNA-based tests is very high, that is, if a sequence variant is determined to be present or not present, that result is probably accurate, barring human error such as sample mix-up. Clinical validity and clinical utility, on the other hand, may be less straightforward.

Clinical validity is defined as the likelihood that the presence of a sequence variant correctly diagnoses a condition, or its absence indicates that the condition will not occur. The clinical validity of tests such as a DMD deletion is very high – virtually all males with a DMD deletion will be affected. This is not the case, however, for many other tests. In some instances, non-penetrance is known to occur, so the presence of a mutation does not necessarily indicate the presence of disease. In other cases, a sequence variant may be of unknown significance. A unique sequence variant in an individual might be a pathogenic mutation or could represent a rare benign variant that has no affect on the function of the gene or the gene product. Sometimes there are clues to help decide: Is the variant ever found in the general population? Does the variant segregate with the disease phenotype in a family? Does it occur at a site that is conserved in evolution? Does it affect gene or protein function in a measurable way? In some cases, however, the significance of a sequence variant may be unclear, and therefore needs to be interpreted cautiously. Clinicians and patients may be confused by a result that is highly *accurate*, that is, the mutation is indeed present, yet of *uncertain significance*.

Clinical utility is defined as the degree to which the test result informs clinical decision-making. Does the mutation diagnose disease, or indicate risk that an individual will someday develop disease? Does it facilitate family planning or prenatal diagnosis? Is there a medical intervention available that will modify the course of disease or prevent the onset of symptoms that can be implemented based on the results of testing? These questions need to be considered before embarking on testing. There may be tangible benefits derived from performing a genetic test, but there may also be risks, and these risks may apply both to the individual being tested and to other members of the family. Risks can include anxiety, stigmatization, and possible exposure to discrimination, such as loss of employment, health insurance, or life insurance. Most states in the US have laws that offer some degree of protection from discrimination based on genetic testing, but these differ from state to state. There is currently no federal legislation that addresses the issue in the US, and international laws differ from country to country.

In spite of these challenges, genetic testing is likely to increasingly be incorporated into routine medical practice. There are many testing laboratories, both commercial and academic. An internet database, available at www.genetests.org can be used to identify a testing laboratory for any particular genetic disorder.

REVIEW QUESTIONS

10.1 In the pedigree below, a woman (arrow) has had two brothers with Duchenne muscular dystrophy, an X-linked recessive trait. She is pregnant, and the fetus is found to be male. A linkage study is done, using two markers that flank the muscular dystrophy gene. Marker 1 has two alleles, "1" and "2" and marker 2 has two alleles, "3" and "4". Her parents and brothers are all deceased. Based on the genotypes shown (Figure 10.1Q) for the mother (she has the "12" genotype for marker 1 and the "34" genotype for marker 2) and her fetus (allele "1" for marker 1 and allele "3"

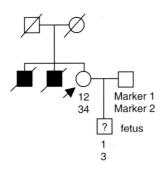

for marker 2), what would you tell her is the risk that the fetus will have Duchenne muscular dystrophy?

10.2 A molecular diagnostic test reveals a single base change in a gene in an individual affected with an autosomal dominant disorder. The change causes an amino acid substitution in the protein. How would you judge whether this is a pathogenic change or a benign variant?

10.3 Some molecular diagnostic tests for large complex genes with multiple exons begin with sequencing of cDNA prepared from mRNA rather than genomic DNA. What is the advantage of this approach?

10.4 A 40-year-old man at risk of inheriting a Huntington disease allele is found to have 74 CAG repeats in his gene. Does this mean that he will definitely develop the disease?

10.5 You are counseling a family with Noonan syndrome. What is the mode of genetic transmission? What is the responsible gene? Is clinical genetic testing available?

FURTHER READING

Burke W. Genetic testing. New Engl J Med 2002;347:1867–1875.

Burke W, Zimmern RL. Ensuring the appropriate use of genetic tests. Nat Rev Genet 2004;5:955–959.

Muntoni F, Torelli S, Ferlini A. Dystrophin and mutations: one gene, several proteins, multiple phenotypes. Lancet Neurol 2003;2:731–740.

Nowak KJ, Davies KE. Duchenne muscular dystrophy and dystrophin: pathogenesis and opportunities for treatment. EMBO Rep 2004;5:872–876.

11
Newborn Screening

INTRODUCTION

The introduction of newborn screening for inborn errors of metabolism was a major contribution to public health. Early detection of disorders such as phenylketonuria (PKU) permits children to be placed on a phenylalanine-free diet before irreversible neurological damage occurs. Newborn screening is carried out throughout the US and in most of the developed world. Advances in methodology are now stimulating an expansion of newborn screening to an increasing array of disorders. In this chapter we will consider the principles and practice of newborn screening in depth. We will see how screening for PKU is carried out and how a child is managed after a positive screening test. We will then look at general principles of inborn errors of metabolism, and consider various approaches to treatment.

KEY POINTS

- Newborns can be screened for an increasing variety of conditions on the principle that early detection can lead to therapy that prevents severe, long-term medical problems. Technological advances are quickly expanding the scope of newborn screening.
- Children diagnosed with inborn errors of metabolism require lifelong care. An unexpected consequence of PKU is a risk of congenital anomalies in the child of an affected woman due to phenylalanine toxicity if the mother is not maintained on strict dietary control during pregnancy.
- There is a wide variety of pathophysiological mechanisms that underlie inborn errors of metabolism. These include defects in enzymes and coenzymes, with physiological consequences of product deficiency and/or substrate accumulation.
- A variety of approaches to the treatment of inborn errors of metabolism are in use or in development, including dietary management, coenzyme supplementation, removal of toxic metabolites, enzyme replacement, and gene therapy.

PART I December 1965

Jocelyn is born after a full-term, uncomplicated pregnancy. Her birth weight is 3100 g, and she is a healthy and vigorous baby. She is being breast-fed and seems to be feeding well. A few drops of blood are taken from her heel on day 2 of life, just prior to her being discharged from the nursery with her mother (Figure 11.1); the blood is blotted onto a card and sent to the state laboratory. Her parents are told that this is a routine test done for all newborns, and so they put it out of their minds. They take Jocelyn home, and she continues to feed well and seems to be thriving. After 1 week, however, they receive a call from their pediatrician, who explains that an abnormal laboratory result has come back. At first Jocelyn's parents are mystified, unaware that any laboratory test had been done. The pediatrician then reminds them about the heel stick. He has arranged for the family to take Jocelyn to a special clinic at the nearby children's hospital.

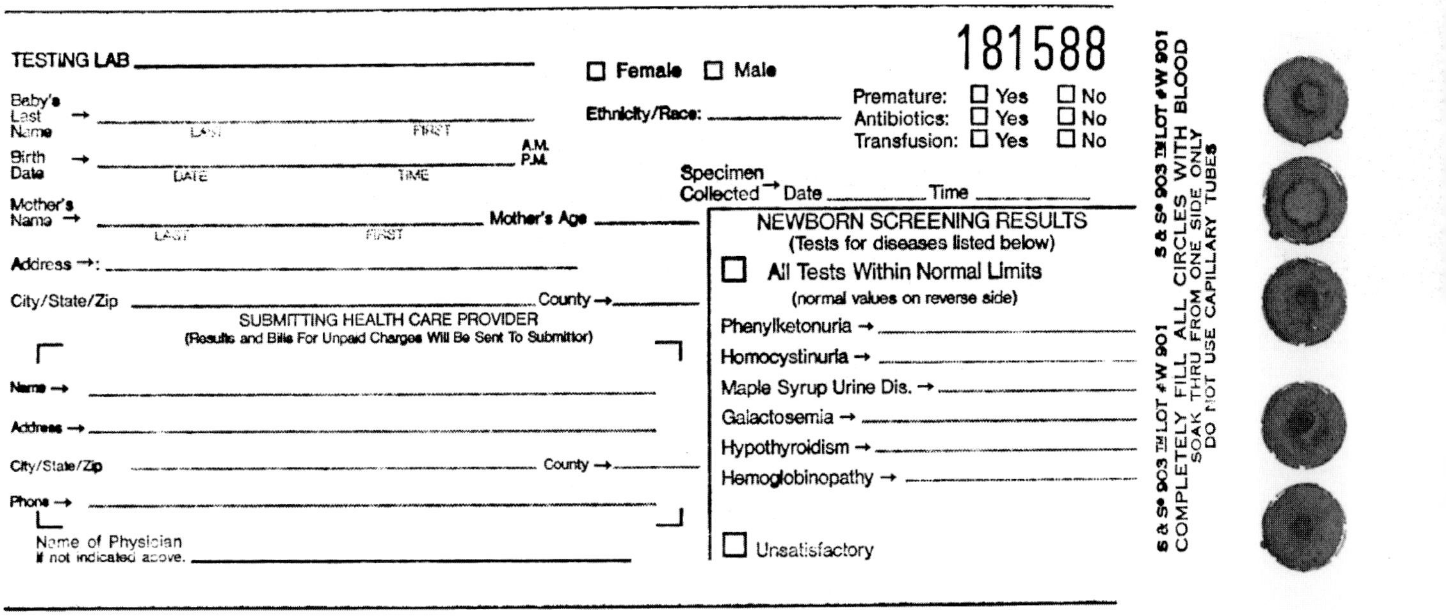

Figure 11.1 • Spots of blood on filter paper card to be sent to a state laboratory.

The concept of the inborn error of metabolism was introduced in Chapter 3. These disorders are the consequence of mutation in genes that encode enzymes required for metabolism or catabolism of specific substances. Enzyme deficiency results in a buildup of substrate and/or deficiency of product, either or both of which can cause disease. Screening of newborns for several inborn errors of metabolism is standard throughout the United States and in most of the developed world. The rationale is that identification of infants with inborn errors can lead to institution of treatment prior to the onset of clinical signs of the disorder. This can prevent otherwise irreversible neurologic damage and other medical problems.

Screening generally is performed by obtaining a blood sample by heel stick just before the baby is discharged from the nursery. The specific disorders included in the testing panel varies from state to state in the US. Screening began to be introduced in the 1960s, and disorders commonly included are PKU (MIM 261600), maple syrup urine disease (MIM 248600) (disorder of branched-chain amino acid catabolism), galactosemia (MIM 230400) (disorder of galactose catabolism), and homocystinuria (MIM 236200). In some areas, newborns also are screened for biotinidase deficiency (MIM 253260) (lack of enzyme required to recycle the cofactor biotin), sickle cell disease (MIM 603903), congenital hypothyroidism, congenital adrenal hyperplasia (MIM 201910), and congenital toxoplasmosis. The criteria for screening for a particular disorder are as follows: (1) The disorder produces irreversible damage if untreated early in life; (2) treatment prevents the damage but only if begun in the newborn period when the infant is asymptomatic; (3) the natural history of the disease is known; (4) a suitable screening test is available; (5) facilities for diagnosis and treatment are available.

The technology for newborn screening has recently undergone major changes. For decades, the mainstay of testing for PKU was a bacterial inhibition assay. Dried blood samples on disks of filter paper were placed onto an agar plate seeded with bacteria and with an analog of phenylalanine that inhibits bacterial growth. Phenylalanine in the blood sample would compete with the analog, permitting a halo of growth around the disk. The size of the halo was related to the concentration of phenylalanine in the sample. Similar assays were developed for many other metabolic disorders. The tests were simple, reliable, and inexpensive, but had to be performed separately for each disorder.

Recently, a new approach to newborn screening has been developed that uses mass spectrometry to detect abnormal levels of metabolites (Figure 11.2). This promises to allow diagnosis of a much larger number of metabolic disorders and is rapidly replacing the bacterial inhibition assay. The principle is that metabolites in blood samples are broken into fragments

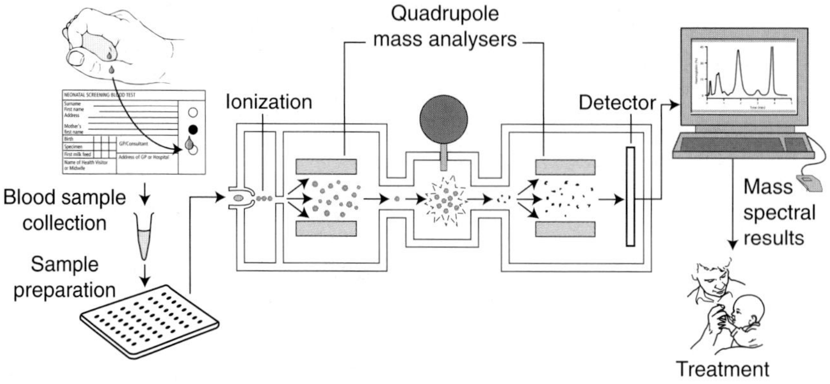

Figure 11.2 • Tandem mass spectrometry. Blood samples are obtained from a standard newborn screening filter paper. The blood is passed through two consecutive mass spectrometers, and the resulting spectrum is read to identify various metabolites in the blood.

and then the fragments analyzed by mass spectrometry. Tandem mass spectrometry, involving two consecutive rounds of analysis, can be used to identify and quantify dozens of metabolites in a single analysis. Efforts are now underway to standardize the approach to newborn screening using tandem mass spectrometry. Some of the disorders that can be detected do not fit standard criteria for newborn screening, perhaps because the natural history is not well defined or there is no known treatment. Current efforts are focusing on a subset of disorders that are appropriate to include on a screening panel, with the hope that a similar set of tests will be accepted as standard across all regions of the US and abroad.

Regardless of the testing method, when a sample is found to have a high concentration of phenylalanine, the baby's physician is notified. The child is referred to a specialty clinic, where blood is drawn for quantification of phenylalanine. A value greater than 20 mg/dL is indicative of classic PKU. Some newborns have phenylalanine values in an intermediate range (7–20 mg/dL), which is indicative of atypical or mild PKU. Either form of PKU is treated by reducing phenylalanine intake. Elevated levels of less than 7 mg/dL correspond with non-PKU benign hyperphenylalaninemia and require no treatment. Benign hyperphenylalaninemia mutations are missense mutations. PKU mutations also are usually missense mutations but might be mutations that lead to deficient production of protein (e.g., stop codons, splicing mutations, deletions).

PART II   December 1965

The next day, Jocelyn is taken to the metabolism clinic. Her parents are told that the laboratory result indicates that Jocelyn probably has phenylketonuria. Jocelyn is examined and the results are normal. Both blood and urine specimens are obtained. Jocelyn's parents are informed about PKU and, in particular, taught about the phenylalanine-free diet (Figure 11.3). Jocelyn will be fed with a special low-phenylalanine formula. Her parents are reassured that Jocelyn can be expected to achieve essentially normal cognitive development if this diet is adhered to. Nevertheless, they are in a state of shock, and are frightened. They spend considerable time talking with the clinic social worker and are introduced to other parents who have children with PKU. This somewhat reassures them. The next day, they get a call from the clinic nurse, telling them that Jocelyn's phenylalanine level was 25 mg/dL (the normal level being less than 2 mg/dL), confirming the diagnosis. Two weeks later, the urine pterin analysis is reported as normal, indicating that Jocelyn has classic PKU and not a cofactor deficiency in which the increased phenylalanine would be a secondary finding.

The frequency of PKU is approximately 1 in 10,000 births. Prior to the advent of newborn screening and treatment, PKU was one of the most common causes of mental retardation. The enzyme responsible for the disorder is phenylalanine hydroxylase, which catalyzes the hydroxylation of phenylalanine to tyrosine (Figure 11.4). In the absence of this reaction, phenylalanine builds up to high levels. Phenylalanine is believed to be toxic at high concentrations. A major phenylalanine metabolite, phenylpyruvic acid, may also be toxic. The major target for

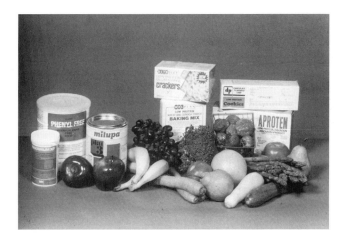

Figure 11.3 • Example of foods permitted in a phenylalanine-restricted diet.

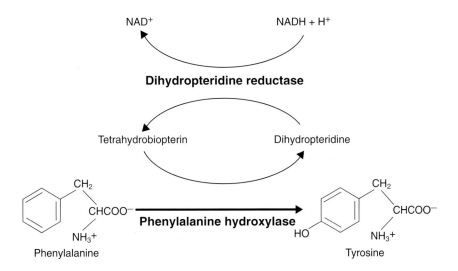

Figure 11.4 • Pathway of phenylalanine metabolism.

toxicity is the nervous system. Also, there is relative deficiency of tyrosine, the precursor for the neurotransmitters dopamine and norepinephrine. A deficiency of these neurotransmitters is likely to be deleterious for the developing brain. Children with untreated PKU exhibit profoundly delayed cognitive development. They also tend to have fair hair and skin owing to relative deficiency of melanin (normally derived, in part, from tyrosine).

Although the majority of those with PKU are affected owing to mutations in the phenylalanine hydroxylase gene, a few have mutations in a different enzyme, dihydropteridine reductase (DHPR) (MIM 261630), or in the synthesis of biopterin. DHPR is involved in the reduction of H2 biopterin into H4 biopterin; H4 biopterin is a cofactor required for the hydroxylation of phenylalanine to tyrosine. It also is required for hydroxylation of tyrosine and tryptophan, which are critical in the synthesis of vital brain neurotransmitters. Absence of DHPR activity results in deficient phenylalanine hydroxylation in the presence of normal phenylalanine hydroxylase enzyme and also in deficient neurotransmitter production. Defects in the synthesis of biopterin, which produce the same effects as DHPR deficiency, are identified by a urine assay of biopterin and neopterin.

Treatment of PKU is based on restriction of dietary intake of phenylalanine. The major protein source is a preparation of individual amino acids excluding phenylalanine and containing supplemental tyrosine as well as carbohydrate, fat, and minerals. Low-protein foods are allowed in measured quantities, but foods that contain significant amounts of protein (e.g., meat, fish, cheese, ice cream) are prohibited. Compliance with dietary treatment is monitored by testing blood phenylalanine levels. The goal is to maintain the level at less than 7 mg/dL, an amount considered safe for normal development. DHPR deficiency and biopterin synthesis are treated with H4 biopterin and supplements of neurotransmitter precursors (DOPA, carbidopa, and 5-OH-tryptophan), perhaps in conjunction with a low-phenylalanine diet.

The care of a child with PKU imposes many demands on a family to maintain compliance with the diet. It is best to provide care in a multidisciplinary clinic, where a physician, a nutritionist, and a social worker, as well as (in some cases) other professionals might be involved. The family is likely to require considerable education and support.

PART III   April 1973

Jocelyn is now 7 years old. She is in first grade and doing well in school. Increasingly, however, she is rebelling against her special diet, mainly because it is not pleasant-tasting, and she sees others her age eating tastier foods at school. After discussion with the metabolism clinic staff, her parents are told that strict adherence to the diet is less important by this age, because the brain is now fully developed. They take this as a sign that Jocelyn's diet can be liberalized. Over time, Jocelyn is less and less compliant, and gradually the family drifts away from the clinic.

The first few years of life are a critical time in terms of brain development. Compliance with the low-phenylalanine diet is especially important during this time. Formerly, it was considered safe to relax the diet later in childhood. The current view is that dietary relaxation during childhood or even in adolescence can lead to cognitive loss and emotional problems. Consequently, most centers now recommend at least some degree of compliance with a low-phenylalanine diet throughout life.

PART IV   March 1986

Jocelyn is now 20 years old. She has completed high school, although her grades were quite poor. She has also had a history of psychological and behavioral problems. Jocelyn has just given birth to a baby boy. His birth weight is only 2000 g, although he was born at term. He is microcephalic and has a congenital heart defect (tetralogy of Fallot). His physicians are optimistic that they can repair the cardiac problem but are concerned that microcephaly predicts that his cognitive development will be delayed. His blood phenylalanine level is in the normal range at 2 weeks of life. He is being breast fed. There is no history of PKU in his father's family. Jocelyn is afraid and confused. She is not married and relies on her parents for emotional support.

There are many possible causes of the birth of a child with microcephaly (small head size) and a congenital heart defect. In the child of a woman with PKU, however, by far the leading cause is a syndrome called **maternal PKU**. If the mother has not adhered to the low-phenylalanine diet, there will be high levels of phenylalanine in the fetal environment owing to the mother's defect, and the fetal phenylalanine hydroxylase activity will not be high enough to deal with this load. The consequence is an ironic outcome of treatment of a genetic disorder – toxicity in the next generation. In this case, the effects of high phenylalanine are particularly devastating. The fetus is exposed at a time when major organ systems, including the brain, are developing rapidly. It is common for these infants to have low birth weight, congenital heart disease, and inadequate brain development at the time of birth.

PART V   Epilogue – September 1988

Jocelyn is pregnant again, by a different partner. Her son is now 2½ years old (Figure 11.5), and Jocelyn and the boy live with Jocelyn's parents. His heart defect has been surgically repaired, but he is severely developmentally impaired. He began walking only recently, and he is not yet talking. For this pregnancy, Jocelyn was counseled to start a phenylalanine-restricted diet prior to trying to conceive and to continue the diet throughout the pregnancy. Her compliance, which has been good, has been monitored by following blood phenylalanine levels. She is reassured that fetal damage from maternal PKU is very unlikely to occur in this pregnancy.

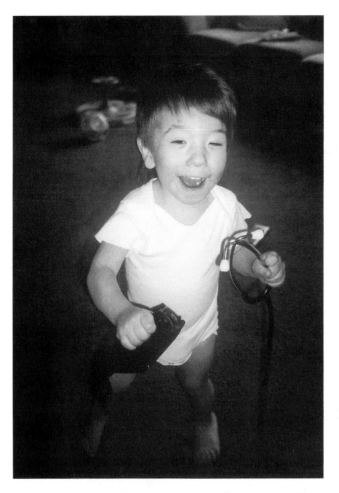

Figure 11.5 • Child with dysmorphic facial features (broad nasal bridge, small nose) and microcephaly due to *in utero* effects of maternal phenylketonuria. (Courtesy of Dr. Harvey Levy, Children's Hospital, Boston.)

Maternal PKU is largely a preventable disease. The woman with PKU should be placed on a low-phenylalanine diet prior to the time of conception. The rationale for preconceptual treatment is that major events in organogenesis occur at a point very early in pregnancy when a woman may not realize that she is pregnant. Preconceptual treatment and continued close adherence to the diet throughout the pregnancy, on the other hand, have been shown to prevent the teratogenic effects of maternal PKU syndrome. Major efforts now are under way to identify women of childbearing age with PKU, to educate them regarding the need to maintain the diet, and to monitor them throughout pregnancy.

INBORN ERRORS OF METABOLISM

Inborn errors of metabolism may result from mutations in enzymes or coenzymes, as is the case of PKU, and may involve toxic buildup of substrate or product deficiency. There are, however, other pathophysiological mechanisms that apply to other biochemical genetic disorders. In addition, there are therapies that extend beyond dietary manipulation.

Another major cellular dysfunction associated with some metabolic disorders is the gradual accumulation of substances within the cell due to hereditary deficiency of enzymes required for their breakdown. This occurs in **lysosomal storage diseases**, in which one or another of the enzymes required to metabolize cell membrane components in the lysosome is missing. A hallmark of these disorders is the progressive buildup of membrane debris in the lysosome, leading to progressive loss of cell function. An example of a lysosomal storage disorder is Tay–Sachs disease (MIM 272800) (see Clinical Snapshot 7.2).

The defect underlying an inborn error need not reside in the gene for the enzyme or the coenzyme. Genetic defects may upset the mechanisms by which cellular proteins are targeted for specific organelles, leading to deficiencies of multiple enzymes. Such is the case for I-cell disease (mucolipodosis II, MIM 252500), in which there is a failure in the trafficking of

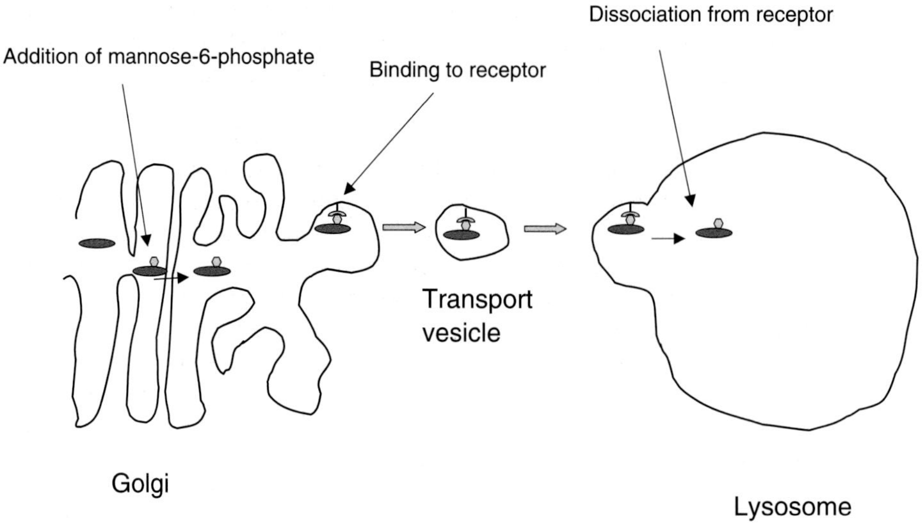

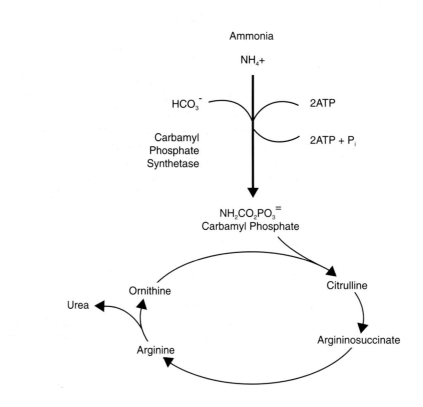

Figure 11.6 • Protein trafficking to lysosome. Lysosomal enzymes are tagged with a mannose-6-phosphate that binds to a receptor within the Golgi. A vesicle pinches off from the Golgi and transports the enzyme to the lysosome. Within the lysosome the enzyme dissociates from the receptor and the phosphate group is removed.

Figure 11.7 • Major steps of the urea cycle. Ammonia is converted to carbamyl phosphate by the enzyme carbamyl phosphate synthetase, which reacts with ornithine to enter the urea cycle.

enzymes to the lysosome (Figure 11.6). Lysosomes become packed with undigested inclusions (hence the term *I-cells*). Lysosomal enzymes are glycoproteins that are targeted to lysosomes by binding mannose-6-phosphate residues to a receptor that transports the enzymes from the Golgi within vesicles. Children with I-cell disease have mutations that disrupt one of the enzymes required to phosphorylate mannose, resulting in the enzymes being secreted from the cell rather than incorporated into lysosomes. The disorder results in growth failure and severe neurological dysfunction and is generally lethal.

Treatment of inborn errors of metabolism is aimed at reduction of the toxic substrate and/or replacement of missing product. This can be done, as we have seen, by dietary manipulation, but there are other approaches as well. One is to provide an alternative system to remove a toxic substrate. Deficiency of any of the enzymes in the urea cycle (Figure 11.7) can lead to buildup of ammonia, which is highly toxic. This can be removed emergently by dialysis, but chronic treatment involves administration of sodium phenylacetate and sodium benzoate, which complex with ammonia to form compounds able to be excreted safely in the urine.

Organ transplantation has been used to treat some metabolic disorders. Liver transplantation has been performed for some children with blocks in the urea cycle, for example. Advances in surgical technique and immunosuppression have vastly improved the safety and success of liver transplantation. Likewise, bone marrow transplantation has been used to treat some lysosomal storage diseases. The rationale is that macrophages from transplanted bone marrow function as scavengers to engulf and digest membrane components that cannot be digested by the enzyme-deficient host cells. This has been tried with a set of disorders known as **mucopolysaccharidoses**. These disorders lead to buildup of proteoglycans (protein molecules with attached sugars) and are manifested clinically as progressive neurologic deterioration, growth failure, skeletal deformity, coarse facial features, and heart failure. Reduction in circulating mucopolysaccharide has been demonstrated in transplant recipients.

Because the pathogenesis of inborn errors of metabolism is based on deficiency of an enzyme, enzyme replacement would seem a reasonable therapeutic approach. Substantial progress toward enzyme replacement has been made in lysosomal storage diseases. The first to be treated in this way was Gaucher disease (MIM 230800), a disorder in which the enzyme glucocerebrosidase is absent. Macrophages become swollen with storage material and cause enlargement of the liver and spleen. In addition, the presence of engorged macrophages in bones leads to bone and joint pain. The missing enzyme can be purified in quantity from placenta, but initial efforts at treatment of patients by enzyme infusion were disappointing. It then was found that there are mannose receptors in the macrophage's cell membrane that are responsible for targeting mannose-containing substances for the lysosome. Chemical modification of purified glucocerebrosidase to expose mannose residues leads to efficient transport of the enzyme into the lysosomes of macrophages. Infusion of this modified enzyme, now produced by recombinant DNA methodology, has been demonstrated to be highly effective in reducing the size of the liver and spleen and reducing bone pain. A similar approach has been used more recently for treatment of other lysosomal disorders, including Fabry disease (MIM 301500), and for some mucopolysaccaridoses, and recently for Pompe disease (MIM 232300), a disorder of glycogen metabolism.

The ultimate approach to treatment would be to replace the defective gene with an intact copy. Gene therapy protocols have also been tested on an experimental basis. These offer the possibility of replacement of the defective gene, effecting a "cure" for the disorder. Most approaches are based on insertion of the gene encoding an enzyme into a virus, which then is used to infect cells, thereby inserting the gene into the cells. Major challenges include targeting the recombinant virus to the correct cells, obtaining physiologically appropriate levels of expression, and avoiding an immune response to the virus. Gene therapy is not yet in routine use for treatment of individuals with inborn errors of metabolism.

REVIEW QUESTIONS

11.1 Why are children with PKU not born with damage to the nervous system?

11.2 Why are children with lysosomal storage disorders usually not symptomatic at birth?

11.3 Enzyme replacement therapy for lysosomal storage disorders involves treatment with an enzyme preparation with exposed mannose-6-phosphate residues. Why is this modification necessary?

11.4 How does tandem mass spectrometry permit newborn screening for a larger number of disorders than previously used bacterial assays?

11.5 What are the general approaches used in the treatment of inborn errors of metabolism?

FURTHER READING

Kayler SG, Fahey MC. Metabolic disorders and mental retardation. Am J Med Genet C Semin Med Genet 2003;117:31–41.

Levy HL. Historical background for the maternal PKU syndrome. Pediatrics 2003;112:1516–1518.

McCabe LL, McCabe ER. Genetic screening: carriers and affected individuals. Annu Rev Genom Hum G 2004;5:57–69.

McCabe LL, Therrell BL Jr., McCabe ER. Newborn screening: rationale for a comprehensive, fully integrated public health system. Mol Genet Metab 2002;77:267–273.

National Institutes of Health. Phenylketonuria (PKU): screening and management. NIH Consensus Statement 2000 Oct 16–18;17(3):1–33.

12

Developmental Genetics

INTRODUCTION

We have introduced the concept of multiple congenital anomalies, and seen how the birth of an affected child can have major impact on the entire family. Establishing a diagnosis for a child with congenital anomalies can be important for counseling of the family, both regarding future medical problems that may be anticipated and for risk of recurrence in future offspring. Diagnosis has been historically based on clinical criteria, but advances in molecular genetics are rapidly revealing the genetic basis for congenital anomaly syndromes. This enables more precise diagnoses to be made, in some cases predicts specific complications, and allows prenatal diagnosis to be offered. It is also revealing the underlying mechanisms of congenital anomalies, shedding light on normal development, and perhaps leading to future advances in prevention or treatment. In this chapter we will consider the story of a child with multiple anomalies that include disparate systems, including the skeletal system and genitalia. We will see how identification of the gene has improved the ability to provide diagnostic testing and counseling, and how the developmental mechanisms of genital development are coming to be understood. We will then look at the discipline of human dysmorphology, and glimpse some of the genetic systems that underlie human development.

KEY POINTS

- The discipline of dysmorphology involves the use of clinical and laboratory approaches to establish the diagnosis underlying congenital anomalies.
- Establishing a diagnosis can provide a basis for counseling a family about the natural history and genetics of a disorder and may suggest specific approaches to management.
- Some congenital anomaly syndromes involve effects on widely varying organ systems. This may reflect the effects of disruption of multiple genes, or the possibility that a single gene participates in developmental processes common to various systems.
- Normal development is dependent on the activation or repression of genes under tight temporal and spatial control. Many of the genetic systems that underlie embryological development are coming to light.

PART I

The pregnancy has proceeded uneventfully right through the time of delivery. Jane and Albert were offered ultrasound examination during the pregnancy but did not choose to do this, as they would not terminate a pregnancy regardless of the outcome. Labor begins spontaneously, but the baby's head fails to engage in the pelvis, necessitating Cesarean section. It is obvious at the moment of birth that there are problems. The baby, a girl, has a large head and short neck and chest, with markedly bowed lower legs. Although she breathes spontaneously in the delivery room, it is immediately apparent that she is having respiratory distress. She is intubated in the

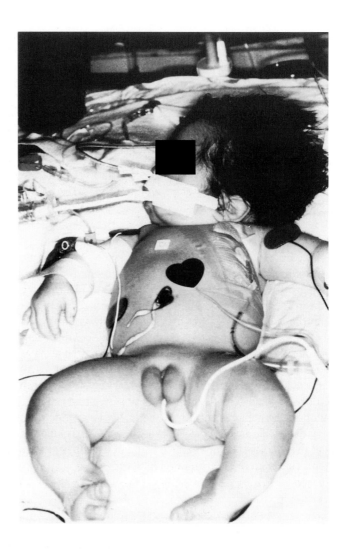

Figure 12.1 • Photograph of child showing pretibial dimples (best seen in right leg) and hypertrophic labia majora. (Courtesy of Dr. Kathryn North, University of Sydney)

delivery room and brought to the special care nursery. Jane and Albert barely have time to see her. Within hours, the baby is transported to a nearby academic medical center. Jane and Albert are confused and frightened.

It is common to offer ultrasound examination as a component of routine prenatal care. In addition to helping to recognize fetal malformations, ultrasonography provides accurate assessment of gestational age. Many couples find that having information about their baby's health prenatally helps them to plan, even if they do not choose termination of pregnancy in the event of fetal problems. The stressful environment of the delivery room is not a good place in which first to learn that a baby is in trouble. This baby apparently has multiple congenital anomalies, including orthopedic problems and respiratory distress. Such problems require assessment and care outside the purview of a community hospital, necessitating transfer to an intensive care nursery in a tertiary medical center.

PART II

A geneticist is called to see the baby soon after her arrival at the medical center. On examination, she is found to have a very short thorax and neck. Her head circumference is 41.5 cm (much greater than the ninety-fifth percentile), and she has a flat facial profile, low nasal bridge, and bilateral epicanthal folds. Her ears are low-set and posteriorly rotated. She has a cleft palate and small lower jaw. There is marked shortening of both lower limbs, with pretibial skin dimples (Figure 12.1). The upper limbs appear to be normal. Genital examination reveals enlarged and pigmented labia majora and cliteromegaly (see Figure 12.1). A vaginal opening is present.

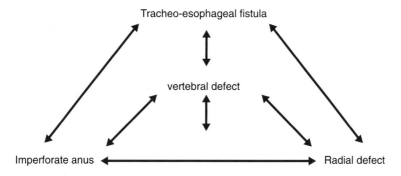

Figure 12.2 • Diagram indicating association of tracheo-esophageal fistula, imperforate anus, vertebral defects, and radial defects. These malformations tend to occur together more often than might be expected due to chance. (Redrawn by permission from Quan L, Smith DW. The VATER association – vertebral defects, anal atresia, t-e fistula with esophageal atresia, radial and renal dysplasia: a spectrum of associated defects. J Pediatr 1973;82:104.)

The physical findings in this infant are indicative of a skeletal dysplasia – that is, a congenital disorder of bone formation. The baby has a large head but small neck, thorax, and lower limbs. Although the skull is large, the bones of the face are small, leading to the low nasal bridge and flat facial profile. It is likely that the large head is responsible for the baby's inability to traverse the birth canal, leading to the cesarean section. Low-set, posteriorly rotated ears, epicanthal folds (extra folds of skin at the inner canthi of the eyes), cleft palate, and small lower jaw (micrognathia) are features found in a large number of syndromes of multiple congenital anomalies. The genital findings are not necessarily abnormal, and there is no doubt that the phenotype is female. The lower-limb anomalies are striking owing to the bowed tibias and skin dimples.

The clinical dysmorphologist tries to recognize patterns of abnormal development, with the goal of establishing an etiologic diagnosis. Major classes of anomalies are malformations, deformations, and disruptions. A malformation is the result of abnormal development of tissue. Developmental mechanisms somehow are interfered with, and the tissue does not form properly. Deformation is defined as the distortion of a normally formed tissue by extrinsic pressure. An example is asymmetry of the skull due to pressure from a benign uterine tumor called a fibroid. Disruption is the damage of a normally formed tissue. For example, a tear in the amniotic cavity can trap a limb, amputating part of the extremity. Disruptions tend to be asymmetric, whereas malformations are more often (but not always) symmetric.

Various patterns of malformations are seen. Some compose syndromes, such as Down syndrome. These are sets of congenital defects that are the consequence of some defined, ultimate cause. Down syndrome results from having an extra copy of chromosome 21. Syndromes can also result from exposure to teratogenic agents such as thalidomide. Whatever the cause – abnormality of one gene or a group of genes or exposure to a teratogen – the outcome is perturbation of multiple developing systems in a reproducible way.

A second pattern of malformations is called a sequence. A sequence generally arises as the consequence of a single primary event, for example, underdevelopment of the lower jaw in the Pierre–Robin sequence. Other anomalies that comprise the sequence are secondary effects of the primary malformation. In the Pierre–Robin sequence, the tongue is too large for the small mouth and interferes with closure of the palate, resulting in cleft palate. Here, cleft palate is not a primary malformation but a secondary consequence of underdevelopment of the jaw.

The third pattern is referred to as an association. It has been observed that particular sets of congenital anomalies tend to occur together more often than expected due to chance. These do not comprise syndromes; the causes are unknown, and many associations are etiologically heterogeneous. Indeed, the majority occur sporadically. One example is the VACTERL association, the major components of which are vertebral anomalies, anal atresia, cardiac anomalies, tracheo-esophageal fistula, renal anomalies, and limb defects (Figure 12.2). Various combinations of these features occur in different babies, reflecting the nonrandom association of these malformations. It is not known why these associations occur. They may reflect processes that have some molecular or morphologic event in common or processes that all occur at the same time in development.

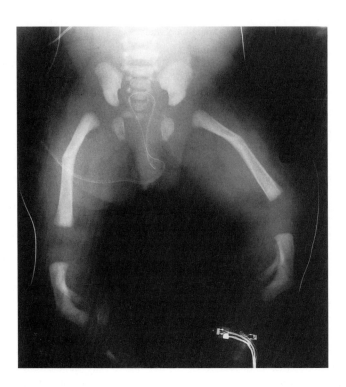

Figure 12.3 • X-ray showing dysplastic femurs, tibiae, and fibulae.

The medical practice of dysmorphology is partly science and partly art. A dysmorphologist examines for both subtle and major anomalies, looking for recognizable patterns. Correctly establishing a diagnosis can help one to provide anticipatory guidance: What does the future hold? Is the child likely to have additional anomalies that are not obvious on cursory examination? It also permits accurate genetic counseling. Sometimes the recurrence risk will be high; other times the family may be surprised to learn that recurrence is unlikely.

PART III

> *The geneticist suggests that a number of investigations be performed. These include X-rays of the entire skeleton (Figure 12.3), head and abdominal ultrasonography, and chromosomal analysis. Albert meets with the neonatologist later that evening, who explains that the baby is very sick but that no definite diagnosis has been made so far. The plan has been to provide maximum support as further information is collected. The orthopedic service has been called to see the baby, but has not sent someone by yet. Albert tells the care team that he and Jane have decided to name the baby Lisa.*

The X-rays reveal hypoplastic scapulae, curving of the femurs and tibiae, dislocation of the hips, and abnormal cervical vertebrae. There are 11 ribs bilaterally. Head and renal ultrasound examinations are normal. A uterus is seen by pelvic ultrasonography. It is likely that the short thorax accounts, at least in part, for the respiratory distress, although the baby might also have tracheomalacia.

There are a large number of skeletal dysplasia syndromes that may present at birth. They are classified by clinical and radiologic features. One of the most common and easily recognized is achondroplasia. Affected babies have a large head but have short arms and legs. There are usually no other congenital anomalies or respiratory problems. Thanatophoric dysplasia (MIM 187600) has been found to be allelic to achondroplasia, both being due to mutations in the gene *FGFR3* (MIM 134934), one of a family of fibroblast growth factor receptor genes. Thanatophoric dysplasia is characterized by extremely short, bowed limbs, large head with hydrocephalus, and small thorax. Unlike achondroplasia, it is lethal in the newborn period.

Chondrodysplasia punctata includes a set of disorders in which there is stippling of the epiphyses, the cartilaginous growth plates. Other congenital skeletal dysplasias have characteristic radiographic features. In diastrophic dysplasia (MIM 222600), there are broad metaphyses and the ears become swollen in infancy. In metatropic dysplasia (MIM 250600), the vertebral bodies are markedly flattened, and limbs are deformed. Kneist dysplasia (MIM 156550) consists of flat facies, myopia, flattened vertebrae, and club-like metaphyses.

This baby's features do not fit these syndromes but fit very well with a rare disorder called **campomelic dysplasia** (MIM 114290). The bowed tibiae with pretibial skin dimples are pathognomonic. The facial features, cleft palate, large head size, hypoplastic scapulae, 11 ribs, and respiratory insufficiency also are compatible with this diagnosis.

PART IV

Lisa is now almost 24 hours old. The geneticist meets with Albert and explains that Lisa has campomelic dysplasia. It is explained that this disorder is most often lethal in the early days of life, due to respiratory insufficiency. On the other hand, many children have been known to survive for long periods, although some require continued respiratory support. Among long-term survivors, prognosis for intellectual function is variable, with cognitive problems noted in some. A family history is obtained, revealing no prior history of similar problems. This is Jane and Albert's first child. Jane had one previous miscarriage at 8 weeks' gestation. Jane and Albert are not related to one another. The geneticist notes that the syndrome is usually sporadic, although recurrence in families has been reported in rare instances.

The major medical complication associated with campomelic dysplasia is respiratory insufficiency. Some babies are stillborn and are unable to make any initial respiratory efforts. The respiratory problems are attributable to a combination of factors, including small trachea and larynx, short thorax, and small lower jaw with airway obstruction by the tongue. Virtually all these babies require intensive ventilatory support at birth. Those who survive may need continued ventilation and tracheostomy.

The prognosis for central nervous system function has been difficult to assess, mostly because of major respiratory problems at birth; there are few long-term survivors. Some infants with this disorder have central nervous system malformations, including absence of the olfactory bulbs, dilated ventricles, and abnormalities of neuronal migration. However, there is relatively little experience with intellectual outcome of infants who were provided aggressive respiratory support from the time of birth.

In addition to the skeletal and cerebral malformations, there can be anomalies involving other organ systems. These include renal anomalies, congenital heart defects, and gastrointestinal malformations. Finally, a proportion of phenotypic females with campomelic dysplasia are found to have a 46,XY karyotype and have partial or complete absence of testes, with varying degrees of abnormality of the external genitalia.

The vast majority of cases of campomelic dysplasia occur sporadically, without prior family history. The existence of families with recurrence in siblings had suggested possible autosomal recessive transmission in some cases. Some consanguineous families have been reported, although overall the segregation ratio has been lower than the expected 25%. The genetics of campomelic dysplasia were explained only after the responsible gene was identified.

PART V

Jane comes in with Albert the next day and both speak with the neonatology staff and with the geneticist. They have decided to continue aggressive treatment. Lisa is currently still ventilator-dependent, having failed one attempt at extubation. The chromosomal analysis is reported later that day and provides another setback: Lisa is found to have the 46,XY karyotype. The geneticist explains that sex reversal has been reported before in campomelic dysplasia. Eventually, Lisa will require exploratory surgery to remove gonadal tissue to protect her from possible tumor formation, assuming that she survives her respiratory problems. The geneticist also notes that the gene responsible for campomelic dysplasia has been discovered. Studies have revealed that affected individuals generally have mutations in just one allele, indicating that the trait is dominant and so most affected individuals represent new mutations. Blood is drawn from Lisa and sent to a laboratory for testing.

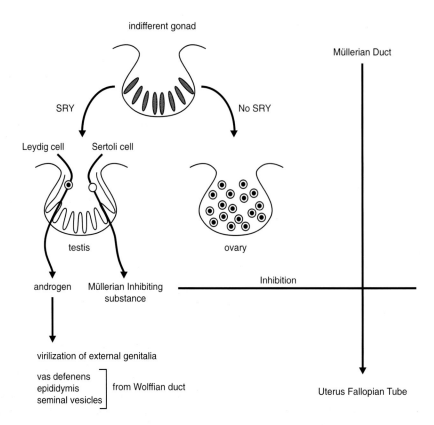

Figure 12.4 • Pathway of sexual differentiation.

Females with campomelic dysplasia generally have normal genitalia, but males may have genital phenotypes ranging from normal male through female-appearing external genitalia. Internal genitalia can be either male or female in XY infants with campomelic dysplasia and, finally, gonads can be either testes or undifferentiated gonads. Understanding the basis for these abnormalities requires a review of normal sexual differentiation. Herein also lies the key to discovering the gene responsible for campomelic dysplasia.

Differentiation of the internal and external genitalia begins with the development of the gonad into either an ovary or a testis (Figure 12.4). Up to 8 weeks of gestation, the gonad, which contains germ cells, is undifferentiated and can become either an ovary or a testis. After that time, a testis forms in the presence of a Y chromosome, and an ovary forms if a Y is absent. The specific gene on the Y chromosome has been identified and is referred to as *SRY*. *SRY* is a transcription factor; its binding to other genes sets into motion a cascade of events that lead to differentiation of the testes.

If a testis forms, Sertoli cells in the testis secrete a peptide hormone, Müllerian inhibiting substance, which leads to regression of the Müllerian ducts. Testosterone produced by the testis leads to growth of the Wolffian ducts into epididymes, vas deferens, and seminal vesicles. The external genitalia also are stimulated by testosterone to grow into a penis and scrotum.

In the absence of *SRY*, an ovary forms instead of a testis. The Müllerian ducts become Fallopian tubes, uterus, and part of the vagina. The Wolffian ducts degenerate due to lack of androgen stimulation, and the external genitalia remain in the female form.

Disorders of sexual differentiation can be explained in terms of this basic process. Presence of *SRY* generally results in formation of a testis. In some instances, *SRY* is deleted from, or mutated on, an otherwise normal Y chromosome, resulting in an XY female; other times, *SRY* is present due to translocation to a chromosome other than Y, leading to an XX male. Y chromosome abnormalities resulting in mosaicism for an XY cell line and a 45,X cell line can lead to phenotypes ranging from normal male, if testes form bilaterally, to Turner syndrome if the 45,X cell line predominates in the gonads. In some cases, a normal testis may form on one side and a "streak" gonad on the other if one side has a Y chromosome and the other only 45,X cells. Müllerian inhibiting substance functions locally, so there will be a Fallopian tube and uterus only on the side with 45,X cells.

The external genitalia depend on androgen stimulation for normal formation. If testes are not present, or do not function normally, the external genitalia will be female. Conversely, if there is exposure to androgens in a 46,XX fetus with ovaries, the external genitalia will appear male, although there will be no gonads in the scrotum. This occurs in females with congenital adrenal hyperplasia, in which deficiency of an enzyme required for adrenal hormone synthesis results in excessive androgen synthesis due to shunting of precursors proximal to the enzyme block into the androgen biosynthetic pathway. Testosterone binds to a cytoplasmic receptor that is encoded by a gene on the X chromosome. Deficiency of the receptor leads to androgen insensitivity, associated with normal testes and no Müllerian structures but female external genitalia.

The gene responsible for campomelic dysplasia was identified through a combination of positional cloning and candidate gene approaches, using knowledge of the association with gender reversal to provide a clue to the nature of the candidate gene. The probable location of the gene was determined by the finding of several individuals with campomelic dysplasia who had chromosome rearrangements involving region 17q24.1–q25.1. In December 1994, two groups reported the isolation of a gene, referred to as *SOX9*, from the region of the translocations and found mutations in individuals with campomelic dysplasia who did not have chromosomal abnormalities (Foster JW, Dominguez-Steglich M, Guioli S, et al. Campomelic dysplasia and autosomal sex reversal caused by mutations in an *SRY*-related gene. Nature 1994;372:525–530. Wagner T, Wirth J, Meyer J, et al. Autosomal sex reversal and campomelic dysplasia are caused by mutations in and around the *SRY*-related gene *SOX9*. Cell 1994;79:1111–1120).

SOX9 is a gene that has a region of homology with *SRY*. The region is a stretch of 80 amino acids called the **high-mobility group domain**, which is believed to bind to DNA and stimulate transcription. Genes that include this domain are called *SOX* genes (for SRY box). *SOX9* was mapped to a region of mouse chromosome 11 that is homologous to human 17q24, making it a candidate for campomelic dysplasia. The two groups independently cloned translocation breakpoints in different individuals with campomelic dysplasia and found that *SOX9* mapped to the region. Inactivating mutations were found in *SOX9* in others with campomelic dysplasia.

SOX9 is involved in testis formation as part of the cascade of activated genes. Its expression appears to be regulated by *SRY*. Why some XY individuals with mutations experience gender reversal and others do not is not understood. Those with gender reversal have dysplastic gonads rather than normal testes. These gonads do not produce Müllerian inhibiting substance, so fallopian tubes and uterus are present. There is deficient androgen production, however, so virilization of the external genitalia is incomplete. Dysplastic gonads can lead to malignant gonadoblastoma, and so they are surgically removed before adolescence.

The *SOX9* gene is also active in developing bone, consistent with the phenotype of campomelic dysplasia. Affected individuals are heterozygous for *SOX9* mutations, indicating that the disorder is dominant, not recessive. Instances of familial recurrence are accounted for by mosaicism in one parent.

PART VI

Jane and Albert have had more education in genetics during the past few weeks than ever during their years in school. They have agonized over the medical decisions regarding Lisa's care, not wanting to put her through unnecessary suffering if her prognosis is indeed poor. Because no central nervous system malformations have been noted by magnetic resonance imaging of the brain, and the literature indicates a range of cognitive outcomes, they are inclined to continue active support. They are encouraged when they meet with another family with a 3-year-old child with campomelic dysplasia, who is on a ventilator at home and is doing fairly well. They decide to continue ventilatory support, and a tracheostomy is placed. After 1 month, Jane and Albert take Lisa home.

This case illustrates a number of issues commonly encountered in genetic counseling. First, the problems are complex and usually are well outside the knowledge of lay individuals. The parents have never heard of the syndrome and may have little or no understanding of the principles of inheritance, let alone molecular genetics. Counseling is complicated further by the emotional trauma of having a sick child, for whom life-and-death decisions need to be made.

It is often helpful to introduce a family to others who have firsthand experience with a genetic syndrome. Although specific manifestations and severity can differ from individual to individual, such contact provides at least a glimpse of what life may be like for a person with the disorder in question. The long-term prognosis for children with campomelic dysplasia remains in question, largely due to limited experience.

INBORN ERRORS OF DEVELOPMENT

Approximately 3% of all pregnancies end with the birth of a child with a birth defect. Usually, these are isolated defects, such as cleft lip or a neural tube defect; the child is otherwise healthy, although he or she may suffer serious consequences from the presence of the malformation. Most of these malformations occur sporadically and are believed to have a multifactorial etiology. Others are determined by single genes or chromosomal abnormalities. Aside from isolated malformations, some babies are born with a complex of multiple congenital anomalies.

Until recently, the molecular basis of syndromes of abnormal development was largely unknown. This vastly limited the tools available for diagnosis. The identification of genes involved in both normal and abnormal development is rapidly changing this picture. Normal development involves processes of cell replication, migration, and differentiation, tightly controlled in a spatial pattern and temporal sequence. Major developmental events are initiated through cell–cell signaling, with binding of a receptor leading to transduction of a signal to the cell nucleus to initiate a program of transcription of specific genes.

Some of the first genes involved in development to be discovered were initially studied in the fruit fly, *Drosophila*. Over the years, a curious set of *Drosophila* mutants had been identified. *Drosophila* species have the typical arthropod body plan of three segments – head, thorax, and abdomen. Rare mutants, referred to as **homeotic mutants**, have distinctive and often bizarre disruptions of body segmentation. The mutant *Antennapedia*, for example, has legs protruding from the head where antennae should be. Other mutants are characterized by segmentation defects (e.g., conversion of a legless abdominal segment into a thoracic segment with legs).

Many of the genes responsible for these phenotypes have been cloned. It has been found that they share a region of homology that has come to be called the **homeobox** or **Hox**, which consists of approximately 60 amino acids (corresponding with 180 base pairs of DNA) that have DNA-binding properties. Other genes involved in the regulation of development share a different DNA-binding domain called the **paired box** or **Pax**. The Pax box consists of 128 amino acids. In *Drosophila*, there are five *Pax* genes, most of which appear to be involved in body segmentation.

There are several groups of *Hox* genes in *Drosophila* that share sequence homology. One group, referred to as the homeotic complex (HOM-C), consists of eight genes. These genes are expressed in an anterior–posterior pattern in the *Drosophila* embryo, in a spatial order that is the same as their arrangement on the chromosome (Figure 12.5). The gene at the 3' end of the complex is expressed in the head region, and loss of function of this gene causes disruption of development of head structures. Genes located in a 5' direction are expressed in progressively more posterior segments. Areas of expression tend to overlap, however. The overlapping expression explains the transformation of one body segment into another in a homeotic mutant: When one *Hox* gene is not expressed in a segment, persistent expression of another leads to transformation of the segment. *Pax* genes also are expressed in specific segments in the *Drosophila* embryo. Both Hox and Pax proteins bind to DNA and activate the transcription of other genes. They are believed to act as switches that invoke tissue-specific developmental programs.

The discovery of Hox and Pax boxes prompted a search for homologous genes in higher eukaryotes, including humans. Using DNA probes for Hox or Pax boxes, regions of homology

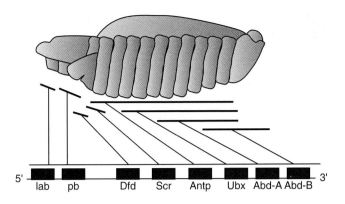

Figure 12.5 • Domains of expression of genes of the *HOM-C* complex in *Drosophila*, with map of region shown at bottom. (Redrawn by permission from McGinnis W, Krumlauf R. Homeobox genes and axial patterning. Cell 1992;68:283–302.)

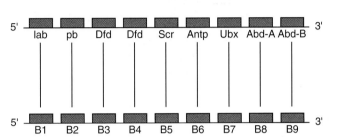

Figure 12.6 • Genes of *HOM-C* complex in *Drosophila* (top) and homologous genes of *Hox-2* cluster in mouse (bottom).

were indeed found. Moreover, mammalian *Hox* genes, like their *Drosophila* counterparts, are arranged in tandem arrays and are expressed in an anterior–posterior direction that mirrors their order on the chromosome (Figure 12.6). There are nine *Pax* genes in the human genome, seven of which also include Hox box sequences.

There are no known natural Hox mutants in the mouse, but study of Hox function has been accomplished by targeted disruption of these genes. A vector containing a mutant *Hox* gene has been introduced into mouse embryonic stem cells. The disrupted segment recombined with the wild-type gene and introduced the mutation into the mouse gene. The embryonic stem cells then were injected into mouse blastocysts, which in turn were implanted into a pseudopregnant uterus and brought to term. Breeding of these chimeric mice resulted in fully heterozygous animals. Mice with Hox mutations tend to have congenital anomalies in the body region where the mutant gene is expressed, indicating that the mammalian *Hox* genes, like their *Drosophila* counterparts, function to regulate the proper morphogenesis of different anterior–posterior regions of the embryo.

In contrast to *Hox*, three natural mouse *Pax* mutations have been identified. One is called *undulated*, the phenotype of which is skeletal deformities. It is due to a single base change in the *Pax1* gene. The second mouse mutant is *splotch*, associated with *Pax3* mutations. *Splotch* has arisen naturally several times, and different *splotch* alleles have been characterized. The third mouse mutant is referred to as *smalleye*, due to *Pax6* mutations. The human homolog of this gene is responsible for the dominant condition Waadenburg syndrome, which consists of deafness, widely-spaced eyes, and a patch of white hair above the forehead.

Identification of the genes involved in development has revealed some unexpected connections between seemingly disparate conditions and has also challenged long-standing diagnostic classification schemes. For example, consider the gene *sonic hedgehog*. The pathway of *sonic hedgehog* action is shown in Figure (12.7). *Sonic hedgehog* mutations occur in some familial or sporadic cases of holoprosencephaly (MIM 142945), a major malformation of the central nervous system in which cleavage of the forebrain into two hemispheres fails partially or completely. Mutations in *patched*, the *sonic hedgehog* receptor, are responsible for basal cell nevus syndrome (MIM 109400). This is an autosomal dominant disorder characterized by large head size, skeletal anomalies, and a predisposition to tumors, including benign basal cell nevi, basal cell carcinomas, and medulloblastomas. The developmental anomalies appear to be due to reduced gene dosage of *patched* (haploinsufficiency), whereas the tumors display loss of

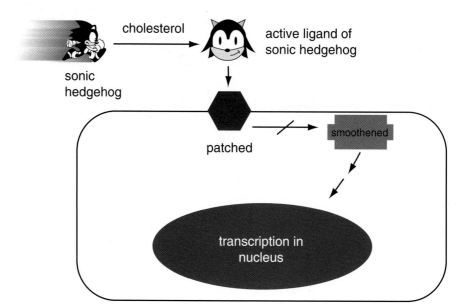

Figure 12.7 • *Sonic hedgehog* signaling pathway. Sonic hedgehog protein is processed into an active ligand by a reaction mediated by cholesterol. The ligand binds a cell surface receptor, *patched*. *Patched* normally inhibits activity of smoothened mutations, but when sonic hedgehog binds to *patched* this inhibition is released, which leads to a signal being transduced to the nucleus to activate transcription of genes involved in cell differentiation.

heterozygosity for *patched*, a classic tumor suppressor mechanism. Some sporadic basal cell carcinomas have been found to have *smoothened* mutations. Finally, the autosomal recessive Smith–Lemli–Optiz syndrome (MIM 270400) (cerebral dysgenesis, sometimes including holoprosencephaly, growth retardation, hypogenitalism, limb anomalies) is due to a block in cholesterol metabolism. Cerebral anomalies in this disorder, and in fetuses exposed to drugs that inhibit cholesterol synthesis, may be due to aberrant *sonic hedgehog* signaling.

REVIEW QUESTIONS

12.1 What is the difference between a disruption and deformation? Would either one be the consequence of teratogen exposure *in utero*?

12.2 Would a uterus and Fallopian tubes be present in an individual with a 46,XY karyotype and a mutation in *SRY* that interferes with testicular development?

12.3 Virtually all mutations responsible for achondroplasia occur at the same site in the *FGFR3* gene. Why is there such a restriction in location of mutations?

12.4 A high proportion of dominantly inherited congenital anomaly syndromes are due to new mutations. Why is this the case?

12.5 What is the relationship between the orientation of *hox* genes on the chromosome and their patterns of expression?

FURTHER READING

Brennan J, Capel B. One tissue, two fates: Molecular events that underlie testis versus ovary development. Nat Rev Genet 2004;5:509–521.

Hunter AG. Medical genetics 2: The diagnostic approach to the child with dysmorphic signs. Canad Med Assoc J 2002;167:367–372.

Prior HM, Walter MA. SOX genes: architects of development. Mol Med 1996;2:405–412.

13

Carrier Screening

INTRODUCTION

We have seen in the chapter on population genetics that some genetic disorders occur at increased frequency in specific populations. The basis for this may reside in phenomena such as the founder effect or balanced polymorphism. The clinical importance is that ancestry may be a clue to the risk that an individual is a carrier for a recessive genetic disorder and that some couples may be at risk of having an affected child. There may not be a known family history of the disorder, so many couples only learn of their risk after the birth of an affected child. The principle of carrier screening is to identify such couples so that they can be counseled about their risk and the options available to deal with the risk. In this chapter we will further explore the principles of carrier screening. We will look at a population-based screening program for thalassemia in Sardinia that has significantly reduced the frequency of this disorder on the island and see how the program has evolved from the premolecular to the molecular era. We will look at other examples of carrier screening programs, some equally successful and others less so. Finally, we will look at general principles of carrier screening programs, and see some of the challenges faced in implementation.

KEY POINTS

- Carrier screening involves testing of individuals for heterozygosity for genes that would produce significant disorders in the homozygous state. Couples found to be at risk if both partners are carriers can be offered counseling regarding their options to deal with the risk.
- An individual may be at increased risk of being a carrier for a particular genetic trait on the basis of ancestry. Many screening programs are targeted towards particular groups known to be at risk.
- Couples found to be at risk have many options, including prenatal diagnosis, adoption, use of an egg or sperm donor, or planning for the medical needs of an affected child.
- The decision to implement a carrier screening program requires careful assessment of risks and benefits and provision of counseling, testing, and management resources. Carrier test results require careful interpretation and counseling of the couple.

PART I 1975

Gino is a 12-year-old boy who lives in Cagliari, Sardinia. When he was 6 months old, Gino was having difficulty feeding and was irritable and listless. He also was noted to be pale, and his abdomen was protuberant. A blood test confirmed his physician's impression that Gino had thalassemia. Gino has been receiving blood transfusions every 4 weeks since he was 18 months old. This has improved his energy level and growth. His spleen was removed when he was 6, and he has required antibiotic treatment for infections ever since. Over the past several years, Gino's major problems have been diabetes mellitus and severe heart failure. He has required

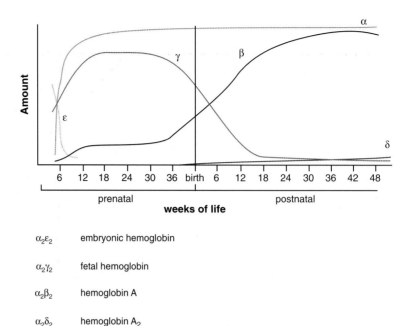

Figure 13.1 • Synthesis of globins in fetal and adult life. Alpha-globin synthesis begins in early fetal life and continues through adult life. The epsilon-chain is made for a short time in the early embryo and contributes to embryonic hemoglobin ($\alpha_2\varepsilon_2$). The gamma-chain is made for a period during fetal life, complexing with alpha-globin to make fetal hemoglobin ($\alpha_2\gamma_2$). Beta-globin synthesis begins in the fetus but achieves predominance after birth. This is the constituent of adult hemoglobin, hemoglobin A ($\alpha_2\beta_2$). A minor adult hemoglobin species, A$_2$, consists of $\alpha_2\delta_2$.

$\alpha_2\varepsilon_2$	embryonic hemoglobin
$\alpha_2\gamma_2$	fetal hemoglobin
$\alpha_2\beta_2$	hemoglobin A
$\alpha_2\delta_2$	hemoglobin A$_2$

hospitalization several times in the past 2 years for management of these problems. His family realizes that probably Gino will not survive much longer. He has normal intelligence, although he is far behind in school as a result of his illness. He is well aware of the seriousness of his medical condition. Recently, Gino has been started on an experimental therapy that requires injection of a new drug. It is too soon to know whether this will help with his problems and prolong his life.

Thalassemia is a form of chronic anemia due to an inherited deficiency in the production of one of the chains of hemoglobin. Hemoglobin, the oxygen-carrying molecule of the red blood cell (RBC), consists of two pairs of globin chains, each of which binds one heme molecule. The major form of hemoglobin in the adult, hemoglobin A, is a tetramer of two alpha-globin-chains and two beta-chains. There are other beta-like chains that can bind to the alpha-chains and are expressed at different times in life (Figure 13.1). Epsilon-chains are produced during early embryonic development and gamma-chains during fetal life. These bind with alpha-globin to produce embryonic and fetal hemoglobins, respectively. Beta-chain synthesis begins during fetal development, but beta-globin does not become predominant until after birth. An additional beta-like chain, delta, is made in small quantities after birth and comprises a minor species of hemoglobin called A$_2$.

Individuals with beta-thalassemia have deficient production of beta-chains, whereas those with alpha-thalassemia have deficient alpha-chain production. The pathophysiology of beta-thalassemia (Figure 13.2) begins with chronic anemia. There may be no problems in the early months of life while fetal hemoglobin ($\alpha_2\gamma_2$) is made. As fetal hemoglobin production declines, however, the anemia begins. This leads to poor growth, lack of energy, and irritability.

The production of RBCs is regulated by the body's need for oxygen. In children with thalassemia, RBC production is stimulated because of chronic tissue hypoxia. The bone marrow expands to increase its output of RBCs, which leads to weakening of the long bones and enlargement of bones in the skull that normally do not contribute to hematopoiesis. Fractures and a characteristic facial deformity result. Hematopoiesis also occurs in the liver, leading to hepatomegaly. The extra production of RBCs, of course, is futile, as the newly made erythrocytes also are deficient in beta-globin. Alpha-chains unite with the few delta- or gamma-chains present, but most precipitate in the cell. These RBCs are removed from circulation by the spleen. The spleen enlarges owing to extramedullary hematopoiesis as well as trapping of defective RBCs. Massive enlargement of the spleen necessitates splenectomy, which in turn leads to susceptibility to bacterial infection.

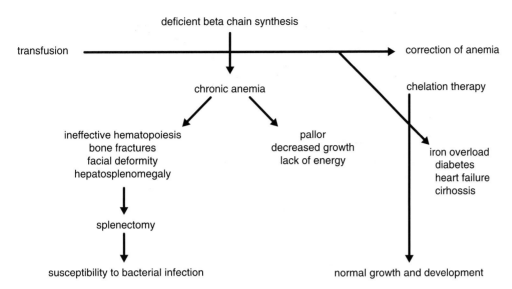

Figure 13.2 • Pathophysiology of thalassemia.

Left untreated, beta-thalassemia is fatal due to the effects of anemia, bone destruction, and rupture of the spleen. The obvious treatment is to replace RBCs by transfusion. Transfusion of intact RBCs corrects the anemia; bone marrow spaces return to normal size, and extramedullary hematopoiesis ceases. Energy and growth resume normally, and quality of life can be vastly improved. Unfortunately, the treatment is not without adverse effects. There is a risk of infection, particularly with hepatitis virus. More significant, though, is the problem of chronic iron overload. Transfused RBCs have a limited life span and, when they degenerate, the iron in heme must be disposed of. The body's capacity to excrete iron is overwhelmed rapidly, and iron accumulates in tissues, where it is toxic, leading to cirrhosis of the liver, diabetes mellitus, and heart failure. The treatment of thalassemia by transfusion, then, is ultimately as bad as the disease.

In the mid-1970s, an approach was developed to deal with iron overload, based on the use of a chelating agent, deferoxamine. Deferoxamine binds iron and renders it soluble, so that it can be excreted in the urine. The drug is not absorbed through the gastrointestinal tract and so must be administered by subcutaneous infusion. This is administered overnight using a pump connected to a needle placed under the skin.

With regular transfusions and deferoxamine, a person with thalassemia can live a productive life. Activity and energy levels can be normal. The therapy, though, is very expensive – tens of thousands of dollars annually. This can strain the finances of a family and of the community. Moreover, thalassemia is particularly prevalent in some areas of the world, many of which can ill afford the burden of this disease on their health-care systems.

PART II 1976

> Gino died earlier this year of congestive heart failure. Although his family had known for a long time of the seriousness of his medical condition, they still were shaken by the loss. The experience has also caused concern among relatives about their chances of having children with thalassemia. In particular, Gino's cousin Rosa was recently married, and she and her husband Antonio are thinking about starting a family. Rosa asks her doctor about her risks of being a thalassemia carrier and about whether Antonio might be a carrier.

Thalassemia is not uniformly distributed around the world. Prevalence is highest in the Mediterranean region, North-Central Africa, the Middle East, India, and Southeast Asia. In Sardinia, where the frequency of the disease was 1 in 213 persons in the mid-1970s, virtually everyone knew somebody – a friend or a relative – who was affected. Thalassemia and its complications consumed a large fraction of funds for health care on the island and were among the most common reasons for hospitalization.

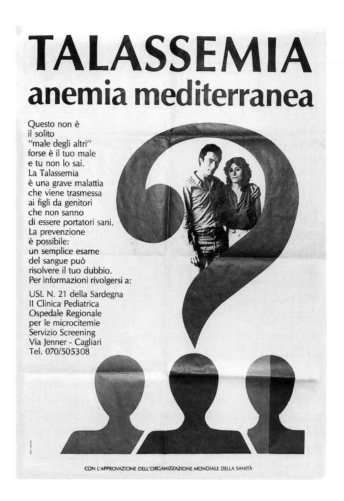

Figure 13.3 • Poster publicizing the thalassemia screening program in Sardinia. (Courtesy of Dr. Antonio Cao.)

Thalassemia is inherited as an autosomal recessive trait; hence, both parents must be carriers to have an affected child. In a population where the disorder is prevalent, such as Sardinia, there is a substantial chance for a person to be a carrier. How can the risk be measured? One way would be to screen the population for carrier status. Unlike many autosomal recessive disorders, carrier testing for thalassemia is possible by fairly simple means. Beta-thalassemia carriers have mild anemia, which is clinically silent but can be detected by blood testing. They also have elevated levels of hemoglobin A_2. Although such testing became the basis for population screening for clinical purposes, as will be described shortly, it was not necessary to go to this extent to estimate the carrier frequency. That could be done easily using the Hardy–Weinberg equation (see Chapter 7).

On Sardinia in 1975, 1 of every 213 individuals was affected with thalassemia. This is a frequency of $0.0047 = q^2$. Therefore $q = 0.0685$ and $p = 1 - q = 0.9315$. The carrier frequency is $2pq = 2(0.0685)(0.9315) = 0.01276$, or 12.76%. Matings between thalassemia carriers on Sardinia indeed were not uncommon in the 1970s.

PART III 1978

Rosa and Antonio are referred to a thalassemia screening program that has begun in Southern Sardinia (Figure 13.3). The two meet with a counselor, fill in a questionnaire about their health and family history, and are told about thalassemia and the screening test. Because there is a history of thalassemia in Rosa's family, she is tested first and is found to be a carrier. Antonio then is tested. The results for both Rosa and Antonio are shown in Figure 13.4. Both Rosa and Antonio are found to be thalassemia carriers. They are counseled that they have a 25% risk of having a child with beta-thalassemia. Rosa is now 18 weeks pregnant. A sample of fetal blood is drawn under ultrasound guidance, and the fetal blood cells are incubated with [³H]-leucine.

	Mean Cell Volume (fl)	% HbA$_2$	Electrophoresis
Rosa	65	6.7	A-F-A$_2$
Antonio	68	7.1	A-F-A$_2$
Normal Range	80-110	1.5-3.5	A-A$_2$

Figure 13.4 • Results of thalassemia screening in Rosa and Antonio. (A = hemoglobin A; F = fetal hemoglobin; A_2 = hemoglobin A$_2$.)

The newly synthesized globin is analyzed for the alpha–beta ratio. The ratio is found to be abnormal, indicating that the fetus is affected with thalassemia. After agonizing over their decision, Rosa and Antonio decide to terminate the pregnancy.

In 1977, a pilot program was launched to screen for thalassemia carriers in Southern Sardinia. Carriers can be easily identified by an accurate and inexpensive blood test, showing reduced RBC volume and relatively increased hemoglobin A$_2$ compared with A (because of a reduction in $\alpha_2\beta_2$ production with normal $\alpha_2\delta_2$). A public education program was initiated using town meetings, posters, pamphlets, and advertising via radio, television, and newspapers. Couples planning a pregnancy were targeted, and one member of each couple was tested first, with the partner tested only if the first partner tested positively. If both partners were found to be carriers, prenatal diagnosis was offered.

In the 1970s, the only way to diagnose beta-thalassemia prenatally was to draw fetal blood from the placenta and to measure the production of beta-globin. Diagnosis was complicated by the fact that very little beta-chain is made early in pregnancy, at which time the majority of globin is fetal hemoglobin ($\alpha_2\gamma_2$). Beta-globin production was determined by incubation of fetal blood in the presence of tritiated leucine. Beta- and gamma-globin were separated by electrophoresis and quantified by measuring incorporation of radioactivity.

During the first 3 years of screening, 4057 individuals were tested. The testing was voluntary and included approximately two-thirds of the population of childbearing age in the region. Six hundred twenty-two thalassemia carriers were detected (for a carrier frequency of 13.6%, which included a few carriers for globin disorders other than beta-thalassemia). An additional 2402 carriers were detected on the basis of a known family history of beta-thalassemia. A total of 694 couples were found to be at risk of having an affected child, and 177 pregnancies were monitored by prenatal diagnosis. The rate of acceptance of prenatal testing changed dramatically during the 3 years of pilot testing, increasing from approximately 73% in 1977 to nearly 93% in 1980. Among the 177 tested pregnancies, five resulted in miscarriage due to fetal hemorrhage or premature labor. Forty-two fetuses were found to be affected with thalassemia, and 39 were electively terminated. The frequency of beta-thalassemia in this region of Sardinia declined from 1 in 213 persons in 1976 to 1 in 290 in 1978 (Cao A, Furbetta M, Galanello R, et al. Prevention of homozygous β-thalassemia by carrier screening and prenatal diagnosis in Sardinia. Am J Hum Genet 1981;33:592–605).

At around the same time, population screening for thalassemia also was initiated on the island of Cyprus, with similar success. It is interesting, though, to compare these programs with two other population screens for recessive disorders begun in the United States in the 1970s – one for sickle cell anemia and one for Tay–Sachs disease.

Sickle cell carrier screening began shakily in the United States in the early 1970s. The test used at first did not distinguish sickle cell carriers from those with the disease and, unfortunately, the same was true for much of the educational material disseminated at the time. Therefore, those who tested positively were, in many cases, subjected to discrimination (e.g., denial of employment or health or life insurance, or raising of insurance premiums). Furthermore, when the screening began, prenatal diagnosis of sickle cell disease was not possible. This vastly limited the options of those found to be at risk of having an affected child. The screening program was poorly organized, overly ambitious, and racially divisive.

Several changes have occurred over the years that have led to a reappraisal of sickle cell screening. First, it has been found that early identification of sickle cell disease is important as affected children are at high risk of developing life-threatening infections. Newborn screening now is offered widely and is performed on all newborns, not just African Americans. Another development is the advent of methods of prenatal diagnosis based on DNA technology. This provides the option of prenatal diagnosis to couples found to be at risk. A study of carrier screening for hemoglobinopathies in New York has demonstrated the wide acceptance of a program in which the testing is readily available and adequate and effective counseling and education are provided.

Screening for carriers of Tay–Sachs disease began in many countries around the world in the early 1970s (Kaback M, Lim-Steele J, Dabholkar D, et al. Tay–Sachs disease – carrier screening, prenatal diagnosis, and the molecular era. JAMA 1993;270:2307–2315). Nearly 1 in 30 Jewish individuals of Eastern European (Ashkenazi) background is a carrier for the infantile form of Tay–Sachs disease, which is a tragically progressive, lethal disorder. Screening has targeted this population with an aggressive program of public education, rigorous quality control of laboratory testing, and ready availability of genetic counseling. Prenatal diagnosis of Tay–Sachs disease is possible with a reliable biochemical test or, more recently, with a DNA-based test. For ultraorthodox Jewish groups in which abortion is not acceptable, confidential screening has been used to avoid marriages between carriers. From 1971 through 1992, almost 1 million individuals had been tested and more than 36,000 carriers detected. Prenatal testing was done for more than 2400 pregnancies at risk. Prior to screening, approximately 60 new Tay–Sachs disease cases were identified around the world each year. Currently, the rate has fallen to three to five cases per year, comparable to the frequency in non-Jewish couples. More recently, screening in the Ashkenazi population has been broadened to include cystic fibrosis, Canavan disease, and other disorders such as Gaucher and Niemann–Pick disease.

These experiences highlight the factors that determine the success of a population screening program. First, the screening must be based on a test that is reliable, accurate, cost-effective, and readily available. Second, the screening must be organized in a manner that is appropriate to the customs of the target population. Third, there must be options available to those found to be at risk that are acceptable in the population. Finally, the goal of screening must be the improvement of the health of individuals, not the improvement of the gene pool of the population. These lessons will likely be increasingly important as the genetic basis for common diseases comes to light and mass screening for other genetic traits is contemplated.

PART IV

Rosa's second pregnancy was in 1980 and was found to be unaffected, resulting in the birth of a healthy boy, Paolo. A third pregnancy in 1982 also resulted in a healthy child, a girl named Maria. Now Rosa is pregnant again. This time, the pregnancy is monitored by amniocentesis, and a DNA test is used (Figure 13.5). Both Rosa and Antonio are found to carry the beta[39] mutation. This same assay is used to test amniotic fluid cells, and the fetus is found to be a carrier. The pregnancy is continued, and a healthy baby girl, Gabriella, is delivered.

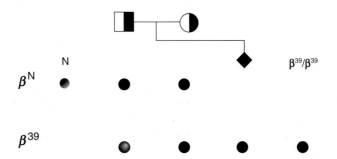

Figure 13.5 • Dot-blot test for beta[39] mutation. The beta[39] region is amplified by polymerase chain reaction, and either normal (top) or mutant (bottom) oligonucleotide is hybridized with the sequence. An individual homozygous for the wild-type allele hybridizes only with the wild-type oligonucleotide (*N* at left). Both heterozygous parents hybridize with both sequences. The fetus, and a beta[39] homozygote, hybridizes only with the mutant oligonucleotide. (Courtesy of Dr. B. Handelin.)

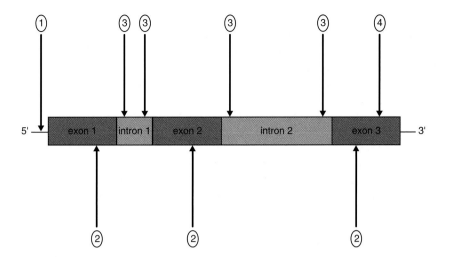

Figure 13.6 • Sites of mutation in the beta-globin gene. [1] Promoter mutations lead to decreased level of transcription. [2] Point mutations within exons cause amino acid substitutions or cessation of translation [stop mutations]. [3] Intron mutations affect the fidelity of splicing. [4] polyA addition site mutations lead to decreased mRNA stability.

By 1987, the frequency of beta-thalassemia in Sardinia had fallen to approximately 1 : 1100, despite the cumbersome method of prenatal diagnosis used in the early years. Because beta-globin is produced only by RBCs, prenatal diagnosis by amniocentesis was not possible. It remained to develop a DNA-based test to simplify the approach to prenatal diagnosis.

Beta-globin was one of the first human genes to be cloned. Characterization of globin gene mutations has revealed the diversity of ways in which a genetic change can alter the function of a gene product and also provides a basis for molecular diagnosis. The most prevalent beta-globin mutation in Sardinia, identified in 1981, is a nonsense mutation at codon 39. This mutation results in a form of thalassemia referred to as *beta*^{0}, because no beta-globin is made. A person who is homozygous for this mutation produces a 39 amino acid beta-globin peptide (full-length beta-globin is 146 amino acids) that is degraded in the cell. More than 95% of Sardinians with beta-thalassemia have this mutation. Another rare mutation was found in approximately 2% of the carriers, this one is a frameshift at codon 6 that also results in a truncated protein. A low proportion of Sardinians with thalassemia have a form referred to as *beta*$^+$, in which a small amount of beta-globin is produced. Two mutations were found to be associated with this phenotype in different individuals. Both interfere with mRNA splicing, one at nucleotide 110 in intron 1 and one at nucleotide 745 in intron 2. These four mutations account for more than 98% of thalassemia mutations in the Sardinian population.

Study of globin mutations around the world has revealed a similar story. In each population, a relatively small number of mutations accounts for the majority of affected individuals, yet these mutations differ widely from one region to another. The entire process of gene expression, from initiation of transcription at the promoter, to RNA splicing, to polyA addition, are vulnerable to mutation (Figure 13.6). Missense and nonsense mutations and gene deletions have been found. We have seen in Chapter 7 that the relatively high frequency of globin disorders in certain parts of the world may be attributed to the effects of a balanced polymorphism. We have also seen how the founder effect causes a specific mutation to be more prevalent in specific regions.

PART V   1994

Rosa's youngest sister, Maria, recently was married, and she and her partner, Alberto, are screened for thalassemia carrier status. While they are waiting for the test results, they ask the genetic counselor what is new in treatment for thalassemia. Maria is found to be a thalassemia carrier, but Alberto is not. The partners are informed that they are not at risk of having a child with thalassemia.

The use of chelation therapy has vastly improved the clinical outcome for persons with beta-thalassemia. Most of the long-term complications of the disease are due to iron overload, but early institution of deferoxamine treatment and faithful compliance have been shown to prevent the accumulation of iron and its consequences. Using the end point of cardiac disease, one recent study has shown that 91% of patients treated with deferoxamine were free of heart disease after 15 years; survival in this study correlated closely with serum ferritin measurements, which reflects stored iron. Transfusion and chelation therapy is not without drawbacks, however. There is risk of developing hepatitis, although donor blood now is screened for this virus. The cost of treatment can be high, in the tens of thousands of dollars per year. Moreover, treatment must be continued throughout life, requiring overnight administration of deferoxamine and transfusions as often as every 3 weeks. Efforts to develop a safe and effective oral chelation therapy have not yet been successful. Investigators have therefore sought alternative means of treatment.

Replacement of hematopoietic cells with new cells that do not have mutant beta-globin genes would provide definitive treatment of thalassemia. This can be accomplished by bone marrow transplantation. In one study, bone marrow transplantation was done using human leukocyte antigen–identical donor marrow for patients with beta-thalassemia who were already suffering from the effects of iron overload. Disease-free survival for 3 years or more was 80%. Another study showed 85% disease-free survival when patients were treated prior to the appearance of signs of iron overload. These are encouraging results, but the treatment also comes at a price, both medical and financial. The bone marrow transplant procedure is expensive and involves major discomfort, a small proportion of recipients suffer complications or rejection, and some die.

A long-term goal might be to replace the defective beta-globin gene in bone marrow cells from an affected individual and to transplant these cells back into that person's marrow. This would avoid the risks of graft rejection or rejection of the recipient by the graft (graft-versus-host disease). Beta-globin cDNA has been inserted into hematopoietic stem cells using retroviral vectors. The challenge has been to obtain adequate quantities of beta-globin synthesis, which has not yet been achieved. Gene therapy for beta-thalassemia is therefore not yet possible.

An alternative form of treatment is suggested by the existence of a cluster of beta-like genes. Individuals with beta-thalassemia do not suffer anemia during fetal life because of the production of fetal hemoglobin, which uses the gamma-chains instead of beta-chains. Gamma-chain production falls to very low levels soon after birth. The genes, of course, still are present, but somehow they are permanently inactivated. Can they be reactivated in individuals with beta-globin mutations? Although fetal hemoglobin has greater oxygen affinity than adult hemoglobin and is best suited to oxygen transport in the oxygen-deprived fetal environment, it might function well enough in the adult to ameliorate many of the effects of beta-thalassemia.

CARRIER SCREENING

Most couples learn that they are both carriers for an autosomal recessive disorder after the birth of an affected child. Carrier screening offers an opportunity to identify couples at risk before this time, allowing them to use this information in their planning. Options for a couple in which both partners are carriers include:

- Choosing not to have children
- Artificial insemination or egg donation
- Prenatal diagnosis and termination of an affected pregnancy
- Prenatal diagnosis and planning for care of an affected child
- No prenatal testing

Screening options are tailored to the disorders for which members of a couple are at risk, generally on the basis of ethnic background. Tests may be based on the detection of a gene product, such as an enzyme assay, or on detection of pathogenic mutations. Gene product tests tend to be highly sensitive but may be subject to false-positive results and may require access to tissue in which the gene is expressed. DNA-based tests are highly specific, but some pathogenic mutations may escape detection. Some of the disorders subject to carrier screening are listed in Table 13.1. In some cases, carrier testing may be offered to the general population, in instances in which there is no specific ethnic predilection. Special care must be exercised in counseling individuals who do not come from a population known to be at risk. On the one hand they might not be aware of having an ancestor who is derived from the group at risk; on the other hand, their carrier risk and the sensitivity of genetic testing may be unknown.

TABLE 13.1 Major disorders subject to carrier screening in specific populations

Population	Disorder	Test	Carrier frequency
Ashkenazi Jewish	Tay–Sachs disease	Enzyme/DNA	1/30
	Cystic fibrosis	DNA	1/29
	Familial dysautonomia	DNA	1/36
	Canavan disease	DNA	1/40
French Canadian	Tay–Sachs disease	DNA	1/70
Asian	Thalassemia	Hematologic	Population-specific
Mediterranean	Thalassemia	Hematologic	Population-specific
African	Sickle cell anemia	Hematologic	1/10
White	Cystic fibrosis	DNA	1/25

TABLE 13.2 Comparison of testing outcomes using a 70% or 90% sensitive mutation screen

Outcome	70% Detection rate		90% Detection rate	
	Frequency	Risk of CF in offspring	Frequency	Risk of CF in offspring
N/N	0.9447	1/30,000	0.929	1/250,000
N/C	0.054	1/300	0.069	1/1,000
C/C	0.00078	1/4	0.0013	1/4

N = Normal result, C = carrier result

Some of the challenges faced in establishing a carrier screening program are illustrated by cystic fibrosis. In 1997, a Consensus Development Conference was held at the National Institutes of Health (NIH) to review the question of cystic fibrosis screening. The panel recommended that cystic fibrosis testing be offered to individuals with a family history of the disorder and for all couples contemplating pregnancy or currently pregnant, but not to the general population. There was concern, however, that the medical community was not well prepared to offer testing and counseling on this large scale. A task force was set up to help establish the resources necessary to implement the NIH panel's recommendations. After several years of discussion, in 2001 a joint committee of the American College of Medical Genetics and the American College of Obstetricians and Gynecologists issued joint recommendations that CF mutation screening be made available to all couples contemplating pregnancy. A standardized mutation panel was defined, consisting of the 25 mutations that occur at a frequency of at least 0.1% of all *CFTR* mutations in a US panethnic panel. Explanatory brochures were created, along with informed consent documents.

The sensitivity of the screening test differs in different populations. No mutation screen detects 100% of possible *CFTR* mutations, and therefore lack of detection of a mutation does not guarantee that an individual is not a carrier. Even if both partners are not found to carry a cystic fibrosis mutation, they are still at risk of having a child affected with a mutation not included in the testing. The impact of this can be seen if one compares the outcomes of a test that detects 70% of mutations and one that detects 90% of mutations (Table 13.2).

With either test, a finding that both partners are carriers leads to a 1 in 4 risk of cystic fibrosis in an offspring, and reliable prenatal testing is possible. Finding that neither partner is a carrier substantially reduces the risk of having an affected child, although that risk still is not zero. Couples need to be informed that this screening test does not detect all possible mutations and that some couples considered to be at very low risk may, rarely, still have an affected child. The most problematic scenario, however, is the middle one: One partner is found to be a carrier, and the other is not. This will be a common occurrence, happening in 5% or so of

Figure 13.7 • (A) Poly T polymorphism in intron 8 consists of three alleles, in which there can be 5T's, 7T's, or 9T's. The 9T allele is the most common and leads to normal splicing of the CFTR transcript. Normal splicing also occurs with the 7T allele, but exon 9 is skipped if the 5T allele is present. (B) Genotypes associated with CBAVD or mild CF associated with the poly T polymorphism and the R117H mutation. R117H acts as a mild CF mutation on the same chromosome with (in cis) a 7T allele, but a has a greater phenotypic effect if in cis with a 5T allele. If there is a CF mutation on the opposite chromosome (trans), R117H in cis with 7T results in CBAVD but in cis with 5T results in mild CF. CBAVD may also occur with R117H in trans with a 5T allele, or with homozygosity for 5T. It is unknown whether the 5T chromosomes carry another, undetected CF mutation.

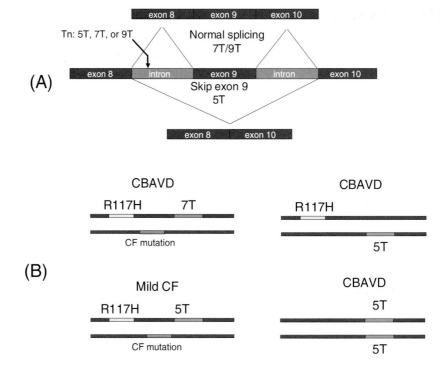

couples with a 70% sensitive screen and in more than 6% of couples with a 90% sensitive screen. In each case, the risk of having an affected child is increased over the population risk, as one partner is known to be a carrier and the other might still be a carrier for an undetected mutation. In such couples, mutation analysis will not identify cystic fibrosis in a fetus, as the second *CFTR* mutation is undetectable. Consequently, mutation screening has alerted the partners to their increased risk yet has offered nothing further in the way of prenatal diagnosis. The sensitivity of mutation screening, moreover, is highly variable among different ethnic groups. Only 30% of cystic fibrosis mutations in the Asian-American population are detected with most commonly used testing schemes, for example. In these populations the level of uncertainty provided by a negative test is even greater.

Aside from the complexities introduced by incomplete ascertainment of mutations, there are also counseling challenges due to genetic heterogeneity. It has become clear that not all *CFTR* mutations lead to the classical syndrome of cystic fibrosis. For example, some mutations lead to the pulmonary complications without the pancreatic insufficiency. An even milder phenotype associated with particular *CFTR* mutations has been identified in some males with infertility due to congenital bilateral absence of the vas deferens (CBAVD). Other syndromes associated with *CFTR* mutations include chronic pancreatitis or chronic sinusitis. The particular phenotype associated with a rare combination of two mutant alleles may be difficult to predict.

Further complication is introduced by the existence of a polymorphism within intron 8 of *CFTR*, in which individuals may have a run of 5, 7, or 9 thymidine bases (5T/7T/9T) (Figure 13.7). The 5T allele is associated with skipping of exon 9 and reduced *CFTR* expression. The presence of the 5T allele may modify the expression of a mild *CFTR* allele on the same chromosome. Some males with CBAVD have been found to have a *CFTR* mutation on one chromosome and a 5T allele on the other; whether the chromosome with the 5T allele includes another undetected *CFTR* mutation is unknown. *CFTR* mutation status must therefore be interpreted in the context of other variants in the gene, at least in some cases, highlighting the importance of careful genetic counseling in reporting results to patients.

REVIEW QUESTIONS

13.1 A couple request screening for globin disorders. One partner is of African descent and one of Mediterranean descent. Are they at increased risk of having a child with a globin disorder?

13.2 Why are some carrier screens done using biochemical testing (e.g., Tay–Sachs disease) and others by DNA testing?

13.3 Why is it important to consider ancestry in interpretation of a carrier screen for a disorder with allelic heterogeneity such as cystic fibrosis?

13.4 One of the pitfalls in carrier screening by testing for specific DNA mutations is that a negative test does not exclude carrier status, since an individual may still carry a mutation that was not included in the screening panel. Aside from cost, why is complete sequencing of a gene not an ideal solution to this problem?

13.5 Is there any point in offering carrier screening to couples who would not terminate an affected pregnancy?

FURTHER READING

Cao, A. Carrier screening and genetic counseling in beta-thalassemia. Int J Hematol 2002;76 Suppl 2:105–113.

Cohen AR, Galanello R, Pennell DJ, Cunningham MJ, Vichinsky E. Thalassemia. In Hematology, American Society of Hematology Education Program, 2004;14–34.

Watson MS, Cutting GR, Desnick RJ, et al. Cystic fibrosis population carrier screening: 2004 revision of American College of Medical Genetics mutation panel. Genet Med 2004;6:387–391.

Weatherall DJ. Thalassemia: The long road from bedside to genome. Nat Rev Genet 2004;5:625–631.

14

Genetic Risk Assessment

INTRODUCTION

One of the major promises of the Human Genome Project is the prospect of understanding the genetic basis of common disorders. This offers the possibility of genetic testing to identify individuals at risk with the hope of providing approaches to reducing that risk or providing treatments to improve outcome. There are many challenges faced in implementation of this approach, however. Common disorders result from a complex interaction of multiple genetic and nongenetic factors. Genetic testing may in some cases reveal only an increased relative risk, and there may be major uncertainty regarding actual risk of disease. There can also be ethical, legal, and social pitfalls, including concerns about stigmatization or discrimination resulting from a positive test in a healthy individual. We will consider these issues in this chapter, focusing first on a relatively common disorder for which screening is possible. We will see how early diagnosis can be a prelude to preventative treatment, but also how genetic testing can be poorly predictive of who will develop disease. We will then look at some general principles in the implementation of predictive or presymptomatic genetic tests.

KEY POINTS

- Predispositional tests can be offered in some cases to identify individuals at increased risk of disease. The risk may be based on family history or the fact that an individual comes from a population known to be at increased risk.
- Predispositional testing can be valuable if an individual found to be at risk can be offered approaches to reduce risk of disease or improve outcome in advance of clinical appearance of symptoms.
- Predispositional tests need to be interpreted with caution, since they do not equate with diagnostic tests. Many individuals found to be at increased risk will not develop symptoms of the disorder.
- Risks and benefits of predispositional tests must be carefully weighed in deciding to implement testing programs, or to offer testing to an individual.

PART I

It is after a Saturday game of softball that George is finally convinced by his wife Nancy that he needs to see a doctor. Over the past 6 months he has had gradually worsening pain in his right knee that gets especially bad after vigorous physical activity. George has nursed the pain – with ibuprofen, with ice packs, or with a warm bath – but although the intense pain usually subsides, it never completely goes away. George is feeling well otherwise, pretty well, he thinks, for a 50-year-old.

Nancy makes the appointment for George with Dr. Chen, and goes with him to the visit. On questioning, George reports that the knee might have been slightly swollen when the pain began a few months ago, but he doesn't think it is anymore. He does not describe hip or ankle pain,

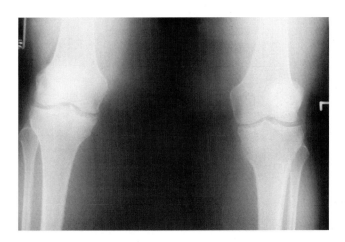

Figure 14.1 • Radiograph of both knees showing calcification in the joint space. (Courtesy of Dr. Daniel Solomon, Brigham and Women's Hospital.)

but the left knee hurts a little. His other joints are without pain and he has no constitutional complaints. George has no history of prior surgery and he has always been thin. He denies any chronic illness in his family except for adult-onset diabetes mellitus in his mother. His children (two boys) are well. He drinks socially, up to six beers per week, and does not smoke.

Dr. Chen does a physical examination, which she finds to be normal. She then orders plain radiographs of the knees (Figure 14.1).

George presents with a history of pain in a single joint (although there is a hint that the other knee may also be involved). The onset is not acute; indeed the pain has been increasing over a period of months. Major conditions in the differential diagnosis are:

- Trauma (no history to suggest that here)
- Bursitis/tendonitis (expect no effusion, but have point tenderness)
- Septic arthritis (diagnosed by aspiration of effusion)
- Crystal-induced inflammation (gout or pseudogout)
- Rheumatoid arthritis (atypical presentation – usually polyarticular)

PART II

The radiographs reveal moderate bicompartmental degenerative joint disease and calcium deposits within the cartilage (chondrocalcinosis). Dr. Chen explains to George and Nancy that it will be necessary to refer George to a rheumatologist. Dr. Chen is not sure what the cause of the joint changes might be. She recommends that George continue to take ibuprofen to help him with the pain.

George sees Dr. Gold, a rheumatologist, about a week later. Examination now reveals a small effusion on the right knee, but otherwise the knee is normal, without joint line tenderness or laxity of the ligaments. George's other joints are within normal limits, he has no organomegaly, his skin is normal, and his review of systems is negative for liver disease or diabetes. A right knee aspiration is performed and 5 cc of yellowish cloudy fluid are obtained. The white blood cell count in the fluid is 10,000 with 70% polymorphonuclear leukocytes, 15% lymphocytes, 10% monocytes. Positively birefringent, rhomboid-shaped crystals are seen on polarizing light microscopy (Figure 14.2) and are determined to be calcium pyrophosphate dihydrate crystals.

The X-ray here shows intra-articular calcification, which would be most compatible with pseudogout. The joint aspiration reveals evidence of inflammation, and the positively birefringent crystals confirm this diagnosis. The crystals represent calcium pyrophosphate dihydrate (CPPD). The term "psuedogout" derives from some overlap in clinical features with classical gout, in which uric acid crystals deposit in joints to cause episodes of acute inflammation. Here, however, the crystals are of different composition (CPPD). The pathophysiology of crystal formation is not well understood. Increased levels of calcium or pyrophosphate may contribute, as well as underlying abnormalities of the cartilage matrix. Clinical attacks may

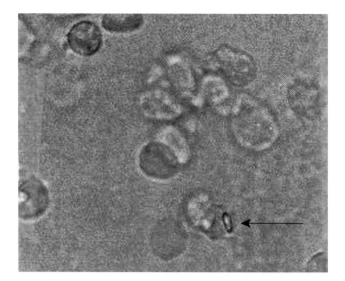

Figure 14.2 • Rhomboid, positively birefringent calcium pyrophosphate dihydrate crystal in a white blood cell from synovial fluid (*arrow*). (Courtesy of Dr. Daniel Solomon, Brigham and Women's Hospital.)

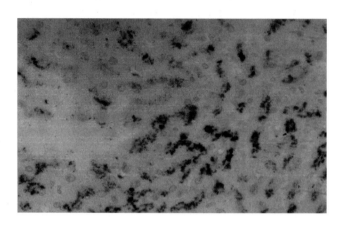

Figure 14.3 • Liver biopsy stained with Prussian blue showing intracellular iron deposition. (Courtesy of Dr. Norman Grace, Faulkner Hospital.)

occur acutely, in a single joint, or can be more chronic and involve multiple joints. Sometimes there are systemic signs, such as fever or elevated white blood cell count. Pseudogout is etiologically heterogeneous. Most cases occur sporadically, but dominant inheritance has been described. There is also an association with several systemic disorders, including:

- Hemochromatosis (increase in iron stores, reflected in elevated transferrin saturation)
- Hyperparathyroidism (elevated calcium)
- Hypophosphatasia (low phosphate)
- Hypomagnesemia (low magnesium)
- Hypothyroidism (low thyroid hormone, high TSH)

PART III

On receiving the results of the joint aspiration, Dr. Gold obtains a blood sample from George. This reveals normal levels of calcium, phosphate, creatinine, parathyroid hormone, and thyroid stimulating hormone. Complete blood count is normal, but his ferritin level is 1500 ng/ml and his transferrin saturation is 70%. After explaining the possible significance of these findings, Dr. Gold refers George to a gastroenterologist, Dr. Pathak. Dr. Pathak performs a liver biopsy, which shows intrahepatocyte iron deposition without fibrosis or active hepatitis (Figure 14.3). Hepatic iron index is calculated to be 2.1.

The laboratory findings in this patient suggest hemochromatosis (based on the high ferritin and transferrin saturation). Ferritin is an intracellular protein that binds iron and serves as a storage site for iron in the cell. Normal values in males range from 15 to 400 ng/ml (values are lower in females due to menstrual blood loss). Transferrin is the major iron transporting protein in the blood. It delivers iron to cells by binding to a membrane receptor (the transferrin receptor). Iron stores are usually expressed in terms of percent transferrin saturation (iron divided by total iron binding capacity). Normal values are 20 to 45%. The findings in this individual suggest elevated iron stores, based on high ferritin and transferrin saturation.

Aside from joints, the liver is a major target for the pathology associated with hemochromatosis. This manifests as iron deposition in the liver, which results in hepatocellular loss and ensuing fibrosis. Hepatic iron index is calculated as the hepatic iron concentration in μmol/g divided by age in years; individuals with hemochromatosis tend to have values greater than 2.

PART IV

> Dr. Pathak explains to George and Nancy that these findings are diagnostic of hemochromatosis. He explains what this is, and points out that George will now require phlebotomy on a weekly basis. George and Nancy are incredulous, and ask whether there is a medication that George can take. Dr. Pathak tells them that there is not, but reassures them that phlebotomy is a highly effective therapy, and can be expected to avoid more serious complications such as cirrhosis. He is less optimistic about the joint pain going away, though. George jokes that at least he will win his company's blood drive, and Dr. Pathak points out that, no, the pint a week that George has removed will be discarded, and not used in the blood bank.
>
> It is Nancy who asks how George got hemochromatosis. Dr. Pathak, who was just coming to that, tells them that hemochromatosis is a hereditary disorder.
>
> "But no one in the family has this," Nancy protests. "At least as far as we know."
>
> Dr. Pathak learns that George has a brother Ron and a sister Cindy, both of whom are well. Ron is 53 and Cindy is 47. George and Nancy have two sons, ages 17 and 21, both of whom are also well. Dr. Pathak explains the inheritance of hemochromatosis, and suggests that George have a blood test that can help in counseling the family.

Hemochromatosis is a disorder of iron absorption. Iron is absorbed in the duodenum, transported across the apical cell membrane by a transporter protein (DMT-1, divalent metal transporter-1), where it binds to transferrin. Transferrin carries the iron to cells, including erythroid cells, where it binds to the tranferrin receptor. This complex is taken into the cell in a clathrin-coated pit, which then fuses with other vesicles to form an endosome. A proton pump reduces pH, the iron disassociates from the transferrin, and is transported by DMT-1, either to be used in iron-containing proteins or to be bound to ferritin. The transferrin-receptor complex is returned to the cell surface, where, at neutral pH, the transferrin is released into the circulation.

The major gene responsible for hemochromatosis is referred to as *HFE*. It is located on chromosome 6 within the HLA complex, and is homologous with a class I HLA molecule. Like such molecules, HFE binds to beta-2-microglobulin. It also binds to transferrin, which is believed to inhibit transferrin binding to iron. It is thought that mutations in the *HFE* gene interfere with the interaction of the HFE protein with transferrin, allowing transferrin to bind a greater quantity of iron, leading to increased iron absorption and delivery to tissues.

The increased iron delivery results in iron deposition in multiple tissues. Cirrhosis is the most common severe complication. Other complications include congestive heart failure, diabetes mellitus, impotence (in males), and bronze discoloration of the skin. The disorder is more common in males; females tend to be protected by menstrual blood loss.

Hemochromatosis is treated by phlebotomy. A pint of blood removes 250 mg of iron; removal of a pint a week will deplete iron stores in 1 to 2 years. Ferritin levels are followed to monitor progress of therapy. Phlebotomy is initially carried out weekly, but gradually the frequency can be decreased to every 2 to 3 months. Although chelators could be used, their use is more complicated (intradermal injection) and expensive. At present, blood removed from individuals with hemochromatosis cannot be used for transfusion. This is not due to medical reasons, but is a rule based on the requirement that blood donation be voluntary (individuals with hemochromatosis are not voluntary donors). There is interest in waiving this rule on a national level, and local waivers can be obtained in some cases.

PART V

> George has an HFE test, which reveals that he has the genotype C282Y/H63D. Dr. Pathak refers him to the Genetics Clinic to discuss the further implications of this finding. George meets with Laurie Thomas, a genetic counselor. Laurie explains the genetics of hemochromatosis, and, specifically encourages George to contact Ron and Cindy.
>
> It is very difficult for George to call his brother and sister to explain all this to them, but he finally does so. Within days, Ron and Cindy have the HFE test done. Ron turns out to have only the C282Y mutation, but Cindy has the same genotype as George. She has iron studies, which reveal a transferrin saturation of 42% and ferritin of 120 mg/dl. Cindy is told that she will need to be followed for signs of hemochromatosis.
>
> It is Nancy who calls their two sons, Tim and Steven. She explains what has happened, reassuring them that George is doing well. She urges both of them to have the HFE test, which is done with Laurie's help. Tim is found to have only the H63D mutation. Steven, however, is homozygous for C282Y. He is brought in to see his primary care physician, who begins an evaluation of clinical signs of hemochromatosis. His transferrin saturation is 40%, but his ferritin is only 250 ng/ml and his liver function tests are normal. It is decided to monitor his ferritin levels and liver function, but treatment is not initiated.

Hemochromatosis is inherited as an autosomal recessive trait. *HFE* mutation is responsible for the most common form in the Caucasian population, but mutations in other genes may also occur. The most common *HFE* mutation, present in 85% of *HFE* alleles, is a cysteine to tyrosine amino acid substitution at position 282 (C282Y). Most affected individuals are either homozygous for this mutation, or compound heterozygotes for C282Y/H63D (histidine to aspartate change at position 63). Interestingly, H63D homozygotes usually do not develop hemochromatosis. The carrier frequency for *HFE* mutations is about 1/10 in individuals of northern European ancestry. This implies a frequency of hemochromatosis of 1/400 in this population, which is higher than the frequency of the disease actually diagnosed in the population. Apparently, even the C282Y/C282Y homozygotes do not always develop clinical manifestations of hemochromatosis. Genetic testing may therefore not be an ideal means of population screening (see below), but has a role in screening members of a family in which hemochromatosis has been diagnosed. Early detection of individuals in the family can lead to a program of monitoring, with institution of phlebotomy for those found to be manifesting increased iron stores. This can be life saving in some, avoiding complications such as cirrhosis and congestive heart failure.

PART VI

> Something has been gnawing at Dr. Chen since she learned that George has hemochromatosis. George is lucky that his disorder was diagnosed before he developed irreversible liver or heart disease. But his diagnosis was made on the basis of other, more benign symptoms. How many other patients is she following are there who will not be so lucky? Her reading has led Dr. Chen to realize that hemochromatosis is a relatively common disorder. She begins to ask her colleagues whether they think that they should screen their patients for hemochromatosis.

The rationale for population screening is the same as articulated above for screening family members: Diagnosis of individuals at risk of hemochromatosis before the onset of life-threatening complications allows institution of a safe and effective therapy that prevents these complications. The availability of such a therapy outweighs many of the concerns often associated with population screening, such as fears of stigmatization and discrimination. There remain many questions, however, for example how many people with elevated ferritin or transferrin saturation will go on to develop cirrhosis if not treated. The reliability of various screening tests is also not fully established.

One of the major questions that must be faced as a population screen is contemplated is whether to base the screening on a genetic or phenotypic test. The **genetic test** is likely to have high sensitivity and specificity, but nonpenetrance means that some individuals deemed to be at risk by genotype will never develop the disease. A **phenotypic test** based on a measure of ferritin or transferrin saturation, for example, avoids this concern. Other considerations include cost effectiveness of both approaches, and the fact that genetic testing only detects hemochromatosis due to specific *HFE* mutations, and misses both rare *HFE* mutations and mutations in other genes responsible for hemochromatosis.

Currently, it is widely agreed that screening should be offered to relatives of patients with hemochromatosis. This can be based on genetic testing, since the mutation testing will identify those in the family who are at risk. These individuals can then be followed phenotypically. The value of screening for the general population continues to he discussed, although the consensus is that, if screening is to be done, phenotypic testing with ferritin or transferrin saturation is preferred to genetic testing.

GENETIC SCREENING FOR DISEASE RISK

The ability to test for risk of disease in an asymptomatic individual is often cited as a major promise for the application of genetics in medical practice. The principle is that those determined as being at risk can be offered intervention either to prevent disease or to avoid serious complications. Genetic testing offers the advantages that it can be done at any time in life, is noninvasive, and does not depend on access to diseased tissue. Pitfalls are that tests may be of limited predictive value and clinical utility.

It is important to distinguish **presymptomatic and predispositional tests**. Presymptomatic tests apply to disorders that display age-dependent but complete penetrance, such as Huntington disease. An individual who tests positive will eventually develop the disorder if he or she lives long enough. The test is essentially deterministic of disease risk, though it may not predict time of onset or severity. A predispositional test determines relative risk of disease but does not insure that an individual will or will not manifest the disorder. A test such as *HFE* genotyping for risk of hemochromatosis is predispositional because of incomplete penetrance of *HFE* mutations. Predispositional tests apply to multifactorial traits, where multiple genes and/or environmental factors contribute to disease. Determining genotype at a single locus is not sufficient to determine absolute risk of disease.

The clinical utility of presymptomatic or predispospositional testing includes the possibility of informing family planning or enabling strategies to reduce risk or institute treatment. Presymptomatic tests for disorders that are transmitted as single gene traits, often dominant traits, can be helpful for reproductive decision-making. An individual who is at risk of inheriting the trait is also at risk of transmitting it. If the disorder displays age-dependent penetrance, however, the individual may not know if he or she has inherited the gene mutation until after reproductive age. This means that the trait may be passed onto offspring before the parent knows that he or she is affected. Genetic testing permits identification of the gene mutation prior to onset of symptoms, informing the decision-making process about having children, and even permitting prenatal testing.

Risk reduction or treatment strategies are based on the idea that the disorder can either be avoided altogether, or the occurrence of complications forestalled, by taking action on the basis of test results. In some cases, for example in testing for the risk of cancer, this may take the form of surveillance. Surveillance can be offered to anyone at risk, of course, but those known to be at risk on the basis of a genetic test might be expected to be more vigilant. In contrast, those found not to be at risk may not require close follow-up. This will only be the case, of course, if the family mutation is known and the individual has tested negative for the mutation. If the family mutation is not known, a negative test is harder to interpret, since there is always the possibility that a mutation is present, but cannot be detected by the particular test employed.

Other forms of risk reduction include preventative surgery (also often used by those at risk of cancer), modification of diet or habits such as cigarette smoking, or use of medication. There may be a compelling reason to pursue such strategies in those found to be at high risk, where the efficacy of risk reduction is well established. In some cases, though, there may only be a modest increase in relative risk on the basis of testing, and evidence supportive of a benefit for risk reduction may be less clear.

There are potential risks of genetic testing to determine liability towards disease. Those who test positive may experience anxiety or stigmatization, or may be at risk for loss of insurance or employment. Those who test negative may erroneously assume that they can continue or resume self-destructive behaviors such as smoking, or forget that everyone is at risk of diseases such as cancer or heart disease and may fail to comply with routine screening procedures.

Some have prophesized that one day a person will go to the doctor and be told in advance of the various disorders for which he is or is not at risk. It is already possible to arrange testing for a number of genetic polymorphisms directly through the internet. Most of the tests offered in this way have not been carefully validated, or are provided with little or no counseling to explain the test limitations and options available to deal with risk. In some cases, the conditions may not be amenable to any form of risk reduction. The degree to which the prophesy of genetic risk assessment will be realized remains to be seen. Testing is most likely to be accepted in instances where there are proven strategies for risk reduction that do not markedly reduce quality of life. The predictive value of tests will have to be high, which may be accomplished by simultaneous testing of several factors, including both genetic and nongenetic tests. Finally, safeguards to insure that individuals who are tested do not suffer negative social consequences will need to be put in place, and resources for counseling and education will have to be increased.

REVIEW QUESTIONS

14.1 What is the rationale for presymptomatic diagnosis of hemochromatosis? What is the major limitation in the use of genetic testing for the two common *HFE* mutations as a screening test?

14.2 What is the difference between presymptomatic genetic testing and predispositional genetic testing?

14.3 What is the potential utility of presymptomatic testing for family planning?

14.4 An individual has a predispositional test that reveals he has a relative risk of 2.5 of developing the disease. What does this mean?

14.5 How might predispositional testing render an individual vulnerable to stigmatization or discrimination?

FURTHER READING

Adams PC, Reboussin DM, Barton JC, McLaren CE, Eckfeldt JH, McLaren GD, et al. Hemochromatosis and Iron Overload Screening (HEIRS) Study Research Investigators. Hemochromatosis and iron-overload screening in a racially diverse population. N Engl J Med 2005;352:1769–1778.

Pietrangelo A. Hereditary hemochromatosis – a new look at an old disease. New Engl J Med 2004;350:2383–2397.

EASL International Consensus Conference on Haemochromatosis. III. Jury document. J Hepatol 2000;33:496–504.

15

Genetic Testing for Risk of Cancer

INTRODUCTION

We have already seen that cancer is fundamentally a genetic disease. Although most of the genetic changes are acquired in somatic cells, some individuals inherit a predisposition. This may be based on mutation of one copy of a tumor suppressor gene or having a DNA repair defect. Risk of cancer in such individuals can be markedly increased, raising the possibility of genetic testing to identify such individuals in the hope of instituting preventative measures or surveillance to insure early diagnosis. An increasing number of cancer predisposition syndromes are being identified. In this chapter we will consider one example associated with increase risk of breast and ovarian cancer. We will see how genetic testing can be used to identify people at risk based on family history, and the various options available to modify that risk. We will also explore some the complexities faced in deciding to be tested, in interpretation of test results, and in deciding on a course of action after a positive result.

KEY POINTS

- Genetic predisposition to cancer is recognized by a pattern of familial transmission, as well as characteristics such as early age of onset and multifocality.
- A number of cancer predisposition syndromes have been identified and some of these are subject to genetic testing.
- A positive genetic test result for cancer predisposition can be helpful in planning a program of surveillance or institution of medical or surgical approaches to risk reduction. It can also provide a basis for genetic counseling of family members.
- Like all predispositional tests, cancer genetic test results must be interpreted with caution, since not all individuals will develop cancer, and there are both risks and benefits to being tested.

PART I

The phone rings Tuesday at dinner time and Elaine almost decides not to get up to answer it. But she does, and her husband Jim sees her face fall and tears come to her eyes. It is Elaine's father, telling her that her mother had a mammogram today and very suspicious mass was found. Elaine's mother is 55 years old and has been in good health. Her father explains that it was a "routine" mammogram, though in fact her mother had been worried about a lump in her breast. Actually, she has had lumps before – her breasts have been described as "cystic." Her physician had recommended that she have a mammogram annually, though in fact it has been more like 3 to 4 years since the last study. In any case, her mother is scheduled for a biopsy of the lesion later this week.

Breast cancer affects about one in nine women in North America. Many come to attention because of a breast mass, often noted by the woman herself. There are many possible causes of breast masses other than cancer. One common cause is "fibrocystic disease," in which there

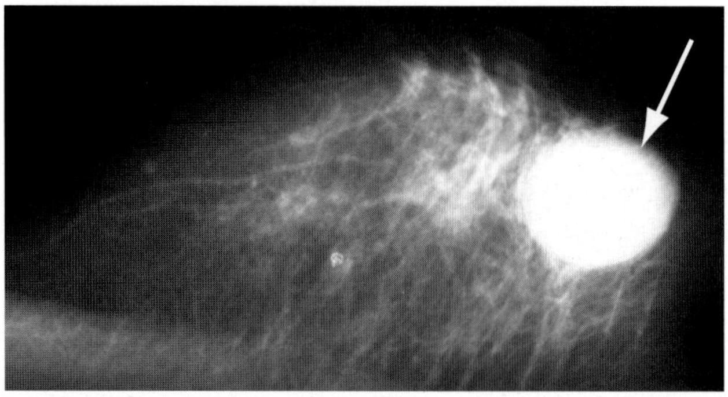

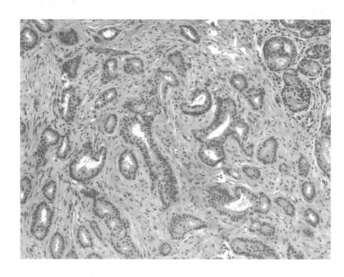

Figure 15.1 • Mammogram showing breast carcinoma (*arrow*). (Courtesy of Dr. Wanda Bernreuter, University of Alabama at Birmingham.)

Figure 15.2 • Photomicrograph showing infiltrating ductal carcinoma of the breast (hematoxylin and eosin stain). (Courtesy of Dr. Amy Adams, University of Alabama at Birmingham.)

are multiple, benign, fluid-filled cysts within the breasts. These can be readily diagnosed by ultrasound; brown bloodless fluid may be aspirated, which can relieve symptoms of pressure. The use of self-examination and mammography as screening tools has led to earlier diagnosis of breast cancer and improved prognosis. Although the issue remains controversial, mammography is now commonly recommended on an annual basis for women 40 years of age and older. Findings such as microcalcifications or densities (Figure 15.1) are followed up by biopsy.

PART II

Elaine goes to see her mother the next day, and stays with her during the coming week. The biopsy is done, and reveals an invasive ductal carcinoma (Figure 15.2). It is recommended that the mass be excised and that a sentinal lymph node biopsy be done. The possibility of modified radical mastectomy is also offered, although it is pointed out that it that there is no evidence that this will improve the outcome. Elaine's mother is very anxious to avoid this extensive surgery and elects to have the "lumpectomy." The surgery is performed, and the lymph nodes are found to be positive for tumor. The family is informed that the tumor is stage IIA, since the tumor is less than 5 cm in diameter and there is evidence for lymph node metastases. The doctor points out that this is associated with a favorable prognosis, more than 80% 5-year survival.

Breast cancers are derived from epithelial cells, and are therefore classified as carcinomas. The most common pathology is referred to as invasive ductal carcinoma. In the past it was common to treat women with breast cancer by removal of the affected breast and dissection of surrounding lymph nodes. The radical mastectomy involves removal of the pectoralis major and minor muscles and axillary lymph nodes. This approach is rarely used today. The modified radical mastectomy leaves the pectoralis major in place. More recently, breast-conserving surgery, followed by radiation therapy of the involved region, has been shown to have similar efficacy to mastectomy for many tumors. Breast cancer staging is based on the size of the tumor,

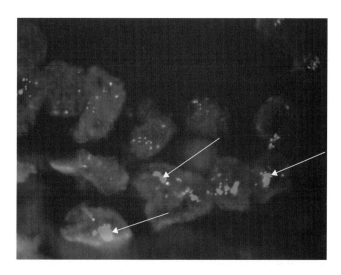

Figure 15.3 • *In situ* hybridization showing amplification of the Her-2/*neu* gene (*arrows*). (Courtesy of Dr. Andrew Carroll, University of Alabama at Birmingham.)

the degree of involvement of lymph nodes, and the presence of metastases to more distant sites. Smaller tumors, with less nodal invasion and no distant metastases are associated with a more favorable prognosis.

PART III

Elaine's mother, and, indeed, the whole family, are relieved to hear this relatively favorable prognosis. They are advised that she should have radiation treatments following the surgery, which are initiated. At a follow-up visit a few weeks later they are informed that the tumor was negative for estrogen receptor and negative for HER-2/neu amplification (Figure 15.3). They are told that the HER-2/neu result is good news: it puts her in a more favorable prognostic category. The lack of estrogen receptors means that she will not benefit from treatment with tamoxifen; instead they recommend a course of systemic chemotherapy.

The approach to therapy depends on a number of variables, including the stage of the tumor, whether the woman is pre- or postmenopausal, and the results of genetic studies done on the tumor cells. Tumors that express estrogen or progesterone receptors tend to respond to treatment with hormone antagonists and are associated with a more favorable rate of long-term survival. Tamoxifen is an estrogen antagonist that has been shown to be effective in preventing recurrence of breast cancer in women whose tumors are estrogen receptor positive. The drug is associated with side-effects such as hot flashes and vaginal dryness, but is, overall, well tolerated. HER-2/neu is an oncogene that is amplified in some breast cancers. The gene encodes a membrane tyrosine kinase growth factor receptor. Overexpression of this gene, usually a result of gene amplification, is associated with poor prognosis. Given that Elaine's mother's tumor is estrogen receptor negative and that she has evidence of spread to lymph nodes, it is recommended that she be treated with chemotherapy.

PART IV

About 6 months have gone by since the initial diagnosis, and Elaine's mother is doing well. She has tolerated the chemotherapy reasonably well, although the treatment has, at times, been grueling. For Elaine, one effect of this experience has been to increase the degree to which she is interested in having for regular breast examinations. She examines herself at least monthly, and has scheduled a visit with her gynecologist. It is while she is in the waiting room that she reads an article about the genetics of breast cancer. The article alarms her: her mother's sister died of ovarian cancer at age 55 and her grandmother's sister was said to have died of breast cancer, although that was many years ago and details are not available. Elaine discusses this with her gynecologist. At first he tries to reassure her, but on further discussion offers to refer her to speak with a cancer geneticist.

It has been clear for a long time that genetics contributes to risk of breast cancer. First-degree relatives of individuals with breast cancer face a two to three times increased risk of themselves developing the disease compared with the general population. Moreover, some families demonstrate transmission of breast cancer in an autosomal dominant fashion. Other members of these families may have ovarian cancer, and, in some, males are affected with breast cancer, a rare occurrence in the general population. These observations prompted a search for a gene or genes that would explain this risk, and culminated in the discovery of two genes that predispose to breast cancer. The genes are referred to as BRCA1 and BRCA2. Since the discovery of these genes, and the ensuing possibility of genetic testing, clinics have been set up to offer genetic counseling and testing for individuals thought to be at risk.

PART V

It takes almost 2 months to get an appointment in the cancer genetics clinic, and it is necessary for Elaine to travel into the city – which she hates to do – for the appointment. She is given a form to fill out prior to the visit that requests detailed family history information. She speaks with her mother and father in an effort to fill in as much detail as she can, though they have only a relatively small amount of knowledge about other members of the family. Elaine is 24 years old, recently married, and has a 2-year-old daughter. Elaine has a sister, Carol, who is 28, and a brother, Michael, who is 30. Both Carol and Michael are healthy, and each has two children. Elaine's mother had a sister who died of ovarian cancer. She also has a brother who is 57 years old and has hypertension, but otherwise is well. Her mother's parents are both deceased: her father died of a heart attack and her mother of an accident at age 48. They confirm that Elaine's grandmother was said to have had breast cancer, but they don't know much more than that. She died more than 40 years ago, so there is no prospect of getting additional records. At the counseling visit, Elaine relates all this to a genetic counselor. The counselor asks about her ethnic background, and Elaine answers that both her parents are Eastern European Jewish.

Given the high frequency of breast cancer in the general population, it is not uncommon for an individual to have an affected relative. How much family history is enough to convey sufficient risk to suggest the possibility of a BRCA1 or BRCA2 mutation? The presence of multiple affected first- or second-degree relatives with any combination of breast or ovarian cancer at any age would suggest a genetic predisposition. Alternatively, if there are fewer affected relatives, young age of onset (<45 years) in an affected relative, the presence of a male relative with breast cancer, a relative with multiple primary cancers (bilateral breast cancer or breast and ovarian cancer), and the presence of both breast and ovarian cancer in different first or second degree relatives would constitute risk factors. There are risk assessment computer programs that are used to determine the probability that an individual carries a BRCA1 or BRCA2 mutation. A commonly used threshold for testing is a risk of 10% or higher.

PART VI

The visit with the genetic counselor goes on for over an hour. The counselor explains to Elaine about the genetics of breast cancer, and about the options available for genetic testing. She explains that testing is available for BRCA1 and BRCA2 mutations, although not all possible mutations are detected with current approaches to testing. She also reviews the potential risks and benefits of testing. Elaine has done considerable reading prior to the visit and has already decided that she would like to be tested. The counselor suggests that, given her Ashkenazi Jewish background, that she first be tested for the common mutations in that population. She also suggests that Elaine's mother be tested first, to determine if she carries one of these mutations prior to testing Elaine herself. Elaine agrees to discuss this with her mother and get back in touch with the counselor by telephone.

The decision whether to undergo genetic testing for breast/ovarian cancer is a complicated one, and involves both technical and psychosocial issues. Both the BRCA1 and BRCA2 genes are large, and a wide variety of mutations has been found in affected individuals. Detection of all possible mutations is technically challenging and expensive, requiring complete sequence analysis of the coding region and intron – exon borders. It is estimated that 15% of mutations are missed even by complete sequencing. In the United States, this is done by one laboratory – Myriad Genetics, Inc., which owns the patent on testing for mutations in this gene. There are some mutations, however, that are particularly common in specific populations. Within the Ashkenazi Jewish population, for example, two BRCA1 mutations (185delAG, a two-base deletion at position 185, and 5382insC, a one-base insertion at nucleotide 5382) and one BRCA2 mutation (6174delT) are particularly common. Searching for these mutations can be done at relatively low cost and might obviate the need for complete gene sequencing. When possible, it is helpful to test an individual who is known to be affected with breast or ovarian cancer, since a negative test in an at-risk relative could indicate that this is not the family mutation, or that the individual being tested did not inherit the family mutation.

The risk/benefit analysis of testing for cancer risk is at least equally complex. There is no simple treatment that has been proven to completely effective in reducing the risk of cancer in BRCA1 or BRCA2 mutation carriers. The most extreme option, prophylactic mastectomy and oophorectomy, does have proven benefit (as will be explored below), but is a major and traumatic life event. Surveillance for cancer by physical examination, mammography alternating with MRI, transvaginal ultrasound, and serum testing for CA-125, a marker of ovarian cancer, may allow for earlier detection of cancer and improved rate of survival. Prophylactic administration of tamoxifen, though it can lower risk of breast cancer, has not been proven to be effective in BRCA1 or BRCA2 carriers. Many women will opt for testing in the hope of relief of anxiety about their risk, but, of course, face a possibility of confirming their fears of being at risk of cancer. Also, some who test negative for a family mutation have experienced guilt at the fact that they have escaped a fate that affects others in the family, especially siblings. There has been much discussion about stigmatization of cancer gene mutation carriers, and tangible risks of discrimination, including denial of employment, health insurance, disability insurance, and life insurance. Many states in the US and other countries have begun to address this via legislation banning "genetic discrimination." There is currently no federal legislation on this topic in the US, and existing laws vary in their degree of protection against various types of discrimination, for example exempting life insurance from protection. Health insurance companies differ in their willingness to pay for genetic testing for cancer risk, though an increasing number in the US are offering such coverage for individuals with established risk factors.

PART VII

Elaine explains what she has learned to her mother and father, and asks her mother if she would be willing to undergo testing. Her mother gets very upset as the conversation progresses, and tearfully refuses to be tested. She has had enough of breast cancer, and is not interested in knowing whether she has passed a genetic risk of cancer on to her children. Elaine is disappointed and upset, but at some level understands her mother's reluctance. She calls the counselor back and explains that she would like to be tested, but that her mother has refused. The counselor arranges for Elaine to sign an informed consent document and for blood to be drawn for testing. It is arranged for Elaine to come back to the clinic in 3 weeks to hear the results. The time passes slowly, but finally Elaine and Jim come together to the clinic visit. Elaine is not surprised to hear that she has been found to carry a mutation in BRCA1 (185delAG). She had already begun to think through what she would do if she tested positive, and has a long conversation with the counselor about her options.

The risk of cancer to a BRCA1 or BRCA2 mutation carrier is estimated from previous experience with carriers of similar mutations. In some cases the analysis is complicated by the fact that a mutation might be rare, so that there is little experience with cancer risk in carriers. Direct sequence analysis also reveals some genetic variants that are of unknown significance, making it unclear whether they increase cancer risk at all. Risk assessment is more straightforward in carriers of common mutations such as 185delAG. Even here, though, estimates of risk have evolved as more data has accumulated. Initial estimates of risk were as high as 85%, reflecting in part a bias of ascertainment towards testing families where many individuals have developed cancer. A population-based study by Struewing et al. (New Engl J Med

1997;336:1401–1408) estimated the risk of breast cancer by age 70 to be 56% and ovarian cancer to be 16% for Ashkenazi Jewish carriers of the common BRCA1 or BRCA2 mutations.

As noted previously, there is no definitive treatment for mutation carriers that will eliminate the risk of cancer. The least that might be offered is surveillance, but recent studies indicate that prophylactic surgery can substantially reduce the risk of cancer. Bilateral mastectomy reduces the risk of breast cancer, though there is a possibility of cancer developing from small amounts of residual breast tissue. Mastectomy also does not address the risk of ovarian cancer. Salpingo-oophorectomy has been demonstrated to reduce the risk of both ovarian and breast cancer and the benefit appears to apply if done after completion of child-bearing. Whether the combination of mastectomy and salpingo-oophorectomy offers significantly improved protection in spite of the much more significant cosmetic and psychological impact remains to be determined.

PART VIII

Elaine and Jim are very concerned about her risk of cancer and feel that they must do everything in their power to avoid the possibility that she might develop cancer. They have one child, and feel that what is most important to them is protecting Elaine's ability to be there for her, and that they would be satisfied that their family is complete with one child. Elaine therefore opts to have a bilateral mastectomy. She inquires about also having an oophorectomy, and is advised that this is better done after menopause. Meanwhile, Elaine has spoken with Carol and Michael and discussed with them the possibility of their being tested. They both opt to be tested; Carol is negative, Michael is positive. Michael has two daughters, and asks about whether they should be tested. Also, it has been increasingly difficult to keep Elaine's mother from realizing that several members of the family have been tested. The three children together decide to meet with their parents and break the news to their mother.

The news that an individual carries a breast cancer gene mutation has major implications for the family, as well as for the individual. In some cases, testing one person, such as a child, indirectly reveals mutation status in another, such as a parent. Carrier status is of greatest importance to women in the family, who are at risk for breast and ovarian cancer. Males, too, can be at risk of cancer, mainly prostate cancer, and, principally for BRCA2 carriers, breast cancer as well.

Genetic testing of children raises complex ethical issues. There is a long tradition of offering testing for certain disorders in children, such as muscular dystrophy. These studies are done to establish a diagnosis in a symptomatic child, and offer genetic counseling regarding recurrence risk and prenatal diagnosis for family members at risk of having a child with a devastating disorder. The situation is far different for cancer risk testing. Here, children are not symptomatic, and are not really at risk until they grow up. There is no intervention that would be offered to the child to reduce his or her risk. The consensus of opinion in the medical genetics community has been to test children only if they will benefit in the immediate future in terms of improved health care (Am J Hum Genet 1995;57:1233–1241). Children at risk of inheriting a breast cancer mutation should be offered counseling at an appropriate age, when they can make their own informed decision about whether to be tested.

PART IX   EPILOGUE

Elaine has adjusted well following her surgery and life is more or less back to "normal." She has become involved in a breast cancer advocacy group. Part of her role is talking with women who have been diagnosed, or have been determined to carry a breast cancer susceptibility gene. She is also involved in fundraising efforts to support further research in the field.

The mechanism of action of the BRCA1 and BRCA2 gene products is not entirely clear, but it appears that they are involved in the response of the cell to repair of DNA damage. Both genes act via a tumor suppressor mechanism, requiring homozygous mutation in tumor cells.

There are multiple additional genes involved in the pathogenesis of breast cancer, including at least one additional, putative dominantly inherited "BRCA3." In addition, there are genes that function as modifiers of risk of breast or ovarian cancer, as well as genes whose somatic mutation contributes to the progression of the cancers. It is hoped that further study of these genes will lead to improved diagnostic tools as well as insights that may produce more effective therapies.

FAMILIAL PREDISPOSITION TO CANCER

Cancer is a common disorder, affecting at least one in four individuals, so virtually everyone has a family history of cancer. There are, however, families in which the risk is transmitted as a single gene trait with high penetrance. These families are characterized by autosomal dominant transmission of a tendency to develop cancer. The specific spectrum of cancers differs from family to family, but can be sorted into a number of familial cancer syndromes. Affected individuals within these families tend to develop their cancers at an earlier age than sporadically affected individuals, and may develop multiple, independent, primary tumors.

As we have seen in Chapter 8, most instances of familial predisposition to cancer are the result of mutations in tumor suppressor genes. An at-risk individual inherits a germ line mutation and will develop cancer if the remaining nonmutated copy of the gene undergoes mutation in a susceptible tissue. The specific distribution of cancer types depends on the types of tissues in which the gene is normally expressed, and the specific role of the gene in that tissue. The major genes and syndromes are summarized in Table 8.1.

Identification of individuals at risk can be important from a number of points of view. In some cases there may be specific treatments that can be provided to prevent cancer. For example, individuals who inherit a mutation in the *RET* oncogene are at high risk of developing medullary thyroid carcinoma, even in childhood. Prophylactic thyroidectomy in these individuals can be life-saving. As with breast and ovarian cancer, surveillance programs can be instituted to insure early detection and treatment of cancer. Those at risk of colon cancer, for example, will be offered colonoscopy at a younger age than is routine in the general population. In some instances, the information may be used for family planning purposes. This especially true for conditions such as neurofibromatosis, where, in addition to a risk of malignancy, the syndrome causes major physical and developmental problems that may begin in childhood.

The approach to risk assessment begins with collection of family history information. Often, this is the indication for consideration of testing. As far as possible, the history should be documented, to be sure that there is accurate information about types of cancers in affected relatives, age of onset, etc. Information that is obtained second hand is often inaccurate, and can lead to erroneous estimations of risks to relatives. Sometimes a physical examination will be warranted. This is typically the case in disorders, such as neurofibromatosis, where specific signs and symptoms may be used to establish a diagnosis. In other disorders, however, such as breast and ovarian cancer syndrome, no physical signs will distinguish individuals at risk from others in the family.

How much family history of cancer does one need to have to warrant genetic testing? Cancer is common, and virtually everyone will have some family history of cancer. Specific criteria for testing have been developed for the various familial cancer syndromes. For breast and ovarian cancer, computer models have been developed that take into account the number of affected relatives, their degree of relationship to the person being counseled, age of onset of cancer, etc. A risk is calculated, and by convention testing is offered to individuals at 10% risk or greater. Formal testing criteria, such as the Amsterdam Criteria (see Table 15.1) have been developed for identification of individuals who warrant testing for colon cancer.

Ideally, genetic testing should first be performed on a member of the family who is known to be affected with cancer. The reason for this is that virtually all of the tests involve screening for mutations where not all possible mutations can be detected. Testing an affected individual maximizes the chance of finding a mutation if one is present, and provides the possibility of reliable testing for other family members at risk. The affected individual(s) may not be available for testing in some cases. If an unaffected individual is tested a positive test will indicate

TABLE 15.1   Amsterdam 2 Criteria for HNPCC

- At least 3 separate relatives with colorectal cancer (CRC) or HNPCC-related cancer (HRC), i.e. gastric, ovary, ureter/renal pelvis, brain, small bowel, hepatobiliary tract and skin (sebaceous tumours)
- One relative must be a first degree relative of the other two
- At least two successive generations affected
- At least one cancer (CRC or HRC) diagnosed < 50 years
- Familial adenomas polyposis excluded in CRC case(s)
- Tumors pathologically verified

that the person is at risk, but a negative test is harder to interpret. It may mean that the individual did not inherit the family mutation, or that the family mutation could not be detected, or that there is no mutation in the family at all.

These complexities, as well as the ethical, legal, and social issues that were discussed above, warrant formal genetic counseling as part of the evaluation. Usually this involves at least two visits: an initial visit to gather information, make a decision about testing, and arrange for the testing, and a follow-up to report the results of testing. This paradigm is likely to be expanded to include other areas of risk assessment for inherited adult-onset disorders as the genes responsible for these conditions come to light.

REVIEW QUESTIONS

15.1 A fifty-year-old man presents with breast cancer. He has two teenage daughters. Is testing for a genetic cause of breast cancer indicated? If so, which gene or genes would be appropriate to test?

15.2 A 30-year-old woman requests counseling regarding her risk of breast and ovarian cancer. Her mother died of ovarian cancer and her aunt currently has breast cancer. It is suggested that her aunt be tested before testing is done on her. What is the rationale for this recommendation?

15.3 A 40-year-old man has colorectal cancer, which also affected his mother and his mother's brother. His maternal aunt also had endometrial cancer. Does this family history satisfy Amsterdam criteria for HNPCC?

15.4 A 35-year-old man with a family history of colon cancer is found to have multiple polyps in the colon. He has two children, aged 5 and 7 years. An *APC* gene mutation is found in the man. Should his children be tested?

15.5 A woman is found to have medullary carcinoma of the thyroid. What form of genetic testing would be appropriate, and what would be offered to those in the family found to carry a mutation.

FURTHER READING

Dumitrescu RG, Cotarla I. Understanding breast cancer risk – where do we stand in 2005? J Cell Mol Med 2005;9:208–221.

Lee RC, Kmet L, Cook LS, Lorenzetti D, Godlovitch G, Einsiedel E. Risk assessment for inherited susceptibility to cancer: a review of the psychosocial and ethical dimensions. Genet Test 2005;9:66–79.

Narod SA, Offit K. Prevention and management of hereditary breast cancer. J Clin Oncol 2005;23:1656–1663.

16
Pharmacogenetics

INTRODUCTION

The absorption, metabolism, distribution, and reaction to pharmacological agents are all under some degree of genetic control. It should therefore be no surprise that there are individual variations in how people respond to drugs. As the genes that underlie these responses come to light, it becomes possible to offer genetic tests that will predict adverse reactions, enable customization of dosing to insure optimal therapeutic levels, and to tailor the choice of drug to individual needs. In this chapter we will explore the principles of pharmacogenetics, considering a specific case of adverse reaction to anesthetics called malignant hyperthermia. We will see how genetic studies are explaining the basis for this condition and how testing can be helpful to identify family members at risk. We will also glimpse the future of pharmacogenetics, which many predict will lead to an individualization of drug therapy.

KEY POINTS

- Individual reaction to a drug can be influenced by genetic traits that affect absorption, biodistribution, excretion, and physiological effects.
- Genetic testing for specific polymorphisms involved in drug metabolism offers the possibility of avoidance of side-effects and customization of treatment to the physiological needs of the individual.
- It is expected that pharmacogenetic testing will increasingly be used as a component of routine medical decision making.

PART I

Eric was not looking forward to this day, though he was looking forward to not having frequent sore throats any more. Finally, though, he was to have his tonsils taken out. At age 10, he was pretty well prepared for the surgery, but nevertheless frightened. His parents were with him right up to the point where he was taken to the operating room. The last thing he remembers was a nurse giving him some medication and his mother . . .

In the operating room, things were going smoothly. Eric was given a dose of succinylcholine to prevent coughing and then an endotracheal tube was inserted. Anesthesia was halothane and nitrous oxide. The surgery was begun, and the anesthesiologist settled in to his routine of close monitoring. About 10 min into the operation, though, he began to become concerned. The first sign was an increase in CO_2 levels monitored in Eric's exhaled air. Within minutes, Eric's heart rate increased to over 150 beats per minute and he began to stiffen. Rate of ventilation was increased, but his pCO_2 remained elevated. Eric's temperature was also rising, now at 38°C. The anesthesiologist called for the surgery to be stopped, and for additional help. He administered a dose of dantrolene and obtained a blood gas. Eric was found to have a mixed metabolic and respiratory acidosis. The halothane was stopped, and medications administered to maintain anesthesia. Over the next half hour the tachycardia resolved and Eric was transferred to the intensive care unit.

TABLE 16.1 Trigger agents and safe agents for individuals susceptible to malignant hyperthermia (modified from Ali SZ, Taguchi A, Rosenberg H. Malignant hyperthermia. Best Pract Res Clin Anesthesiol 2003;17:519–533)

Trigger agents
  Depolarizing muscle relaxants (e.g., succinylcholine)
  Halogenated anesthetics (e.g., halothane)

Safe agents
  Nondeplorizing muscle relaxants (e.g., vecuronium)
  Nitrous oxide
  Intravenous anesthetics (e.g., ketamine, propofol)
  Vasopressors (e.g., epinephrine, dopamine)
  Other sedatives (e.g., opiates, benzodiazepines)

The signs and symptoms are typical for malignant hyperthermia. Malignant hyperthermia is a syndrome that occurs in rare, susceptible individuals who are exposed to one of several drugs ("trigger agents") (Table 16.1). These drugs include depolarizing muscle relaxants such as succinylcholine and halogenated anesthetics such as halothane. Both are commonly used in general anesthesia. The muscle relaxant facilitates intubation, avoiding coughing and choking, and halothane is a widely used and generally safe anesthetic. Susceptible individuals are rare – 1:15,000 children in Europe and the US – but when exposed to a trigger agent, a life-threatening event may ensue.

The pathophysiology of malignant hyperthermia begins with a sudden and massive release of calcium from the sarcoplasmic reticulum into the muscle sarcoplasm. Normally, calcium release causes actin molecules to engage with myosin, leading to muscle contraction. The massive calcium release leads to sustained muscle contraction. There is a sudden increase in muscle metabolism, depleting ATP and leading to increased oxygen consumption. CO_2 production increases, leading to a respiratory acidosis, while the rise in muscle metabolism with depletion of oxygen causes an increase in lactic acid, leading to lactic acidosis. The increased CO_2 production is often the first sign of malignant hyperthermia. Heart rate increases to keep up with the increased oxygen demands. The acidosis is accompanied by increased blood potassium, which can lead to cardiac arrhythmia, and ventricular fibrillation or cardiac arrest may occur. The sustained muscle contraction and hypermetabolic state leads to increased body temperature, which may exceed 46°C, and itself may be lethal.

Anesthesiologists are trained to recognize malignant hyperthermia and to react emergently. The anesthesia will be stopped immediately, substituting "safe" drugs that do not trigger malignant hyperthermia. Ventilatory rate is increased to remove CO_2. If necessary, antiarrhythmia drugs are administered and acidosis may be corrected. The mainstay of treatment, however, is administration of dantrolene. Dantrolene works as a muscle relaxant, and specifically acts to inhibit calcium release in the muscle. It can be used to abort an attack, and can be life-saving. The drug is continued for 24 to 48 hours, since repeat episodes are possible.

PART II

Eric did not awaken until the next day, and he was surprised to find that he was connected to more tubes and lines than he had ever seen before. He expected his throat to be sore, which it was, but did not expect his whole body to be aching. His parents were at the bedside, and seemed very relieved to see him awake. He asked what happened, and his mother began to cry.

In fact, both his parents by now understood that Eric had very nearly died. The night of the surgery, both the surgeon and the anesthesiologist spoke with them, and explained that Eric had experienced an episode of malignant hyperthermia. They were confused at first – they never expected to hear the word "malignant" following Eric's surgery. They were reassured to hear that Eric did not have cancer, but when the anesthesiologist explained what had happened they were not so reassured. But then they were relieved to hear that the episode had been effectively treated. Eric's body temperature, they were told, peaked at 39.5°C, requiring a cooling blanket, but his

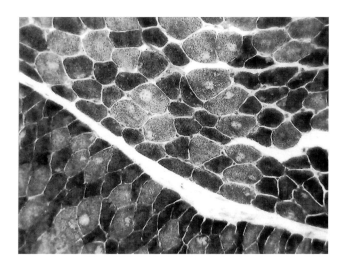

Figure 16.1 • Photomicrograph of muscle showing central core disease. Pale areas within muscle cells are the pathological central cores. (Courtesy of Dr. Shin Oh, University of Alabama at Birmingham.)

temperature did come down and it does not appear that any permanent damage was done. They were told that he will need to be kept on medication for several days. They also are asked if anything like this has ever happened to anyone else in the family.

Malignant hyperthermia was first described in 1960, in a study of an extended family in which multiple relatives of an affected individual were found to have elevated creatine phosphokinase (CPK) values. CPK is a muscle enzyme that leaks out of damaged muscle cells. The trait was found to segregate in the family as an autosomal dominant. Since then, it has become apparent that malignant hyperthermia is a classic dominant trait with incomplete penetrance. Although the trait is inherited as a dominant, the actual syndrome only occurs in individuals who are exposed to one of the trigger agents. Otherwise, an individual may go through life never experiencing an episode. Moreover, not all at-risk individuals have an episode even if exposed to a trigger agent. This makes it difficult to be sure whether a relative of a known affected has inherited the trait. Those who have the trait usually enjoy good health other than having a risk of the catastrophic event of malignant hyperthermia. Some may be at greater risk of heat stroke, and some have some degree of chronic muscle weakness. In some cases, individuals may have a myopathy referred to as central core disease, based on the appearance of muscle through the microscope (Figure 16.1). Most, however, have normal muscle function.

PART III

The answer to the question about family history was no, at least not to the knowledge of either of Eric's parents. Eric's subsequent hospital course was uneventful. His muscle aching took weeks to fully resolve. His doctor had mentioned that a test he called CPK was very abnormal – as high as 30,000 the day of the surgery, and still 1000 a week later. Nevertheless, things went well, although Eric was upset to realize that he still had his tonsils. Arrangements were made to have them removed many months later. This time, a different anesthesia regimen was used without incident. Eric's parents were warned, though, that, if Eric ever should need surgery in the future, his doctors should be informed about this event. Otherwise, though, both Eric and his family put the incident behind them.

If the patient survives the acute episode, complete recovery can occur. There can be a massive breakdown of muscle, which leads to a release of muscle protein, especially myoglobin, into the blood. Myoglobin can overload the kidney and lead to kidney failure in some instances. CPK also may leak out of the muscle, causing massive elevation in the blood. CPK itself is harmless, but is a marker of muscle breakdown. Individuals who have experienced an episode of malignant hyperthermia obviously need to avoid exposure to trigger agents in the future. This means that alternative "safe" agents must be used for surgical procedures. It is recommended to wear a bracelet warning of the risk, since it is possible that emergency surgery could be required at some point where the patient's prior medical history might not be available. The risk may apply to other family members as well, who should be advised to raise the issue if they should require surgery in the future.

PART IV

> *Eric never did forget the incident, but over the next 15 years he did not require surgery again. He has told his doctors about the event, which has been noted in his medical record. Now, however, his mind is on his own son, Jonathan, who is 3 years old. Jonathan has a hernia, and Eric and his wife have just learned that he will require surgery. As the surgeon is explaining the procedure, it is Eric's wife, Jean, who brings up Eric's history. She thinks that she was told that this can run in families – could Jonathan be at risk? The surgeon requests additional information, and speaks with the anesthesiologist. They ask Eric for details about the episode. Of course, Eric doesn't remember much, and the hospital where the surgery was performed was closed years ago. Eric has no idea who the surgeon was. He calls his parents, though, who look through old papers, and they retrieve the information that Eric's episode was labeled "malignant hyperthermia." The anesthesiologist explains that they may need to use an alternative approach to anesthesia in Jonathan, to be on the safe side. He says that it is possible to do a test for malignant hyperthermia, but it will be difficult to do on a young child. He promises to look into testing more thoroughly though, before the surgery is scheduled.*

Testing for susceptibility to malignant hyperthermia is not easily done. The classical test involves biopsy of a relatively large sample of muscle, and test of the muscle for contraction on exposure to halothane and caffeine. The muscle must be tested within hours of biopsy, which means that the biopsy can only be done in a center that is properly equipped and experienced. There are only a few such centers anywhere in the world. As a result, testing is cumbersome and expensive. The test is 97 to 99% sensitive and about 90% specific. An at-risk individual may be treated as though affected, using safe anesthetics, rather than undergo the expense and inconvenience of biopsy. Moreover, it is difficult to remove a large enough sample of muscle from a child, making it unlikely that a young child will be tested.

PART V

> *A few days later, Eric and Jean get a call from the anesthesiologist, who has spoken with a colleague in the genetics clinic. He says that genetic testing for malignant hyperthermia may be possible, and arranges for Eric and Jean to be seen in the genetics clinic. They speak with a genetic counselor, who explains that genetic testing is possible, although there are no laboratories in the US that offer the testing on a routine clinical basis. There are, however, laboratories in Europe that offer the testing, and it is possible to send a blood sample for analysis. It is arranged for a sample to be sent from Eric, with the understanding that Jonathan can be tested if Eric's test is positive.*

The major gene responsible for malignant hyperthermia is designated *RYR1* (*MIM180901*); it is located on chromosome 19 and encodes a muscle cell membrane ion channel, referred to as the ryanodine receptor. Interestingly, its relationship with malignant hyperthermia was first discovered in a natural porcine model of the disease. In swine, the trait is referred to as porcine stress syndrome (PSS). PSS is inherited as an autosomal recessive trait, and is of economic importance because susceptible animals who experience the disorder under conditions of stress, such as crowding, undergo changes that devalue the meat. The porcine gene encoding the ryanodine receptor was found to be responsible for PSS, and in humans with malignant hyperthermia, the most common site of mutation is the corresponding *RYR1* gene.

The ryanodine receptor is so-called because it binds a toxic substance ryanodine. It encodes a membrane protein that controls calcium release from the sarcoplasmic reticulum in muscle. Muscle contraction is initiated when acetylcholine is released from a motor nerve synapse at the muscle membrane. The depolarizing current is transmitted through membrane channels, T tubules, which make contact with the sarcoplasmic reticulum, a modified endoplasmic reticulum. The ryanodine receptor resides at the junction between the T tubules and sarcoplasmic

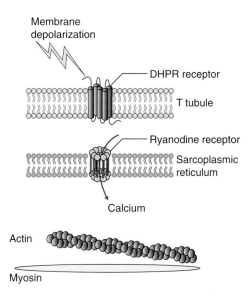

Figure 16.2 • The ryanodine receptor resides in the sarcoplasmic reticulum membrane and is juxtaposed to the DHPR receptor in the T tubule, which is an invagination of the muscle cell membrane. Depolarization of the membrane results in opening of the ryanodine receptor, leading to entry of calcium into the cytoplasm. This, in turn, causes actin to interact with myosin, leading to muscle contraction. In individuals susceptible to malignant hyperthermia, mutation in the ryanodine receptor, or, more rarely, the DHPR receptor, leads to excessive calcium entry into the sarcoplasm.

reticulum (Figure 16.2) and triggers calcium release into the sarcoplasm upon depolarization of adjacent calcium channels, referred to as dihydropyridine receptors (DHPR). The increased calcium causes actin to engage with myosin, initiating muscle contraction.

The mutations responsible for malignant hyperthermia appear to lead to excessive calcium release, either as a consequence of exposure to succinylcholine, which elicits a large scale membrane depolarization, or halothane, which interacts directly with the receptor. The two drugs acting together behave synergistically to trigger malignant hyperthermia episodes. Individuals who are not exposed to trigger agents may never have an episode. Most have normal muscle function, but some have a chronic myopathy, indicating some degree of calcium leakage without exposure to a trigger agent.

PART VI

More than 2 months pass before the test results are available. Eric has been found to have a mutation at codon 2434, in which a leucine is substituted with proline. A cheek swab is taken from Jonathan. Four weeks later Eric and Jean learn that Jonathan did not inherit this mutation, which is a great relief. They are told, however, that other family members should be tested for the mutation. Eric speaks with his sister and brother, both of whom have children. His sister is found to have the same mutation, as does one of her children. Eric's brother does not have the mutation.

Molecular diagnosis of malignant hyperthermia poses many challenges. The *RYR1* gene is not the only one responsible for malignant hyperthermia (though it is the cause of the disorder in more than half of affected individuals). Other genes, including one that encodes one of the subunits of DHPR, can also be involved. The gene includes 106 exons and encodes a protein of 5000 amino acids. Molecular testing is hampered by the complexity of scanning a large gene for mutations, and potential ambiguity in the interpretation of mutation data. A variety of different mutation types has been found in different affected individuals. Because of these challenges, mutation analysis is not used as the primary diagnostic screen for malignant hyperthermia, in spite of the difficulties posed by the muscle contraction assay. Failure to find a mutation would not rule out the diagnosis, whereas false negative results cannot be tolerated in a potentially lethal disorder. Genetic testing can be useful in family counseling, however. If a known affected individual is tested and the mutation is found, testing can be offered to other relatives to determine whether they are at risk. Those found to be at risk would be managed with safe agents for anesthesia, whereas those who have not inherited the trait do not require such special treatment.

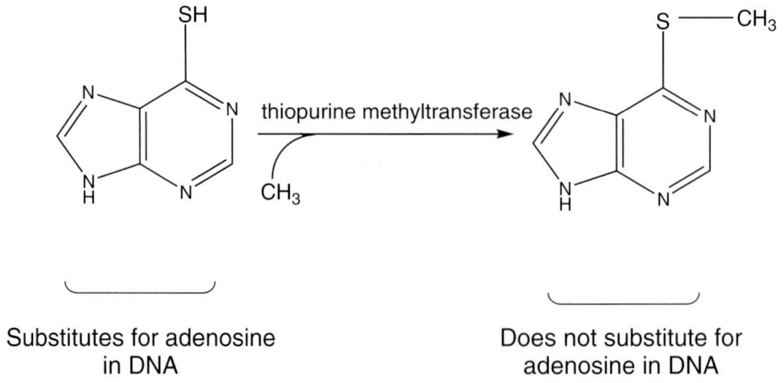

Figure 16.3 • Thiopurine methyltransferase (TPMT) catalyzes methylation of 6-mercaptopurine and other sulfur-containing purines. The nonmethylated form is incorporated into DNA in the place of adenine, whereas the methylated form is not. In effect, then, TPMT inactivates the drug. An individual with low TPMT activity will accumulate a high concentration of active drug, and be at greater risk of toxicity.

PHARMACOGENETICS AND PHARMACOGENOMICS

Malignant hyperthermia represents an example of a **pharmacogenetic trait** – a genetic trait in which expression of the phenotype requires exposure to a pharmacological agent. The effects of a drug in an individual are dependent on multiple variables: drug absorption, biochemical reactions that activate or inactivate the drug, distribution in the circulation, excretion, and interaction of the drug with its cellular target(s). Any of these variables can be subject to modification by genetic factors. The result is that the concentration of active drug can differ from person to person in spite of administration of the same dose, and the efficacy of the drug at any given serum concentration can likewise differ. These differences can include rare toxic reactions, such as is the case in malignant hyperthermia. Awareness of these inherited traits can be life-saving, as we have seen, and can also avoid needless toxicity, or, conversely, inadequate dosing in some individuals.

An important example of a drug metabolism pharmacogenetic trait involves the enzyme thiopurine methyltransferase (TPMT). TPMT is responsible for transfer of a methyl group to thiopurines, including the cancer chemotherapeutic agents 6-mercaptopurine and 6-thioguanine (Figure 16.3). Methylation of these drugs interferes with their ability to bind to DNA, and therefore effectively inactivates the drug. Approximately 1/300 individuals is homozygous for a polymorphism that leads to deficient TPMT activity. These individuals fail to inactivate the drug, and therefore experience an exceptionally high level of activity from a standard dosage. 6-mercaptopurine is commonly used in the treatment of childhood leukemia. If drug dosage is not reduced in homozygous children, they will likely die from toxicity, since a standard dosage to them is, in effect, an overdose.

Another example is polymorphism of the gene *CYP2D6*, which encodes the enzyme debrisoquine hydroxylase, one of the P-450 family of hepatic oxidases. Oxidation by the debrisoquine hydroxylase can modify a drug, either to an active or an inactive product (Figure 16.4). Common polymorphisms within the gene are associated with either excessive activity or diminished activity. Variants with decreased activity occur in 5 to 10% of whites in North America and 1 to 2% of African Americans. Gene duplications that result in rapid metabolism occur in 5 to 10% of whites and 29% of Ethiopeans. For a drug that is inactivated by debrisoquine hydroxylase, an individual with rapid metabolism will fail to achieve a therapeutic level and one with slow metabolism will accumulate the drug to the point of toxicity. For a drug that is activated by CYP2D6, rapid metabolism will lead to excessive activity, slow metabolism to deficient activity. Testing for *CYP2D6* genotype is beginning to be introduced into the repertoire of the routine clinical laboratory, since knowledge of genotype can alter drug dosing. The polymorphisms are common, and the list of drugs influenced by the polymorphism includes many in common use (Table 16.2).

Malignant hyperthermia is a prime example of a genetic variation that influences how a drug interacts with targets at the cellular level. Succinylcholine and halothane will induce malignant hyperthermia only in individuals with an at-risk genotype. Another example is a variant in a gene that encodes a sodium channel, *SCN5A*. The variant is present in 13% of African Americans, and places an individual at risk of cardiac arrhythmia when exposed to any of a number of commonly used medications, including some antibiotics.

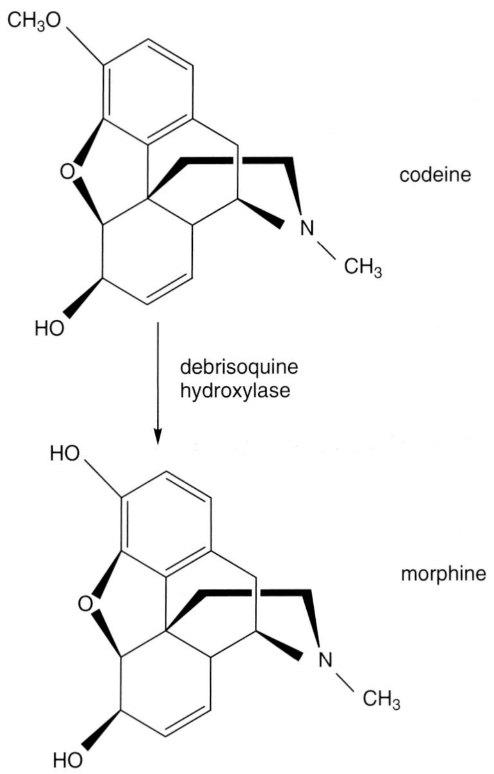

Figure 16.4 • Conversion of codeine to morphine by debrisoquine hydroxylase. The pain-killing effects of codeine are dependent upon this reaction. Low debrisoquine hydroxylase activity will result in reduced efficacy, whereas high activity will cause excessive pharmacological effect.

TABLE 16.2 Example of drugs metabolized by debrisoquine hydroxylase

Drug class	Examples
Analgesics	codeine, hydrocodone, tramadol
Antiarrhythmics	encainide, flecainide, mexiletene, propafenone
Antidepressants	amitriptyline, desipramine, fluoxetine, fluvaxamine, imipramine, nortriptyline, paroxetine
Antihistamines	chlorpheniramine, diphenhydramine, promethazine
Antipsychotics	haloperidol, perphenazine, thiridazine
Beta blockers	carvedilol, metoprolol, propranolol, timolol
Cough suppressants	dextromethorphan

Pharmacogenetic testing is not only used to adjust drug dosage or to predict individuals at risk of adverse reactions. We have seen this with prediction of response to gefitinib in individuals with non-small cell lung cancer (see Hot Topics 8.1). The concept of disease stratification – separating groups of patients into subsets who may respond differently to treatment based on genotypic differences – offers great promise to improve treatment outcomes, but has also generated some controversy. The use of combination therapy of isosorbide dinitrate and hydralazine in treatment of heart failure has been shown to be of particular benefit to those self-identified as black. Traditional definitions of "race" are viewed as social and political designations, rather than biological (see Ethical Implications 7.1). There are genetic differences among groups of people of differing ancestry, although there is substantial genetic admixture in modern populations and any individual group exhibits a wide degree of genetic variability. The use of "race" as a criterion to modify treatment has been viewed with substantial suspicion by many, given the long history of discrimination against African Americans. Designation of race is undoubtedly a surrogate for other genetic factors that predispose some individuals to benefit from this treatment disproportionately, but at present, the genetic factors have not been identified.

It is expected that pharmacogenetics will play a major role in the integration of genetics into routine medical practice. Testing for drug metabolism polymorphisms will permit individualization of drug dosing, avoiding side-effects and increasing the likelihood of efficacy. Such testing need only be done once in a lifetime, and can serve as a guide for future therapy thereafter. As genetic and genomic studies further reveal the pathogenesis of disease and provide tools for disease stratification, there will be an increasing array of drugs that target relatively narrow subsets of patients. Some have predicted the routine use of genetic testing, perhaps using gene chip technology, to provide a patient profile that will customize treatment, insuring the use of the correct medication at the correct dose in an individual patient. The day may be coming when virtually all treatment decisions are based on information obtained from genetic testing.

REVIEW QUESTIONS

16.1 Why is genetic testing for *RYR1* mutation not offered to all individuals as a prelude to surgery to avoid malignant hyperthermia?

16.2 What is the clinical utility of *TPMT* testing in individuals about to undergo chemotherapy with 6-mercaptopurine?

16.3 What is the value of *CYP2D6* testing in clinical practice?

16.4 What is the drug-exposure risk associated with polymorphisms of sodium or potassium channel genes?

16.5 What is the principle behind disease stratification by genetic testing as a prelude to pharmacotherapy?

FURTHER READING

Benkusky NA, Farrell EF, Valdivia HH. Ryanodine receptor channelopathies. Biochem Biophys Res Comm 2004;322:1280–1285.

Evans WE, McLeod HL. Pharmacogenomics – drug disposition, drug targets, and side effects. New Engl J Med 2003;348:538–549.

Evans WE, Relling MV. Moving towards individualized medicine with pharmacogenomics. Nature 2004;429:464–468.

McCarthy EJ. Malignant hyperthermia: pathophysiology, clinical presentation, and treatment. AACN Clin Issues 2004;15:231–237.

Roses AD. Pharmacogenetics and drug development: The path to safer and more effective drugs. Nat Rev Genet 2004;5:645–656.

Tate SK, Goldstein DB. Will tomorrow's medicines work for every one? Nat Genet 1004;36:S34–S42.

17
Gene Therapy

INTRODUCTION

Understanding the molecular basis of genetic disease offers major hopes for diagnosis, prevention, and treatment. Treatment may take many forms, including surgery and pharmacological therapy. In some cases actual repair of a genetic defect or replacement of a defective gene may be possible. This has generated considerable excitement, but also faces daunting challenges. A variety of approaches are in development, with some modest successes and significant setbacks having been encountered along the way. In this chapter, we will look at one of the disorders for which genetic therapy is being explored. We will look at some of the major approaches being developed for insertion of genetic material into cells, and at both the challenges and potential long-range prospects for this approach.

KEY POINTS

- Gene therapy involves either the replacement of a defective gene in a cell or the insertion of a genetic element to deliver a specific product to a specific cell type or site in the body.
- A variety of systems are in development aimed at the delivery of genetic material to specific cell types and achievement of physiologically meaningful levels of expression.
- There remain significant technical and ethical challenges to be overcome in the clinical implementation of genetic therapy, though the area remains a major promise for future development.

PART I[1]

Ethan's parents bring him to the emergency room at 8 months of age. They explain that he acquired only a minor bump on the head while learning to crawl. During a discussion of Ethan's medical history, the attending physician in the ER learns that he has had several, fairly severe nosebleeds. Although the physician suspects a coagulation disorder, he would have expected that this would have come to the attention of his physicians sooner, for example after Ethan was circumcised. Upon physical examination and a discussion with the family, he learns that Ethan's parents elected not to have him circumcised after birth. Screening is ordered to evaluate Ethan for a coagulation defect. Ethan is treated for the bump to his forehead and the physician arranges for the family to follow-up with their pediatrician to discuss the results of the screening tests.

Bleeding disorders are a heterogeneous class of conditions in which blood clotting is defective. They include both inherited and acquired disorders. The process of blood coagulation is typically initiated by injury to endothelium lining the blood vessel. The clot consists of a matrix derived from polymers composed of the protein fibrin, onto which cell fragments called platelets adhere. Fibrin is produced by action of the enzyme thrombin on the substrate fibrinogen (Figure 17.1). The fibrin molecules are then cross-linked by action of the enzyme factor XIII. Thrombin is activated by another clotting factor, factor Xa, which acts on prothrombin.

---

1 This case was modified from a case written by Theresa Strong, MD, and Sandra Prucka, MS, University of Alabama at Birmingham.

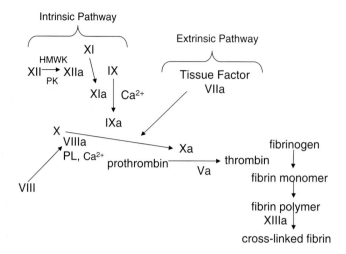

Figure 17.1 • A clot forms when prothrombin is converted to thrombin, which in turn causes conversion of fibrinogen to fibrin, which then polymerizes. Factor X can be activated via the extrinsic pathway, through tissue factor and factor VIIa, or the intrinsic pathway, starting with factor XII. PK = prekallikrein; PL = phospholipid; HMWK = high molecular weight kininogen.

Factor Xa is activated from factor X by either of two pathways, referred to as extrinsic and intrinsic. The extrinsic pathway involves tissue factor and factor VII, whereas the intrinsic pathway begins with factor XII.

Clotting disorders can result from defects in platelet function or from defects in the cascade of events that leads to fibrin formation. Platelet disorders are more likely to produce small punctuate hemorrhages (petechiae) or larger bruises (ecchymoses) on the skin and mucous membranes. Coagulation factor deficiency disorders typically result in bleeding episodes into joints and soft tissues.

PART II

> *The results of Ethan's coagulation screening show a normal prothrombin time (PT) and platelet function analysis. However, studies reveal a prolonged activated partial prothromboplastin time (aPTT), prompting his physician to order a coagulation factor assay. The final results of testing demonstrate that Ethan has less than 1% factor IX clotting activity, a result that is consistent with a diagnosis of hemophilia B. After discussing this diagnosis with the family his pediatrician refers them to a hematologist and genetics team to explain the features of this disorder, its X-linked inheritance pattern, and treatment options in more detail.*

Studies of platelet function include inspection of the blood smear for abnormalities of platelet number or structure and measurement of bleeding time, that is the time to formation of a platelet plug following vascular injury. The PT measures the activity of the extrinsic pathway from factor VII through production of fibrin, whereas the aPTT measures the activity of the intrinsic pathway through fibrin production. Finding an abnormality in aPTT but not PT or platelet function implicates factors XII, XI, IX, or VIII. Some people have inhibitors to clotting factors (e.g., antibodies), which can be determined by mixing patient's plasma and normal plasma. If the patient has a clotting factor deficiency, the clotting will be restored to normal in the mixture. If there is an inhibitor in the patient's plasma, however, the inhibitor will continue to interfere with clotting in the mixture. Finally, the specific deficiency can be determined using assays for the individual factors.

Hemophilia A (factor VIII deficiency) and hemophilia B (factor IX deficiency) are clinically indistinguishable disorders characterized by prolonged bleeding after injury, tooth extractions, or surgery; bleeding into joints or soft tissues, and frequently renewed bleeding after bleeding has stopped. Severe hemophilia is usually recognized in the first year of life, frequently upon circumcision in males, but patients with milder disease may not be diagnosed until they are more than 5 years old. The incidence of hemophilia A is 1/5000 while that of hemophilia B is 1/30,000. The differential diagnosis of hemophilias A and B includes von Willebrand disease, fibrinogen disorders, platelet function disorders, and the recessively inherited factor XI and factor XII deficiencies. These disorders involve deficiency of various components of the clotting cascade, a pathway that seals off a vascular leak following injury to the blood vessel wall.

PART III

> *The family decides to first meet with a hematologist to learn about the treatment of hemophilia. They learn that hemophilia B can be treated using an intravenous infusion of recombinant or plasma-derived clotting factor concentrates. They spend some time with the hematologist as she explains the benefits and risks associated with i.v. infusions. The hematologist refers them to the genetics team where they get a better understanding of the inheritance of the disorder. They learn that there is a possibility that Ethan's mother is an unaffected carrier of a gene mutation for hemophilia B. Genetic testing is performed to find the gene mutation for Ethan and his mother is indeed found to be a carrier of a nonsense mutation that leads to premature termination of translation of the protein.*

The degree of severity of hemophilia is related to the degree of factor deficiency. Severe disease, in which spontaneous bleeding occurs, is associated with less than 1% of normal activity. Levels of greater than 5% lead to bleeding in response to trauma or surgery. Intermediate levels lead to a moderate course. The major sites of bleeding are into joints and soft tissues. Hemarthroses are due to bleeding within the joint capsule, and cause swelling and severe pain. Recurrent bleeds can lead to deformity of the joint. Soft tissue bleeds can lead to hematomas and damage to deep tissues. Bleeding can also occur at mucous membranes, including the gastrointestinal and genitourinary tracts.

Hemophilia is most commonly treated by intravenous infusion of clotting factors, either prophylactically if bleeding is expected, as for a surgical procedure, or in response to bleeding episodes. Although generally effective, there are several limitations to this treatment. The use of plasma-derived coagulation factors has provided therapy where there previously was none, but it has come with its own problems; namely, an extremely high incidence of blood-borne diseases. Hepatitis B, hepatitis C, and HIV all occur in more than half of patients with hemophilia. The use of recombinant DNA-produced protein products has eliminated the risk of transmission of human and animal infectious agents, but the expense of protein replacement therapy (currently $50,000 to $100,000 per year) is considerable. In addition, approximately 20% of individuals with hemophilia A and 3% with hemophilia B develop neutralizing antibodies (referred to as "inhibitors") to the replaced protein, reducing the therapeutic effect.

Both factor IX deficiency and factor VIII deficiency are X-linked disorders. More than 2100 different mutations have been described that result in factor IX deficiency. The majority are point mutations that lead to amino acid substitutions or the introduction of a stop codon. Approximately 10% of mutations are structural alterations of the gene, including deletions, additions, and complex rearrangements. Female carriers have low levels of factor IX and some may exhibit symptoms of mild hemophilia.

PART IV

> *Eighteen years have passed since Ethan was first diagnosed with hemophilia B. Ethan has been in and out of the emergency room for factor infusions, and has been admitted to the hospital many times. He and his parents have become very involved with their local area hemophilia support group. They recently attended a national meeting where experts offered information regarding current research for hemophilia. Ethan and his parents were excited to learn about the prospects of gene therapy. They eagerly approach his hematologist about enrolling him in the clinical trial that was described at the conference. In this trial the therapy is being injected directly into muscle. After discussing the potential risks of gene therapy with his physician, both Ethan and his parents decide to it would be a good idea to try enrolling him in the clinical trial. Unfortunately, though, Ethan is not accepted into the trial, but his physician promises to keep him informed about the success of the trial and will notify him of any new research opportunities for treating hemophilia.*

The concept of gene therapy involves insertion of a gene into a tissue that will lead to permanent production of the missing factor. Gene therapy for hemophilia may offer significant advantages compared to conventional therapies. Continuous production of the therapeutic gene, mimicking the normal situation, is expected to produce optimal prevention and control of

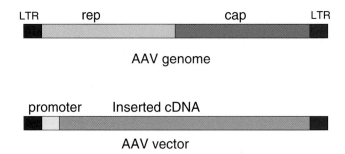

Figure 17.2 • The AAV genome consists of the *rep* and *cap* genes flanked by long terminal repeats (LTR). The gene therapy vector consists of the LTR, a promoter sequence, and a cDNA for the gene of interest. Both viral genes are deleted, and therefore the virus needs to be grown in cells that provide the rep and cap proteins in order to replicate.

bleeding episodes. It is not necessary to achieve normal levels of factor IX activity to achieve a therapeutic effect, as evidenced by carrier females with low factor IX levels but few or no symptoms. A variety of animal models and **gene delivery vectors** have demonstrated the potential long-term therapeutic benefit of factor IX gene delivery. Although the protein is normally produced in the liver, other tissues, such as readily accessible muscle, may be able to act as a factory for the production of factor IX. Gene therapy vectors evaluated for hemophilia B have included adeno-associated virus (AAV), retrovirus, adenovirus, and others. Of these, AAV offers long-term stable expression. One limitation of AAV is that current vectors can only accommodate small genes; however, the small size of the factor IX coding sequence permits use of this vector.

AAV is a single-stranded DNA containing virus that does not cause human disease. The viral genome consists of two genes, *rep* and *cap*, flanked by long terminal repeats, which includes a promoter sequence (Figure 17.2). The rep gene encodes proteins required for replication of the virus and its integration into the genome. The cap gene encodes structural proteins for the viral capsid. Both of these genes can be removed and replaced with a gene of interest when the virus is used as a gene therapy vector. In this case, the products of the rep and cap genes must be provided by another virus in order to replicate the vector. AAV ordinarily integrates into a specific site on chromosome 19, but when used as a gene therapy vector it may integrate at random into the host chromosome or exist outside the chromosome as an **episome**.

Although gene therapy for hemophilia offers the promise of long-term therapy, there are several potential risks that patients must carefully consider prior to enrolling in a clinical trial. Risks include the possibility of **germ line transmission** or **insertional mutagenesis** leading to the development of cancer. This involves integration of the virus adjacent to an oncogene, which would activate the oncogene. AAV vectors used in clinical trials do not efficiently integrate and can direct gene expression from the episomal state, and therefore may be associated with lower risk than retroviral vectors. Gene therapy may also cause an immune response to the encoded protein, factor IX in this case, although individuals will be exposed to factor IX in the course of conventional treatment as well.

PART V

Ethan is still eager to participate in gene therapy and the following year he and his family attend a conference where a new approach to gene therapy using liver directed AAV-FIX is discussed. After a discussion with his physician Ethan is enrolled in the clinical trial. Researchers explain that Ethan is a good candidate for this research therapy because he is free of hepatitis, making it less difficult to determine the effectiveness of gene therapy.

Early clinical trials have shown no significant toxicity in treated patients. In addition, some results have suggested the production of functional factor IX protein following gene transfer; however, therapeutic levels of factor IX have not been reliably achieved. This may be in part due to the size of humans, as compared to the preclinical animal models, making therapeutic doses difficult to achieve. New AAV serotypes have been described that infect cells with considerably improved efficiency, and incorporation of these vectors into clinical trials may improve outcome. Expression of the vector may be targeted to the liver by incorporation of liver-specific promoter sequences adjacent to the factor IX gene and injection of the virus into the portal vein. Preclinical studies have been done in a canine model of factor IX deficiency, and clinical trials in humans have begun.

PART VI   EPILOG

Ethan receives an infusion of recombinant AAV, which requires a brief hospitalization. He is now being followed closely for production of factor IX, which requires repeated blood studies. So far, there is a slight increase in his factor IX levels, though not to a degree that would protect him against major bleeding episodes. Ethan understands that he may not benefit from this treatment, but he is hopeful that perhaps he will, or that further advances in gene therapy will eventually reduce his dependence of factor infusions and his risk of major bleeds.

GENE THERAPY

Gene therapy involves the insertion of a gene into target cells with the hope of achieving stable expression of the inserted gene at levels sufficient to produce physiologically significant quantities of gene product. Gene therapy has major potential applications in the treatment of genetic disorders, where the goal is to replace a missing or mutated gene with an intact copy. In principle, it could be used in nongenetic disorders as well, providing a way to deliver a protein to a highly targeted group of cells. The overall approach has been the subject of high public expectations, but also major challenges. There have been areas of impressive progress to date, as well as significant frustrations and setbacks.

The basic principle of gene therapy is to introduce a gene into a group of cells that will express the gene and deliver the gene product at a site where it will achieve therapeutic benefit. The inserted gene consists of an "**expression cassette**" that includes the gene, a flanking promoter sequence, and other signal sequences, such as a polyA addition site, necessary to achieve expression in the cell. Introduction of the cassette into the cell can be achieved by physical means or through the use of modified viral vectors. Some vectors require that cells be tranfected *ex vivo*, that is cells must be isolated, treated outside the body, and then reinserted. Others can be use *in vivo*, that is administered directly to a patient, for example by intravenous infusion.

Plasmids containing expression cassettes can be introduced into cells in the form of "naked DNA," but efficiency of uptake is low. To improve uptake, plasmids can be complexed with positively charged lipids to form liposomes, which fuse with the cell membrane, or with other polymers such as polylysine. Particles containing the cassettes can be forcibly introduced into cells using a "DNA gun."

Viral vectors are produced by the modification of viruses that naturally infect the target cells. The general concept is that some or all viral genes are replaced by the expression cassette. In some cases the recombinant viral genome will integrate into the target cell genome, resulting in stable expression. Other times, the inserted DNA exists as an episome. In this case, it will be expressed in the cell but will not be transmitted as the cell replicates.

Many different types of viral vectors have been developed for use in gene therapy (Table 17.1). Retroviruses contain single-stranded RNA that is copied into double-stranded DNA in the cell. This DNA can enter the nucleus during cell division and integrate at random sites into the host genome. This offers the advantage of stable, long-term expression in a dividing cell population. One danger, however, is that the inserted DNA may disrupt a host gene, including activation of an oncogene if the inserted gene integrates nearby. This has occurred in some children treated for X-linked severe combined immune deficiency.

Adenoviral vectors contain a double-stranded DNA which can infect both dividing and nondividing cells. The inserted DNA is not integrated into the genome, so the therapeutic benefit is not permanent, but insertional mutagenesis does not occur. Adenoviral vectors have been used in clinical trials, but there have been problems due to toxicity and immune response to viral proteins. Adeno-associated virus has been discussed above. It offers advantages of long-term expression and low toxicity, but its use is limited by the relatively small size (up to 4 kb) of DNA that can be inserted.

Other viral vectors include Herpes virus and lentivirus. Herpes vectors can introduce large genes or even multiple genes as double-stranded DNA. The viruses tend to infect nerve cells, so have been used in experimental treatment of neurological disorders. Lentiviral vectors are derived from the HIV retrovirus, and can infect both dividing and nondividing cells.

TABLE 17.1　Comparison of major vectors used in gene therapy

System	Characteristics	Advantages	Disadvantages
Nonviral Naked DNA	Plasmid DNA exposed directly to target cells	Simplicity; lack of viral toxicity	*Ex vivo* Low efficiency of transfection
Cationic complexes	DNA complexed with cationic lipids or polylysine	Simplicity; lack of viral toxicity	*Ex vivo* Low efficiency of transfection
Gene gun	DNA forced into cells	Simplicity; lack of viral toxicity	*Ex vivo*
Viral Retrovirus	Single-stranded RNA vector that creates double-stranded DNA inside cell and integrates into chromosome	Stable integration of transfected DNA; wide range of susceptible cell types; relatively large capacity for inserted DNA	Insertional mutagenesis; only infects dividing cells
Adenovirus	Double-stranded DNA inserted into cell	Targets dividing and nondividing cells of many different types; relatively large capacity for inserted DNA; can be targeted to specific cell types	Lack of stable transfection; host immune response possible; possible toxicity of viral proteins
Adeno-associated virus	Single-stranded DNA with no viral genes; requires helper virus to package vector	Nonpathogenic; stable transfection as episome or integrated into chromosome; infects dividing and nondividing cells	Small capacity for inserted DNA; difficult to prepare
Herpes virus	Double-stranded DNA inserted into cell	Large capacity; tropism for nerve cells	Limited range of cells can be infected
Lentivirus	Retrovirus derived from HIV	Like retroviruses, but infects nondividing cells	Safety issues not clearly defined

In the US, gene transfer clinical trials supported by the National Institutes of Health are reviewed by the Recombinant DNA Advisory Committee (RAC). Both genetic and nongenetic disorders have been targeted in different trials. Among the genetic disorders are severe combined immune deficiency, cystic fibrosis, and hemophilia. These conditions have in common the fact that pathogenesis is based on gene mutations that lead to lack of expression of a critical protein made by a specific cell type. Use in nongenetic disorders includes cardiovascular disease, HIV infection, and cancer. The goal in cardiovascular disease has been to introduce genes that will lead to revascularization of ischemic tissue. Application in HIV includes generation of antigens that will trigger an immune response, thereby acting as a means of vaccination. Treatment of cancer is aimed at inducing an immune response by causing cancer cells to express foreign antigens, correcting somatic genetic defects in tumor suppressor genes, or activating cytotoxic pathways in tumor cells.

Another approach to modification of gene expression that may find therapeutic application is the use of RNA interference (RNAi) (see Hot Topics 1.1). Transfection of vectors into cells that result in the production of specific siRNAs is being explored for a variety of purposes, including silencing of genes involved in viral infection, cancer, and genetic disorders.

REVIEW QUESTIONS

17.1 What are the potential advantages to gene therapy for a disorder such as hemophilia A or B, where there already exist treatments to manage complications of the disorder?

17.2 What is the advantage of adeno-associated virus as a vector for treatment of factor IX deficiency, and why is it particularly suitable for treatment of this disorder?

17.3 What approaches are used to insert "naked DNA" into cells?

17.4 What is the major risk associated with the use of retroviral vectors for gene therapy?

17.5 Why are adenoviral vectors not suitable for achieving stable, long-term expression of an inserted gene?

FURTHER READING

Dunn AL, Abshire TC. Recent advances in the management of the child who has hemophilia. Hematol Oncol Clin North Am 2004;18:1249–1276.

High KA. Clinical gene transfer studies for hemophilia B. Semin Thromb Hemost 2004;30:257–267.

Lozier J. Gene therapy of the hemophiliac. Semin Hematol 2004;41:287–296.

Verma IM, Weitzman MD. Gene therapy: twenty-first century medicine. Ann Rev Biochem 2005; 74:711–738.

Answers to Review Questions

Chapter 1

1.1 The G–C base pairs have three hydrogen bonds rather than two for A–T pairs, making them more thermodynamically stable.

1.2 Transcription is required to synthesize short RNA primers that serve as a starting point for DNA synthesis.

1.3 RNA: AUG GUU GAU AGU CGU UGC CGC GGG CUG UGA
Peptide: met – val – asp – ser – arg – cys – arg – gly – leu

1.4 (1) alternative promoters, leading to multiple, different proteins derived from the same gene; (2) alternative splicing, leading to different versions of a protein with or without various exons; (3) RNA editing may cause changes in the mRNA sequence after transcription; (4) post-translational modification of proteins.

1.5 Testing cultured fibroblasts in a heterozygous woman should produce two bands, but if clones of cells derived from a single cell are tested, only one of the two forms will be seen, due to X chromosome inactivation.

Chapter 2

2.1 A silent mutation might affect splicing, either by creating a new splice donor or acceptor sequence, or by affecting an exon splice enhancer. Such mutations would result in abnormal splicing. The hypothesis could be tested by looking at the RNA level, where one might see an abnormally spliced mRNA.

2.2 Stop mutation; frameshift mutation; splicing mutation that juxtaposes out of frame exons; deletion of gene.

2.3 Nonsense-mediated decay might cause degradation of RNA molecules with the stop mutation, leaving only wild type molecules available for analysis.

2.4 The mutation is a deletion. Father has not transmitted an allele to the child, who only received the mother's lower allele. The father must have only a single allele, the upper band; the other allele must be deleted.

2.5 A polymorphism can have phenotypic effects, including effects associated with medical problems. The term "polymorphism" only conveys implications about frequency, not the physiological effects of the change. Some common variants occur within genes and affect their function so that a disease phenotype results. Sickle cell anemia due to beta globin mutation is an example.

Chapter 3

3.1 Bill and Zoe are not at risk of having a child with MELAS, since this is a mitochondrial disorder and Bill would not be at risk of passing it on. Zoe has a family history of developmental delay, however, in her maternal aunt's grandson. If this is an X-linked disorder, there is risk that Zoe could be a carrier and therefore might have an affected son.

3.2 It is possible that this is autosomal recessive, in which case the mutant allele must be relatively common, indicating that both partners of the father would be carriers. A more likely scenario, though, is autosomal dominant with either nonpenetrance in the father or germ line mosaicism.

3.3 $\frac{1}{2} \times 0.75 = 0.375$

3.4 The disorder is only expressed in children who inherit the gene from their fathers. None of the children of an affected female is affected. The gene is probably expressed only in the paternal copy.

3.5 Anticipation is seen in conditions due to triplet repeat expansion. The larger the expansion, the earlier the age of onset and more severe the disorder. Larger expansions are also prone to further expansion in the next generation. As a result, the expansion size increases from generation to generation, and severity increases accordingly.

Chapter 4

4.1 No; the bacteria would not be able to splice the introns out of the transcript to produce a functional mRNA. An insert derived from cDNA, where splicing has already occurred, would produce a functional product, provided that the insert is large enough.

4.2 Child c is recombinant. Allele 1 was inherited with the disease in the father of the sibship. The children who inherited 1 from father are expected to have the disease and those who inherited 2 from father are not affected. Child c inherited 1 from father but is not affected. Assuming complete penetrance, this is best explained by recombination.

4.3 The lod score of $-\infty$ implies that there was a recombination at $\theta = 0$ (i.e., the odds ratio at $\theta = 0$ was 0). This implies that the marker is not the actual disease gene.

4.4 In the past, after linkage was established it was necessary to "walk" along the chromosome to find an expressed sequence that corresponds with a gene of interest. Now, once linkage is established genes known to reside within the region can be directly tested for mutation in affected individuals.

4.5 This would cause mutation of the gene, probably associated with lack of expression of the gene product.

Chapter 5

5.1 This means that genes are not sufficient in themselves to determine the trait. There may be a genetic contribution, but something else, perhaps environmental factors or chance, also play a role. There are also rare examples where identical twins will not share the same gene mutation, if the mutation arose somatically in just one twin.

5.2 For this trait it is always more likely that a female would be affected. The fact that their first child was of the less often affected sex implies that the recurrence risk is higher than if the affected child had been female.

5.3 The fact that the SNP is associated with the disease could be interpreted in many possible ways. It could be that the SNP itself alters function of the gene in such a way as to contribute to the disease. Alternatively, the SNP might be in linkage disequilibrium with another variant that is truly associated. The association also could be spurious, perhaps due to population stratification of the sample.

5.4 Population stratification occurs when a particular allele is seen more commonly in a specific population, and where that population is contained within a sample used in a case–control study. For a transmission disequilibrium test it does not matter whether the allele is rare or common in the population, since its segregation to the offspring will occur in accordance with Mendel's laws and a skew in segregation will indicate transmission disequilibrium.

5.5 The haplotype map will permit "tag SNPs" to be used as a marker for a haplotype block, which may be in the range of 10 kb in length. This will reduce the number of SNPs that must be genotyped by an order of magnitude.

Chapter 6

6.1   The cell would normally pause before replicating DNA to either repair DNA damage or, if the damage is too severe, undergo apoptosis. Loss of *TP53* causes the cell to continue to replicate DNA in spite of the presence of mutations, permitting the cell to accumulate mutations. Although most of such cells might not survive, some that do might become cancer cells.

6.2   Homologous centromeres separate during the first meiotic division. Not all homologous segments separate, since those that have undergone genetic recombination will not separate until the second meiotic prophase.

6.3   Nondisjunction occurred in his mother, since he received two chromosomes with alleles derived from his mother. The alleles are different, however, suggesting that nondisjunction occurred in meiosis I, such that he received both homologous chromosomes, with two different alleles.

6.4   The birth of a child with congenital anomalies is most likely for a pericentric inversion with a large inverted segment. Crossing over within the inversion loop gives rise to unbalanced products. If the inversion is paracentric, though, the products are dicentric or acentric, and are unlikely to be compatible with development. A pericentric inversion results in duplications and deficiencies of the chromosome, but chromosomes will be monocentric and therefore stable. If the inverted segment is large there will be a higher chance for crossover and the imbalance will be less severe, and therefore more likely to be compatible with survival to birth.

6.5   Uniparental disomy (UPD) most commonly arises from a "trisomy rescue" event, that begins with a trisomic zygote with ensuing loss of one copy of chromosome 15 from the parent that did not contribute two copies of 15 from nondisjunction. Nondisjunction is more common in female than in male meiosis, so it is more common to have maternal UPD, which will produce Prader–Willi syndrome than paternal UPD, which would give rise to Angelman syndrome. Angelman syndrome is most commonly due to deletion or point mutation in a specific gene implicated in the disorder.

Chapter 7

7.1   II-3 has a 2/3 risk of being a carrier. The risk for II-4 is derived from the Hardy–Weinberg equation:

$$q = 1/200; \ 2pq \sim 2(1/200) = 1/100$$

Therefore the risk of having an affected child is:

$$2/3 \times 1/100 \times 1/4 = 1/600$$

7.2   The carrier frequency is:

$$2 \times 1/20 = 1/10 \ [\text{more precisely, } 2 \times 1/20 \times 19/20 = 19/200].$$

The risk of hemochromatosis in an offspring is:

$$1 \times 1/10 \times 1/2 = 1/20$$

Increased ability to absorb iron in heterozygotes might confer an advantage, maintaining this gene in the population.

7.3 $q^2 = 1/1600$
       Therefore $q = 1/40$ and the carrier frequency $\approx 2q = 1/20$.
       This most likely represents a founder effect, in which a mutation becomes prevalent in a population which is small at the time when the mutation is introduced and where the population remains relatively inbred.

7.4 Equilibrium is established in the first generation after migration, assuming that all the Hardy–Weinberg conditions are met. This would not be true for a sex-linked trait, however.

7.5 If [a] = p, [b] = q, [c] = r, then the genotype frequencies can be calculated from:

$$(p + q + r)^2 = p^2 + q^2 + r^2 + 2pq + 2pr + 2qr$$

Therefore

$$[bc] = 2pr = 2(0.3)(0.5) = 0.3$$

Chapter 8

8.1 It probably functions as a tumor suppressor gene. The lost allele would be the wildtype allele inherited from the mother. Radiation might stimulate loss of heterozygosity or acquisition of other genetic changes, contributing to tumor formation.

8.2 Such a mutation would lead to tumor formation in all cells of a susceptible tissue congenitally. It would likely be lethal.

8.3 The same two "hits" would occur in a tumor suppressor gene in a sporadic as in a familial cancer. It takes time for these two hits to accumulate in a cell to produce a sporadic cancer. If one hit is present in all cells, only a single additional hit needs to occur, which takes less time.

8.4 Chromosome translocation can activate a proto-oncogene by juxtaposing the gene with another gene that is actively transcribed. It is possible that a translocation could disrupt a tumor suppressor gene and thereby inactivate it.

8.5 Microsatellite instability indicates loss of function of one of the mismatch repair genes. It can be a sign of hereditary nonpolyposis colon cancer, which is a familial disorder inherited as a dominant trait.

Chapter 9

9.1 Interphase FISH may accurately diagnosis trisomy, but would not distinguish free trisomy 21 from trisomy due to a Robertsonian translocation. The latter would be important to identify because of the increased risk of recurrence in future pregnancies if one parent is a carrier.

9.2 The biochemical screen is not a diagnostic test. Depending on the components of the screen, sensitivity is between 60 and 80%. It is not 100% sensitive, however, and therefore some pregnancies at risk will not test positive.

9.3 The fetus would be at risk of uniparental disomy for chromosome 15, which could result in Prader–Willi or Angelman syndromes. Testing for UPD would be indicated.

9.4 Although a balanced reciprocal translocation generally does not cause gain or loss of genetic material, there can be exceptions. Sometimes there will be gains or losses at the site of translocation. In addition, a gene could be disrupted by the translocation, or there could be alteration of the expression of a gene due to "position effect." One way to further explore the significance of the translocation is to perform chromosome analysis on both parents. If the rearrangement is not present in either parent there is a greater likelihood that it is clinically significant, whereas if one parent has the same rearrangement it is less likely that it is the cause of the child's problems. Testing for uniparental disomy of the involved chromosomes also can be useful.

9.5 This individual has signs that could be compatible with velocardiofacial syndrome (VCFS), associated with submicroscopic deletion of chromosome 22. A FISH study should be done. If positive, there would be a 50% risk of transmission of the deleted chromosome to a child, who would also develop VCFS.

Chapter 10

10.1 The risk to the fetus would be 25% of having DMD. The mother of the fetus has a 50% risk of being a carrier, since her mother is an obligate carrier (having two affected sons). We do not know here which haplotype is associated with DMD in this family. It is necessary to study each family individually to learn which alleles are in coupling with the disease in that particular family.

10.2 There are many things that might help to determine whether the change is pathogenic. Has the change been seen before in affected individuals or in controls? If the disorder is present in the family does the mutation track with the disease; if the child is the first affected, is the mutation present in either parent? Is the amino acid that is altered conserved in evolution? What is the predicted effect of the amino acid substitution on the function of the protein?

10.3 Sequencing the cDNA will reveal exon skips or insertions of intron sequence into the mRNA indicative of splicing mutations. These may be due to mutations within introns that would be difficult to detect with genomic DNA sequencing unless the entire genomic sequence, including introns, were studied.

10.4 His repeat size is in the range seen in affected individuals with Huntington disease. HD displays age-dependent penetrance, though, so it is not guaranteed that he will become symptomatic before he might die of other causes.

10.5 Information about Noonan syndrome can be obtained at OMIM or GeneReviews. It is an autosomal dominant trait due to mutation of the gene *PTPN11*. Clinical molecular testing is available.

Chapter 11

11.1 Phenylalanine is cleared *in utero* through the placenta and only begins to build up in the child after birth. Mothers of children with PKU are heterozygous carriers, but their levels of phenylalanine hydroxylase are sufficient to metabolize both the mother's and fetus's phenylalanine.

11.2 Symptoms of lysosomal storage disorders occur due to the gradual build up of undigested material within the lysosome. This requires time, typically months to years, to accumulate to the point where symptoms occur.

11.3 Mannose-6-phosphate enables the enzyme to bind to specific receptors in the cell membrane. Upon receptor-mediated endocytosis the endocytic vesicles fuse with lysosomes, releasing enzyme into the organelle.

11.4 Assays such as the Guthrie bacterial inhibition test needed to be customized for each particular metabolic disorder to be tested. Tandem mass spectrometry provides data about a broad array of conditions in a single test based on mass spectra for a variety of metabolites.

11.5 (1) substrate reduction; (2) removal of toxic metabolites; (3) enzyme replacement; (4) organ transplantation; (5) coenzyme supplementation; (6) augmentation of enzyme. action.

Chapter 12

12.1 A disruption involves the destruction of tissue during development, whereas deformation involves alteration of shape without tissue destruction. Some teratogens are responsible for disruptions, based on tissue toxicity or interference with blood circulation.

12.2 Yes; Mullerian inhibiting substance is produced by the testes.

12.3 The mutation occurs at a specific site where it leads to gain of function of the gene product. Mutations at other sites in the gene would not have this effect.

12.4 Most of these disorders lead to early death or significant cognitive or physical impairment, any of which interferes with ability to reproduce. Parent to child transmission of a mutation will therefore be rare, except in cases of germ line mosaicism. As a result, most cases arise by new mutation.

12.5   *Hox* genes are arranged in tandem arrays on the chromosome. The 3′ most genes are expressed in the most cephalad regions, with a progression of genes located in a 5′ direction being expressed more caudally.

Chapter 13

13.1   Yes. Both sickle cell anemia and beta thalassemia are seen in individuals of African descent, whereas beta thalassemia is common in the Mediterranean region. Compound heterozygotes with a beta thalassemia mutation and a sickle cell mutation do have a clinical hematological disorder (sickle–thalassemia).

13.2   Biochemical screening is offered if the biochemical test is less expensive and if it has higher sensitivity, which would be the case if there is a large diversity of mutations that can cause disease. DNA testing is used if the biochemical test does not accurately distinguish the carrier state or if it is difficult to do a biochemical test from readily available tissue such as blood.

13.3   The frequency of specific mutations differs in individuals of different ancestry. The residual risk to an individual who screens negative for mutation depends on the sensitivity of the mutation screen in that individual, which is largely dependent on ancestry.

13.4   Although complete sequencing will detect all mutations, there is also a possibility that variants will be found that are not pathogenic, or at least whose significance is unknown. Mutation screening panels are generally restricted to testing for mutations of known pathological significance.

13.5   There are many reasons to consider carrier screening aside from termination of an affected pregnancy. Other reproductive options can be considered, for example, such as use of a sperm or egg donor. Couples may also use screening for reassurance, or for planning for the medical needs of an affected child.

Chapter 14

14.1   The rationale for presymptomatic diagnosis is that treatment with phlebotomy is preventative of complications, but these complications cannot be successfully treated once they are established. The major limitation of genetic testing is that penetrance is incomplete; hence, an individual who is found to carry a mutation has a high chance of never developing symptoms.

14.2   Presymptomatic genetic testing determines whether an individual at risk of inheriting a gene mutation has indeed inherited it, prior to onset of signs or symptoms of disease. Predispositional testing determines whether an individual is at increased risk of developing disease as compared with individuals in the general population.

14.3   An individual who is a risk of having inherited a gene mutation may wish to know if he or she has inherited it in order to be informed about risks of transmitting the trait to offspring. For a disorder with age-dependent penetrance, signs or symptoms may not be present at a time when reproductive decisions must be made.

14.4   Relative risk compares his chance of developing the disease with that of the general population. This result indicates that he is 2.5 times more likely to develop the disease than the population risk. If the disease is rare, however, there remains a high likelihood that he will not develop the disease.

14.5   It is possible that an individual who tests positive will be denied health, life, or disability insurance, or may be denied employment. Although not affected by the disorder, if the test result were known, being at increased risk could trigger such responses. There is also concern that the individual may face a change in self-image, or in the way he or she is perceived by others.

Chapter 15

15.1   Breast cancer is rare in males, but occurs with increased frequency in *BRCA2* mutation heterozygotes. Testing of this man would be indicated, at least in part because of implications for his daughters, as well as other family members.

15.2 Testing for *BRCA1* or *BRCA2* mutations does not detect all possible mutations. Therefore, a negative test in the 30-year-old women could either mean that she did not inherit a *BRCA* mutation, or that the mutation test did not detect it. Testing her affected relative offers a greater reliability. If her aunt is negative, it means that the mutation test would not pick up a mutation, or that *BRCA* mutation is not responsible for the cancer in the family. If her aunt is found to have a mutation, the woman can be offered reliable testing to see if she inherited the mutation.

15.3 Yes; there are three cases of colon cancer in the family in two generations affecting first-degree relatives. One affected individual is under 50 years of age at the time of diagnosis.

15.4 Screening for colon polyps in individuals with FAP begins at around 10 years of age. If the children are found to not be carriers of the gene mutation, however, they would be spared routine screening. Testing of children at risk is therefore justified, since the results will change their management.

15.5 Medullary carcinoma of the thyroid can be associated with mutation of the *RET* oncogene. Gene carriers would be offered thyroidectomy to avoid this often lethal cancer.

Chapter 16

16.1 The *RYR1* gene is large and there is a wide diversity of mutations. DNA testing would not be cost effective, and there is a risk of missing some mutations. Testing of muscle requires invasive biopsy and is difficult to perform and expensive.

16.2 Those who have a polymorphism that renders them slow metabolizers are at risk of accumulation of toxic levels of the drug, which can cause bone marrow failure, and may be lethal. In such individuals the drug dosage would be adjusted to avoid toxicity.

16.3 Many drugs are metabolized by the CYP2D6 enzyme. Knowledge of genotype can provide a basis for adjustment of drug dosage to avoid toxic side-effects or to insure therapeutic levels.

16.4 Individuals who carry specific sodium or potassium channel polymorphisms are at risk of cardiac arrhythmia upon exposure to certain drugs.

16.5 Disease stratification involves discernment of genetic differences in pathogenesis of disease that occur among individuals with what seems to be the same disorder. This permits precise matching of treatments with specific individual needs.

Chapter 17

17.1 Gene therapy offers many potential advantages over factor VIII or IX infusion. Factor infusion is expensive and involves exposure to blood products, with a risk of infection. It also is used after onset of a bleeding episode, rather than to prevent an episode. In principle, gene therapy would be a permanent cure, avoiding complications of bleeding episodes and risks of treatment.

17.2 Adeno-associated virus offers stable, long-term expression of factor IX. Although it can only incorporate a relatively small insert, the small size of the factor IX gene is accommodated.

17.3 "Naked DNA" can be taken up directly into cells, albeit with low efficiency. Increased efficiency of uptake can be accomplished by incorporation of the DNA into liposomes, complexed with polylysine, or forceful insertion using a "gene gun."

17.4 Retroviral vectors lead to random insertion of genes into the genome. There is a risk that a gene will be inserted adjacent to an oncogene, leading to activation of the oncogene and, consequently, cancer.

17.5 Adenoviral vectors do not lead to insertion of the gene into the genome, and therefore do not achieve stable expression of the inserted gene.

Glossary

acrocentric   placement of centromere near one end of a chromosome

adenine   one of four bases of DNA; abbreviated "A"; pairs with thymine or uracil

age-dependent penetrance   increasing likelihood of manifesting signs or symptoms of a genetic disorder with increasing age

allele   specific form of a gene

alpha-fetoprotein (AFP)   protein secreted during fetal life; high AFP is indicative of congenital anomalies such as open neural tube defects; low AFP can be a sign of Down syndrome

alpha-satellite DNA   repeated DNA sequence enriched at chromosome centromeres

alternative splicing   different patterns of exon splicing of a transcript, resulting in production of peptides that differ in amino acid sequence

Alu sequence   one of a class of intermediate repeated DNA sequences, concentrated within coding regions of the genome

amino acid   chemical building block of a protein, consisting of an amine group, a carboxyl group, and one of 20 specific functional groups

amino acid substitution   mutation that leads to production of a peptide with a different amino acid at one site

amniocentesis   method of prenatal diagnostic testing in which a sample of amniotic fluid is withdrawn for analysis

amniotic fluid   fluid that bathes the fetus within the amniotic cavity, consisting largely of fetal urine with skin, bladder, and amnion cells

aneuploidy   nonintegral multiple of the haploid chromosome set due to one or more missing or extra chromosomes

anticipation   phenomenon whereby a genetic disorder becomes more severe from one generation to the next; characteristics of triplet repeat expansion disorders

anticodon   tRNA sequence that recognizes codon in mRNA to insert appropriate amino acid into the growing peptide

antisense oligonucleotide   sequence of DNA that is complementary to part of an mRNA, used to specifically inhibit expression of that gene

apoptosis   programmed cell death

A site   site in ribosome that will accept next amino acyl tRNA to bind to growing peptide

autocrine growth control   production of growth factor by the same cell that responds to that factor

autosomal dominant   mode of genetic transmission wherein a single mutant allele is sufficient to produce a phenotype, carried on a non-sex chromosome

autosome   non-sex chromosome

bacteriophage   virus that infects bacterial cells

balanced polymorphism   genetic variant that is maintained at relatively high frequency in a population due to selection against homozygotes for the wild-type or variant sequence, with fitness being highest in heterozygotes

balanced translocation   exchange of segments between chromosomes so that no genetic material is lost or gained

Barr body   condensed chromatin representing inactivated X chromosome in interphase cell

bioinformatics   use of computers to catalog and analyze large sets of biological data

blastomere   pluripotent embryonic cell during the first few divisions following fertilization

branch point   point within intron to which splice acceptor sequence binds during splicing process

candidate gene   gene thought to be involved in a specific genetic trait or disorder on the basis of mapping information or physiologic evidence

carboxyl terminal   last amino acid in a protein (in order of assembly)

carrier   individual who has a mutant gene (usually used to describe individual who does not manifest signs of the trait)

case–control study   study of genetic association in which one compares the frequency of an allele in a cohort of affected individuals with a control cohort

C-banding   chromosome staining technique that produces dark staining at centromeres

cDNA   DNA copy of RNA made using the enzyme reverse transcriptase

cDNA library   collection of cloned DNA sequences, representing a portion of sequences transcribed in the cells or tissue of origin

centimorgan   unit of genetic distance corresponding with 1% recombination

centromere   site of attachment of spindle fibers to the chromosome representing the last point of separation of replicated chromatids

centromeric heterochromatin   highly condensed chromatin near the centromere consisting of repeated DNA

checkpoint protein   protein involved in pausing the cell cycle to repair DNA damage

chorionic villus sampling   method of prenatal diagnosis in which fetal placenta is sampled either transabdominally or transcervically

chromatid   one of two replicated arms of a chromosome

chromatin   DNA with associated proteins

chromosome   structure in a cell on which genes are located, consisting of a highly compacted stretch of DNA with associated proteins

chromosome abnormality   clinically significant change of chromosome number or structure

chromosome banding   means of staining chromosomes to elicit characteristic and specific patterns to aid chromosome identification

chromosome painting   means of staining a chromosome based on hybridization with fluorescent-labeled DNA sequences specific to that chromosome

clone   group of cells derived from a common progenitor; in recombinant DNA denotes a purified sequence of DNA

coactivator   protein that interacts with transcription factor to activate transcription

codon   triplet of bases that encode a specific amino acid

cofactor   substance that participates, along with an enzyme, in a chemical reaction

colchicine   chemical that disrupts the mitotic spindle; used to collect cells at metaphase for chromosome analysis

comparative genomic hybridization   method in which a control and reference DNA sample are competitively hybridized to a reference sequence used to detect deletions or duplications

complementarity   occurrence of sequence of bases in DNA or RNA that will form stable double helix by pairing of A to T (or U) and G to C

complex segregation analysis   analysis of pattern of genetic transmission that tests various models to explain data set, establishing a best fit model

compound heterozygote   individual with two different mutant alleles at a locus

conditional knockout   mouse model in which a target sequence is flanked by repeated sequences that undergo recombinational excision when another element, referred to as *cre*, is activated by a tissue-specific promoter

congenital anomaly   structural abnormality present at birth

consanguinity   blood relationship between a couple

conservative change   substitution of one amino acid for another with similar chemical properties, with little or no effect on the structure and function of the protein

consultand   individual seeking genetic counseling

contig   set of overlapping clones of DNA covering a large region

corepressor   protein that interacts with transcription factor to repress transcription

cosmid   cloning vector consisting of plasmid with sequences that allow packaging in a lambda phage head; used for cloning large segments of DNA

CpG dinucleotides   adjacent pair of nucleotides, with 5′–C–G–3′; the C in this location may be methylated

CpG islands   region in which there are many CpG dinucleotides, often near the 5′ end of a gene

crossover   consequence of genetic recombination

cryptic donor or acceptor   sequence within an intron that can serve as a splice donor or acceptor if the usual site is disrupted by mutation

CVS   abbreviation for chorionic villus sampling

cyclin   protein involved in control of cell cycle

cyclin-dependent kinase   enzyme involved in phosphorylation of proteins involved in cell cycle

cytogenetic   pertaining to chromosomes

cytokinesis   process of separation of two daughter cells at end of mitosis

cytosine   one of four bases of DNA; abbreviated "C"; pairs with guanine

deformation   alteration of developing structure in embryo or fetus due to extrinsic pressure

deletion   mode of mutation due to loss of large chromosomal region

denaturation   separation of double-stranded nucleic acid into single strands

dideoxy sequencing   mode of DNA sequencing using 2′ deoxynucleotides

digenic inheritance   mode of inheritance in which heterozygosity at two separate loci lead to phenotype

dinucleotide repeat   stretch of DNA containing a pair of bases (often C–A) repeated many times; repeat number may by polymorphic

diploid   having two copies of each chromosome (except sex chromosomes)

disomic   having two copies of a specific chromosome

disruption   alteration of developing structure in embryo or fetus due to destruction of tissue

dizygotic twins   twins resulting from separate fertilization events

DNA   abbreviation for deoxyribonucleic acid, the chemical basis of heredity

DNA polymerase   enzyme responsible for replication of DNA

DNA transposon   form of repeated sequence similar to transposable genetic elements in bacteria

dominant   allele that exerts its phenotypic effect whether present in heterozygous or homozygous state

dominant negative   mutation in which the gene product of one allele exerts an inhibitory effect on the function of the system

dosage compensation   mechanism of equalizing X-linked gene expression in males and females by suppression of most genes on one X in females

Down syndrome   complex of congenital anomalies resulting from an extra copy of chromosome 21

duplication   mode of mutation due to repetition of one or more bases of DNA, or of a chromosomal region

dysmorphology   study of structural abnormalities of human development

electrophoresis   separation of chemical substances by differential migration in an electric field

elongation factor   protein involved in process of translation in ribosome

endoplasmic reticulum   subcellular structure representing site of protein synthesis

enhancer element   sequence that binds to proteins that "open" the DNA in the region of the promoter

enzyme   protein that catalyzes a specific chemical reaction

ethidium bromide   fluorescent dye that intercalates into DNA; used to stain DNA

exon   segment of gene that encodes amino acid sequence of protein; adjacent exons are separated by introns, which are spliced out during RNA processing

exon junctional complex   ribonucleoprotein complex remnant of splicing apparatus at junction between exons in spliced mRNA

exon skipping   mutation that alters pattern of splicing and results in splicing out of an exon

expressed sequence tag (EST)   region of unique sequence in cDNA clone used in gene mapping

expressivity   range of phenotypic variability of a genetic trait in a population

extinction   elimination of a genetic trait from a population due to selection or genetic drift

fertilization   union of sperm and egg leading to initiation of embryonic development

fibroblast   cell type prevalent in connective tissue

FISH   acronym for fluorescence *in situ* hybridization

fixation   establishment of an allele as the sole allele at a given locus in a population due to extinction of other alleles

fluorescence *in situ* hybridization   means of localization of cloned segment of DNA on chromosome by binding of complementary DNA and visualization by fluorescence microscopy

founder effect   prevalence of a specific allele in a population due to its presence in one of the original members of the population and tendency of members of the population to be relatively inbred

fragile X syndrome   genetic disorder associated with the expansion of a triplet repeat at the *FMR1* locus; associated with X-linked mental retardation

frameshift   mutation that disrupts the sequence so that the reading frame is altered

fraternal twins   nonidentical twins

G1 phase   portion of cell cycle after mitosis prior to next round of cell division

G2 phase   portion of cell cycle between DNA synthesis and mitosis

G-banding   mode of chromosome staining by Giemsa resulting in characteristic patterns of light and dark bands along chromosome

gene walking   cloning overlapping segments of DNA to isolate large region starting from single cloned site

genetic counseling   means of communication by medical professionals to an individual or family to educate them about natural history and genetics of a clinical disorder, along with available options for testing and treatment

genetic determinism   concept that genetic factors are completely determinant of phenotypic characteristics

genetic drift   fluctuation of frequency of an allele in a small population from generation to generation due to statistical variation

genetic heterogeneity   occurrence of multiple alleles at a gene locus or multiple loci that result in a similar phenotype

genetic linkage   proximity of a set of gene loci on the same chromosome

genetic modifier   gene that alters the phenotype associated with another gene

genome   collection of genes in an organism

genomic library   collection of cloned DNA fragments from random sites in the genome

genotype   set of specific alleles at a gene locus in an individual

germ cell   sperm or egg cell

germ-line mosaicism   occurrence of two or more cell lines derived from a single fertilization event but differing by presence or absence of one or more mutant alleles

guanosine   one of four bases of DNA; abbreviated "G"; pairs with cytosine

haploid   having only one complete set of chromosomes

haploinsufficiency   presence of only a single functional copy of a gene due to mutational loss of the other allele

haplotype   set of alleles at a group of linked genes together on a specific chromosome

Hardy–Weinberg equilibrium   mathematical statement of the relation between allele frequencies and frequencies of corresponding genotypes in a population

helicase   enzyme that unwinds DNA double helix at site of DNA replication

hemizygosity   presence of one copy of a gene at a given locus instead of two; applies to X-linked genes in males, or any gene whose homologous copy has been deleted

heritability   statistical measure of the contribution of genetics to a multifactorial trait

heterochromatin   chromatin that remains highly condensed during interphase and usually contains DNA that is genetically inactive

heteroduplex   double-stranded molecule derived from two similar, but not identical, DNA or RNA sequences

heteroplasmy   occurrence of two or more populations of genetically distinct mitochondrial DNAs in a cell

heterozygote advantage   selective advantage of heterozygous individuals over homozygotes; results in balanced polymorphism

heterozygous   having two different alleles at a gene locus

histones   basic proteins that form a complex with DNA in chromosome

HLA   abbreviation for human lymphocyte antigen region on chromosome 6

homeobox   DNA sequence that encodes a 60 amino acid region that is common to homeotic genes

homeotic genes   genes involved in the control of development, discovered originally in *Drosophilia* mutants, that lead to alteration in structures forming in specific body segments

homologous chromosomes   pair of chromosomes, one inherited from each parent

homozygous   having a pair of identical alleles for a particular gene

housekeeping genes   genes that are expressed in a wide variety of cell types and are involved in common, basic mechanisms of cell physiology

Hox   abbreviation for homeobox

hybridization   formation of double helix from complementary strands of DNA or RNA derived from different sources

hypermutability   genetic trait that leads to high rate of mutation during DNA replication; characteristic of some neoplastic cells

identical twins   monozygotic twins

imprinting   differential expression of maternally and paternally derived genes

informative mating   mating in which one partner is heterozygous such that the polymorphic marker and alleles can be distinguished from those contributed by partner to offspring; used in genetic linkage analysis

informativeness   likelihood of informative mating for particular genetic polymorphism

initiation complex   set of transcription factors and RNA polymerase that bind to promoter to initiate transcription

insertional mutation   mutation resulting from insertion of one or more bases into DNA

***in situ* hybridization**   technique of identifying a chromosome region that contains sequence complementary with a cloned segment of DNA

interspersed repeated sequences   set of repeated sequences interspersed at multiple sites within genome

intron   segment of noncoding DNA between exons, spliced out during RNA processing

inversion   mutation due to reverse orientation of a segment of DNA

isochromosome   abnormal chromosome formed from duplication of either the short or long arms

kb   abbreviation for kilobase

kilobase   one thousand bases

lagging strand   strand of DNA synthesized in a set of smaller fragments (Okazaki fragments) at a DNA replication fork

large scale variation   polymorphism of copy number of segmental duplications

leading strand   strand of DNA synthesized in a continuous fragment from a DNA replication fork

lethal trait   genetic trait that renders an individual unable to reproduce

liability   tendency toward expression of a multifactorial trait, consisting of a combination of genetic and nongenetic factors

library   set of cloned nucleic acid segments (genomic or cDNA)

LINE sequence   type of repeated DNA, concentrated in noncoding segments

linkage   proximity of a set of gene loci on the same chromosome

linkage disequilibrium   nonrandom association of alleles at linked loci

linkage equilibrium   random association of alleles at linked loci

locus   site of specific DNA sequence on chromosome

lod score   logarithm of odds ratio of likelihood of data given specified value of recombination compared with random segregation; often abbreviated z

loss of heterozygosity   phenomenon wherein a polymorphic marker that is heterozygous in somatic cells is homozygous or hemizygous in tumor cells due to loss of one allele

LTR retroposon   form of repeated sequences derived from retrovirus-like elements

Lyon hypothesis   scheme of dosage compensation involving inactivation of one X chromosome in every cell in females; formulated by Mary Lyon

lysosomal storage disease   clinical disorder due to absence of activity of a specific lysosomal enzyme, leading to buildup of substrate in lysosome

malformation   abnormality of the formation of a fetal structure

marker gene   polymorphic DNA sequence used in linkage mapping

maternal transmission   characteristic of mitochondrial genetic traits, passed from a mother to all her offspring

maximum likelihood estimate   value of recombination fracture (θ) at which peak lod score is obtained

Mb   abbreviation for megabase

megabase   one million bases

meiosis   process of reduction division in germ line, leading to formation of haploid germ cells

mendelian trait   genetic trait that follows patterns of simple mendelian inheritance

metacentric   presence of centromere at center of chromosome

metaphase   stage of cell division when chromosomes are aligned at the center of the cell prior to separation

metastasis   spread of neoplastic cells from their site or origin to remote sites

methylation   addition of methyl groups to cytosine bases (usually at CpG dinucleotides)

microarray   grid of multiple DNA fragments fixed to a glass slide for hybridization to test sequence

microsatellite polymorphisms   DNA sequence variants due to different numbers of repeats of a simple sequence

misattributed parentage   finding that stated father or mother is not the biological parent of the child

missense mutation   base change in the coding sequence of a protein that leads to amino acid substitution

mitochondrial DNA   circular double-stranded DNA within mitochondrion that encodes 13 mitochondrial proteins, transfer and ribosomal RNAs

mitochondrion   structure in cell involved in aerobic metabolism

mitosis   process of cell division

mitotic spindle   structure in dividing cells that pulls chromatids to opposite poles to make daughter cells

molecular diagnostic testing   identification of specific nucleic acid sequences for medical diagnosis

monosomy   presence of one rather than two copies of a specific chromosome in an individual

monozygotic twins   genetically identical twins resulting from a single fertilization event

mosaicism   occurrence of two or more genetically distinct cell lines derived from a common progenitor

mRNA   processed gene transcript ready for translation into protein

Müllerian duct   embryonic structure that gives rise to uterus and fallopian tubes

multifactorial inheritance   traits determined by a combination of multiple genetic and/or nongenetic factors

multiplex PCR   simultaneous amplification of multiple sequences in a single reaction using multiple sets of primers

mutation   change in the sequence of DNA at a genetic locus

neoplasm   clone of cells released from normal controls of growth

nondirective counseling   approach to genetic counseling in which the counselor provides information and encourages the consultand to make an individual decision without influence by the counselor's views

nondisjunction   failure of proper chromosome segregation, leading to both copies of a chromosome (or both chromatids) going to the same daughter cell

nonhistone protein   protein associated with DNA, not one of the basic histone proteins

nonpenetrance   the absence of phenotype in a person known to carry a specific mutant gene

nonsense-mediated decay   process whereby mRNA carrying a nonsense mutation is degraded in cell

nonsense mutation   mutation that changes a codon for an amino acid to a stop codon

northern blot   method of identification of RNA separated by electrophoresis, blotted onto membrane, and hybridized with labeled nucleic acid

nucleolus organizer regions   sites on acrocentric chromosomes containing ribosomal DNA

nucleosome   knoblike structure consisting of approximately 140 base pairs of DNA and associated histones, forming a structural unit of chromatin

nucleotide   base of DNA or RNA

Okazaki fragments   short segments of newly synthesized DNA on lagging strand at replication fork

oligonucleotide   segment of several bases of DNA or RNA

oncogene   gene that confers some neoplastic properties on a cell, usually derived by activation of a proto-oncogene

oogonial cell   immature egg cell, prior to meiosis

open reading frame   region of cDNA sequence starting with an AUG codon that initiates protein synthesis and including a region that encodes protein, ending at a stop codon

P1 phage vector   cloning vector derived from P1 bacteriophage that can accommodate large inserts of foreign DNA

paired box   DNA-binding domain of set of gene products involved in development, consisting of 128 amino acids

paracentric inversion   inversion of chromosome region not involving centromere

p arm   short arm of a chromosome

pathogenic mutation   mutation responsible for a genetic disorder

Pax   abbreviation for paired box

PCR   abbreviation for polymerase chain reaction

pedigree   diagram of family using standard symbols

penetrance   expression of genetic trait in an individual with mutant genotype

peptidyl transferase   enzyme involved in formation of peptide bond in translation

pericentric inversion   inversion of chromosome region involving centromere

phage lambda   bacterial virus used as a cloning vector

pharmacogenetics   genetic traits that influence the way drugs are absorbed, distributed, excreted, or react physiologically

pharmacogenomics   use of genomic information to develop new drugs and identify new drug targets

phenotype   physical manifestations resulting from specific genotype

phytohemagglutinin   substance derived from kidney beans that stimulates division of T cells; used to culture cells for chromosomal analysis

plasmid circular double-stranded DNA capable of autonomous replication in bacterial cells; used as a cloning vector

pleiotropy diverse physical characteristics resulting from a single genetic trait

point mutation single base change of DNA sequence

polyacrylamide gel electrophoresis method for high-resolution separation of nucleic acids or proteins

polygenic inheritance traits determined by two or more separate genes

polymerase chain reaction means of amplification of a DNA sequence by multiple cycles of replication starting from the pair of primers that flank the sequence

polymorphism occurrence of at least two alleles at a locus each having a frequency of at least 1%

population genetics study of the factors that influence the frequency of genetic traits in a population

positional cloning means of cloning a gene based on its location in the genome

predispositional test genetic test used to determine if an individual is at increased risk of disease

preimplantation diagnosis genetic diagnosis from early embryo, prior to implantation in uterus

premutation sequence variation that predisposes to mutation; usually moderate expansion of a triplet that leads to further expansion, such as in fragile X syndrome

prenatal diagnosis diagnosis of a medical problem in an embryo or fetus

presymptomatic test genetic test to determine if an individual carries a gene mutation to determine risk of disease prior to the onset of symptoms

primer oligonucleotide used as the point of intitiation of DNA synthesis

proband individual in a family who brings the family to medical attention

probe cloned nucleic acid sequence used to identify homologous sequence by nucleic acid hybridization

prokaryote primitive micro-organism lacking cell nucleus

promoter site of initiation of transcription at which RNA polymerase and regulatory factors bind

prophase stage of mitosis when nuclear membrane disappears and chromosomes condense

proposita female proband

propositus male proband

proto-oncogene cellular gene that, when appropriately altered, becomes an oncogene

pseudoautosomal gene located on both the X and Y chromosomes, and hence segregating as an autosomal locus

pseudodominant pattern of transmission of a recessive trait in which one partner is homozygous and one is heterozygous, leading to apparent vertical transmission of the trait

pseudogene DNA sequence with substantial homology to a gene, but not encoding protein

pseudomosaic chromosomally abnormal cell line found in cultured prenatal sample that is believed to have arisen during the culture process

P site site in ribosome that carries the growing peptide chain

purine chemical structure of adenine and guanosine

pyrimidine chemical structure of thymine, cytosine, and uracil

q arm long arm of a chromosome

Q-banding method of chromosome banding using the fluorescent dye quinacrine

quinacrine fluorescent dye used to elicit Q-banding

random segregation independent segregation of nonlinked genes to gametes

R-banding method of chromosome staining that produces bands that are the reverse of G-bands

reading frame set of triplet codons in a gene that encode the protein

recessive allele that exerts its phenotypic effect only if present in homozygous state

reciprocal translocation exchange of segments between two or more chromosomes

recombination association of new set of alleles in coupling on a given chromosome due to crossing over in meiosis

recombination fraction (θ)   probability of recombination between two genetic loci

release factors   proteins involved in release of complete peptide from ribosome during protein translation

renaturation   reannealing of separated single strands of nucleic acid into a double helix

reproductive fitness   relative ability of individuals with a specified genotype to reproduce

response element   sequence in promoter region that binds transcription factors

restriction endonuclease   enzyme that cuts DNA at a defined sequence, usually consisting of four to eight bases

restriction fragment-length polymorphism   genetic polymorphism involving a base change that affects the ability of a specific restriction endonuclease to cut the site

reverse transcriptase   enzyme present in retroviruses that copies RNA into DNA

RFLP   abbreviation for restriction fragment-length polymorphism

ribosome   cellular structure involved in translation of mRNA into protein

ring chromosome   chromosome abnormality in which ring forms following breakage of both long and short arms

RNA   abbreviation for ribonucleic acid

RNA interference   process whereby small single stranded RNA molecule binds to mRNA and inhibits translation

Robertsonian translocation   translocation involving fusion of the long arms of a pair of acrocentric chromosomes

rRNA   ribosomal RNA; RNA component of ribosome

segmental duplication   blocks of 10 to 300 kb of homologous DNA sequence repeated at multiple sites in the genome

selection   impairment of reproductive fitness of individuals with a specific genotype

semiconservative replication   mode of DNA replication in a parent strand is used as template to copy a complementary daughter strand

senescence   phenomenon wherein a cell can undergo a limited number of rounds of division

sequence tagged site (STS)   set of PCR primers that amplify unique sequence in genome, used as marker in genetic map

sex chromosome   X or Y chromosome involved in sex determination

sex-linked gene   gene present on X or Y chromosome

short interspersed element (SINE)   form of repeated sequence 100 to 400 base pairs in length

short tandem repeat   DNA sequence of tens to hundreds of bases tandemly repeated multiple times

simple sequence repeat   stretch of di-, tri-, or tetranucleotide repeated multiple times

single nucleotide polymorphism (SNP)   polymorphic single base change

small nuclear RNA (snRNA)   RNA molecules less than 200 base pairs in length, having a role in the splicing process

somatic mosaicism   presence of two or more genetically distinct cell lines in an individual, derived from a common progenitor

Southern blot   method of identification of DNA fragments separated by electrophoresis, blotted onto membrane, and hybridized with labeled nucleic acid

SOX   acronym for *SRY* box

S phase   part of cell cycle when DNA synthesis occurs

splice acceptor   sequence at 3′ border of intron

splice donor   sequence at 5′ border of intron

splice enhancer   sequence that increases likelihood that an intron will be spliced out of mRNA

splice silencer   sequence that reduces likelihood that an intron will be spliced out of mRNA

splicing   process of removal of introns and ligation of exons during processing of RNA

splicing mutations   mutations that change the patterns of RNA splicing, usually by altering splice donor or acceptor sites

SR proteins   proteins involved in selecting sites for initiation of splicing

SRY   gene on Y chromosome required for differentiation of the testes

stop codon   codon that leads to termination of translation

submetacentric   location of a centromere between the middle of the chromosome and one end, producing a short and long arm

synaptonemal complex   protein–DNA complex involved in pairing of homologous chromosomes during meiosis

syndrome   set of reproducible clinical features due to a common underlying mechanism

systems biology   integrated approach to study of complex biological phenomena

telomere   specific DNA structure at the ends of chromosomes

teratogen   substance that interferes with normal embryonic development

tetraploidy   four complete chromosome sets

theta (θ)   abbreviation for recombination fraction

threshold model   theory of multifactorial inheritance stating that a trait occurs when liability exceeds a threshold

thymine   one of four bases of DNA; abbreviated "T"; pairs with adenine

transcription factors   proteins that bind to DNA and either activate or repress transcription

transfection   introduction of segment of foreign DNA into a cell

transformed cell   cell capable of unlimited number of rounds of replication

transgene   cloned gene inserted into foreign genome

transgenic mouse   mouse into which a foreign gene has been inserted into germ line

transition   mutation that substitutes a pyrimidine for a pyrimidine (e.g., G to A or A to G), or a purine for a purine (e.g., T to C or C to T)

translation   process of production of protein from mRNA

translocase   enzyme involved in moving ribosome along mRNA to next codon in protein translation

translocation   exchange of segments between chromosomes

transmission disequilibrium testing   approach to determining the association of an allele with a multifactorial trait by searching for nonrandom segregation of the allele in families with an affected child

transposon-derived repeats   repeated sequences derived from integration of transposable genetic elements at various sites in genome

transversion   mutation that substitutes a purine for a pyrimidine (e.g., T to G, etc.) or vice versa

triple test   measurement of levels of alpha-fetoprotein, human chorionic gonadotropin, and unconjugated estriol as a screen for Down syndrome

triplet repeat expansion   type of mutation in which a gene segment containing multiple copies of a triplet of bases is expanded in length

triploidy   three complete chromosome sets

trisomy   presence of three copies of a chromosome rather than two

tRNA   RNA molecule that carries a specific amino acid and recognizes the corresponding codon, inserting that amino acid into a growing peptide

tumor suppressor gene   gene that when both alleles are mutated leads to transformation of a cell towards a neoplastic phenotype

two-hit hypothesis   hypothesis formulated by A. Knudson, postulating that malignant transformation occurs following a two-step process

ultrasound   mode of imaging using high-frequency sound waves, used to visualize a developing fetus for prenatal diagnosis

uniparental disomy   inheritance of both copies of a chromosome from the same parent

uracil   base that substitutes for thymine in RNA and pairs with adenine; abbreviated "U"

vector   DNA sequence that conveys an inserted segment into a cell

wild type   most common allele in a population at a particular gene locus

Wolffian duct   embryonic structure that gives rise to epididymis vas deferens and seminal vesicle

X chromosome   one of the sex chromosomes
X-inactivation center (Xic)
    region on X chromosome at which X-inactivation is initiated
Xist   gene on X chromosomes believed to be involved in the initiation of X-inactivation

Y chromosome   one of the sex chromosomes
yeast artificial chromosome (YAC)   cloning vector that allows replication of inserted DNA
    in yeast cells, enabling cloning of very large segments

zygote   sperm or egg cell

Index

Numbers in italics refer to Figures or Tables